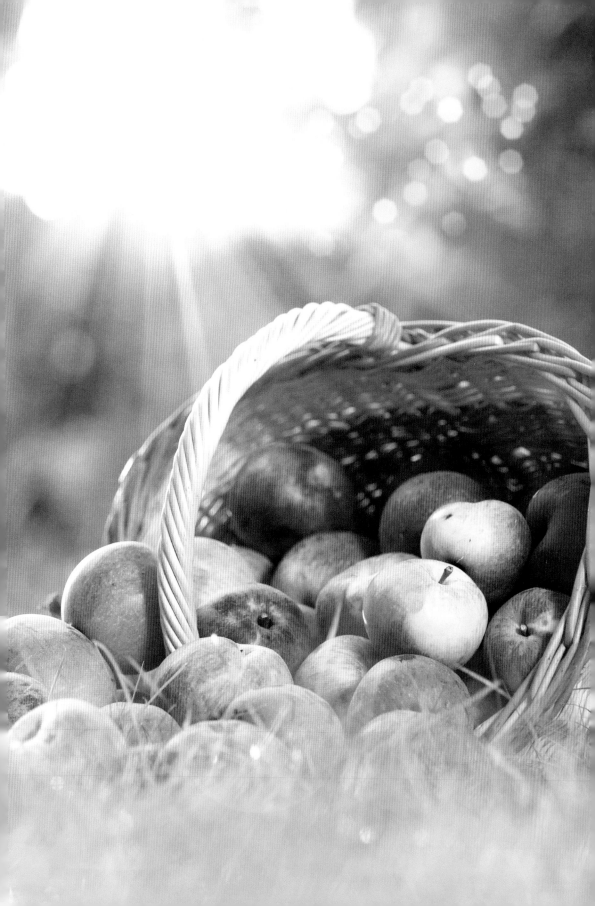

NUTRITION BROUGHT TO LIFE
A THOROUGH GROUNDING IN NOURISHMENT WITH 50 DELICIOUS RECIPES

First edition published September 2020

Alchimia Publishing
2 Farleigh, Ramsden Road, Godalming,
Surrey, GU7 1QE, England, U.K.

www.alchimiapublishing.com

DISCLAIMER
This book is a general guide to nutrition, and is not intended to treat, diagnose, or
give specific medical advice, nor to replace the advice given by your GP or medical
specialist. Each individual person and situation is unique, and while the information
provided in this book draws on the author's extensive research and experience,
there is no guarantee of results associated with this information. The publisher and
author are not liable for any damages or negative consequences to any person reading
or following the information or recipes in this book. All efforts have been made to
ensure the information contained in this book is accurate and up-to-date at the time
of going to press. References are provided for informational purposes only and do not
constitute endorsement of any sources.

A CIP catalogue record for this book is available from the British Library.

ISBN 978-1-9993061-2-0

Printed in the Czech Republic

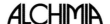

NUTRITION
Brought to Life

A Thorough Grounding in Nourishment
with 50 Delicious Recipes

Kirsten Chick

CONTENTS

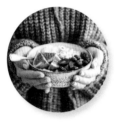
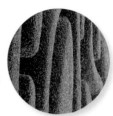
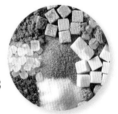
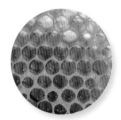
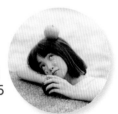
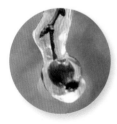
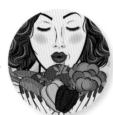
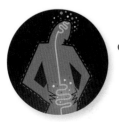
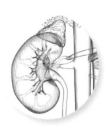

CONTENTS

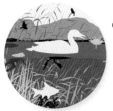
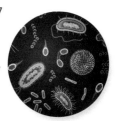
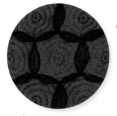
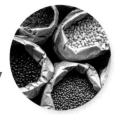
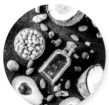
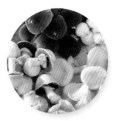
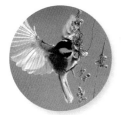
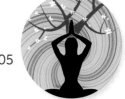
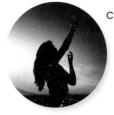
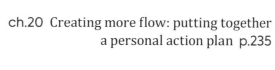 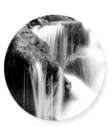
PART TWO: RECIPES p.241

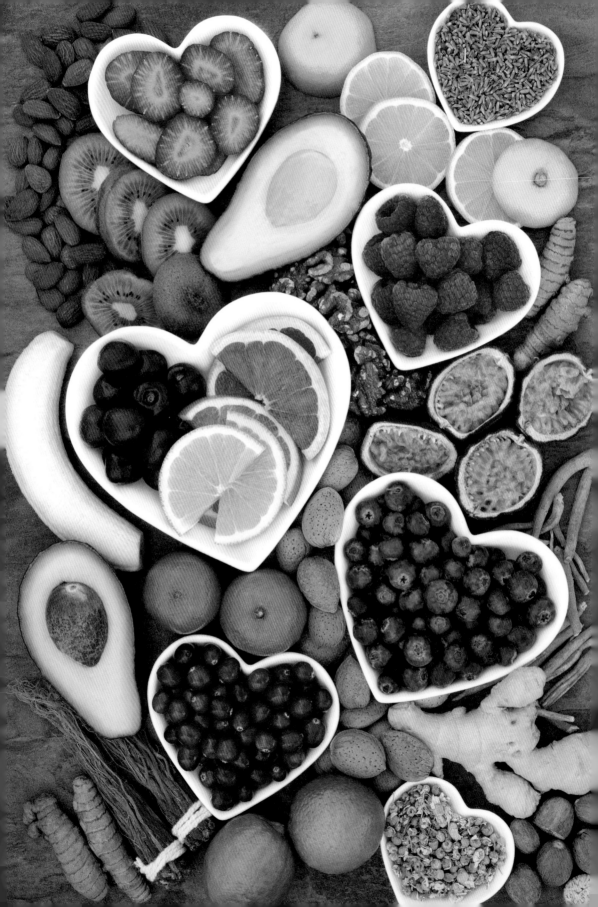

Introduction

Many years ago, nutrition helped bring me back to life. In return, I have spent the intervening years bringing nutrition to life.

Firstly, by bringing the science of nutrition to life, in consultations, workshops and colleges. Describing how the sunshine that energises the planet finds its way into every cell of your body, making everything that you think and do possible. Recounting which parts of your food make up your bricks and mortar, and which form the workers that make everything happen. How each of your body systems work (your heart, intestines, liver, hormones, immune system), how they interact with and form part of each other. And how what you eat can influence all of that. All in ways that are easy to understand, and that celebrate the wonder of it all, while keeping as true to the science and up-to-date with the research as I can.

Secondly, by bringing nutrition more fully into people's lives, in practical and realistic ways. With tips, ideas, recipes and positivity. Encouraging an awareness and appreciation of nutrition in everyday shopping, cooking, eating, snacking and living. Bringing delicious, simply prepared, wholesome food to the table. Easing nutrition off the page into your kitchens and onto your plates.

The passion behind all of this is a strongly held conviction that food is meant to nourish you. Not just give you fuel. Not make you feel inadequate, or lacking in willpower. But truly nourish you.

Nourish:
to provide (someone or something) with food and other things that are needed to live, be healthy, etc. to cause (something) to develop or grow stronger
(merriam-webster.com)

The word nourish summons up feelings of being loved and cared for, being wrapped in a blanket of flavours and colours, and given deeply fulfilling sustenance.

For too long we have been treating our bodies like a slot machine. We count calories like we count our money, and feed them in regardless of quality. We load up with sugar and carbohydrates as if they were tokens for energy, and deprive ourselves of fat if we see too much on our bodies. It's all very black and white, very mechanical – but you aren't a machine! You are much more vibrant, dynamic and colourful than that, and deserve a whole lot more.

You deserve to be nurtured, suckled, fed, given everything you need to live, be healthy, develop and grow stronger. You deserve to enjoy the textures and tastes of different foods, the sensations they evoke and the different ways they make you feel. You deserve to absorb the nutrients and vitality they offer, carry them through every blood vessel, flowing to your brain, your heart, your lungs, your toes, helping you move through and interact with life to the full. You deserve to be nourished.

In order to nourish yourself, you need to understand nutrition and you need to understand your body. So over the course of this book, I'm going to explain the fundamentals of nutrition, examining each nutrient in a way that makes it relevant to how your body works and how you feel. Along the way, I'll be painting clear pictures of how your digestion works, your hormones, your immune system and your detoxification systems. How stress impacts your body, and how you can get everything relaxed, flowing and full of vitality again.

I'll also provide opportunities for you to reflect, make gradual changes, and try out some truly delicious, tried and tested recipes. You'll be forgiven for jumping straight to the recipe section at the back! And then I hope you'll enjoy not just the food, but also exploring why it's so fundamental to your physical and mental health.

My wish is that this book brings nutrition to life for you, and helps you weave nourishment into your everyday life.

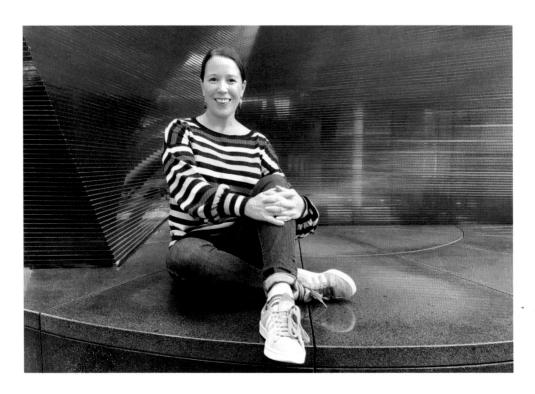

PART ONE

NUTRITION

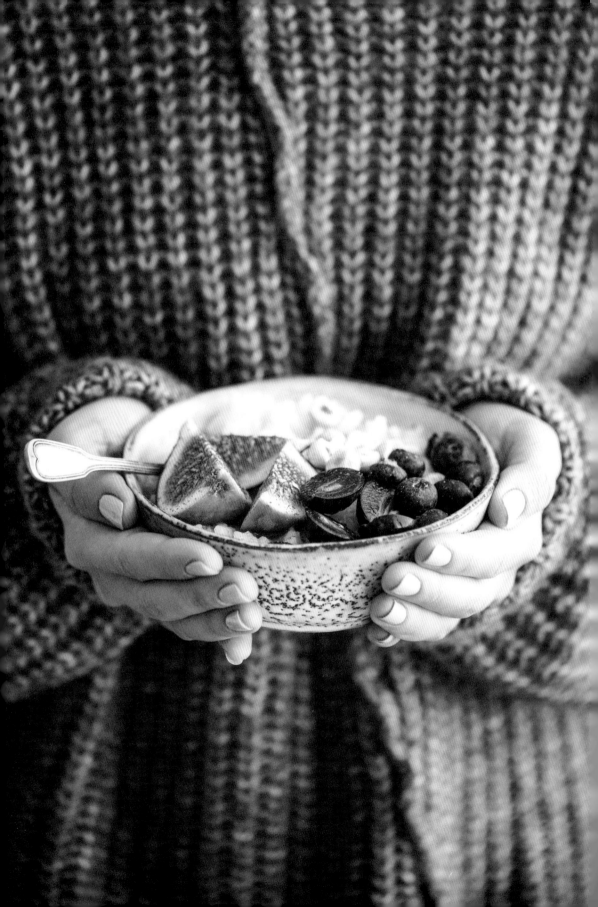

Chapter 1

Why aren't we nourishing ourselves?

"You deserve." There's issue number one for many people. Do you really feel like you deserve all this? There are so many reasons for this that one could spend hours analysing – perhaps you were told you weren't good enough as a child, or bullied or abused in some way, maybe life has let you down too many times to dare to want something, or it may even be an inherent part of our social structure – whatever the reason, low self-esteem is a pattern I've noticed a lot both in my consultation room and among people I've met generally in life.

A list of things that nourish you

The result is often a drive to self-deprive. A sense that you have to eat less, enjoy less, take up less space to be a really good or really healthy person. Or more subtly, not quite getting round to doing those things that really soothe your soul and fire your passions. Filling your life with work/exercise/doing things for other people, and feeling guilty when you do something for yourself, or when you just relax and do nothing for a while.

I'm not saying everyone should live a life of total self-indulgence, but for many, the balance seems to have gone too far the other way. And that's hard to sustain.

It can sometimes be nice to make an honest list of all the things that nourish you, on any level. My list sometimes looks something like this:

- Walking in the woods or on the beach
- Reading a good book in the bath
- Gardening
- Taking time to cook and enjoy a really delicious meal
- Meeting a good friend for tea and cake
- Eventually finding time to have that clear out, or spring clean a room – i.e. a job on my to-do list that I really want to do, not a duty thing or something someone else wants me to do
- Dancing

Then assess how often you are including all of these in your life. Sometimes you might find you tick all the boxes, and at other times you might need to start timetabling a few in.

The trick is to allow yourself time to nourish yourself each day or each week – *guilt-free*. This means without judging what you're doing to be "good" or "bad", or worrying about whether you should be doing something else instead. It means recognising that the things on your list are there because they nourish you on some important level and you need them as much as you need air to breathe. It means valuing yourself enough to put yourself high on your list of priorities. That doesn't mean you have to neglect your children, partner, job, friends etc., it just means that you may need to rebalance how you are spreading out your time and energy.

I can already hear some of you thinking: "Tea and cake? Really?!!" Well this is an area I intend to explore in more detail, but as a starter: if you enjoy a spot of afternoon tea every now and then, and I mean really let yourself enjoy it, then you are less likely to fall into the trap of yo-yoing between cravings, self-recrimination and comfort eating.

So for the time being, accept what's on your list, and reassess every now and then: "Is this still nourishing me, or is it just a habit now – or something that used to energise me or help me relax but doesn't anymore?" Taking the judgement out removes a lot of the stress and emotion, which can help you to feel more clearly what's going on and respond more easily.

So if what feels nourishing right now is to spend five minutes staring out of the window with the sun on your face, then give yourself that five minutes. Spending the whole time nagging yourself with "I should be doing such and such" or "Why can't I get going right now?" denies you that time which you may actually need to recharge, so that you have the energy and clarity to get on with everything else. So bathe in that five minutes, fully immerse yourself in relaxation, knowing that in five minutes you will get going again with renewed vigour and motivation.

Being fully present

There is also commonly a need to keep busy and distracted, because being present is too uncomfortable. To stop and nourish yourself fundamentally involves settling into yourself, being fully present in your body in this moment. So many ancient practices aim for this: meditation, yoga, chi kung, dance... and yet we often find it so difficult. We can sometimes go really out of our way to avoid being fully present. Why is that?

I believe it's partly because there is an aspect of being present that means fully feeling and accepting yourself for who you are. Loving yourself for who you are. Turning off that critical voice that tells you you're too fat, too thin, too lazy, too selfish, too stupid, too boring, not fit enough, not beautiful enough, not healthy enough, not productive enough: inadequate. That in itself is a profound process that may take some work.

In addition, being present can be quite uncomfortable. Most of us are living with some kind of inflammation and discomfort, whether we are aware of it or not. It may be a physical issue, it may be psychological pain or anxiety, or more likely it's both. So we seek distractions that stop us from feeling what's going on, by taking us out of the present moment and away from that deep connection with ourselves. We rush from one distraction to another, from work to the gym to the bar, from television to social media, or running errands for everyone but ourselves.

In terms of food, it's often wolfed down, ignored, or obsessed and worried over. As we shall see, any of this will make digestion and absorption of nutrients more difficult. And in fact, your stress response may already have instructed your digestive system to downgrade its activity in order to save resources. A combination of stress, poorly digested food and related factors will create often inflammatory conditions in the digestive tract that make the very act of eating difficult to be fully present with. There may be actual pain or discomfort, or it may be just enough irritation for the gut to signal the brain to avoid food, or only eat foods that don't require much digestion – such as sugar and refined carbohydrates. The relationship between stress and eating habits is both physical and psychological – and so needs an approach that addresses both.

Practising being present, even for just brief moments, can be a useful part of this. It sends a neurological message to your body that it's safe enough to feel what's going on now, the trauma or threat has gone away. In turn, everything relaxes, helping to free up movement in your body in a way that has untold benefits, including reducing inflammation, helping your body to absorb the nutrients from your food and enabling those nutrients to circulate.

In some cases, trying to be fully present is not yet appropriate, in particular where there is deep trauma. In such a situation, the person will need professional guidance to arrive at a place where they can feel "safe enough" to fully feel everything again.

However, most people who try mindfulness practices of any kind will find them beneficial. And you may well be surprised at how little of each day you are · actually completely present for. It can be interesting to assess every now and then both this and how much you are giving to yourself, on all kinds of levels. You may need to look below the surface a little here. I have met countless people who are "doing everything right": they eat a healthy diet, go to the gym or yoga, meditate, take regular breaks and holidays, spend time with friends – and yet they are still far from nourished. There is a big difference between following the programme and allowing it to nourish you, just as there is a big difference between eating wholesome food and actually absorbing the nutrients from it.

Trust your body

It's important to understand how this all works in order to change it, but you also don't want to get too stuck in your head with it. This isn't an intellectual exercise, it's your body and your life. So you need to include your body, and not just your mind, in the experience and in the decision-making processes. So throughout this book, I'm going to encourage you to check in with your body, find out how it feels, and trust what it's telling you. The more you work on calming down inflammation and stress, the easier that should be.

Our heads can be very clever, but they can also tie us up in knots. We read and hear different things and get confused about what's right. We can also be very judgmental, especially towards ourselves, and give ourselves a hard time if we don't "get it right". We end up trying to do what we think we "should", rather than what feels right. That adds in more stress, which creates more inflammation and constriction, which gets in the way of how well we can digest foods and hydrate ourselves.

Much of this may stem from fear: fear of getting ill or weak, fear of dying, fear of being overweight or underweight, fear of standing out, of not being accepted – and there can be so many levels and nuances to that fear. Instead, a healthier approach might be *commitment to good health from a sense of self-love*, which brings us back full circle to the opening question: why aren't we nourishing ourselves? Working on self-esteem and self-acceptance may be an integral part of this whole process.

So I'm going to ask you to approach your health and nutrition with a playful curiosity, and judge your success by how nourished you feel.

The fundamentals of nutrition and health

In this book we will explore together the fundamentals of how your body works and how nutrition might affect or support it. This includes *how your body digests and absorbs nutrients, how it makes energy, how it protects itself, how it regulates inflammation, how it sends internal messages and how it gets rid of toxins and waste.* Much of this relies on how well things can flow, as opposed to being stagnant or stuck.

It's these fundamentals that are primarily responsible for good health, and working on this level can be beneficial in surprising ways. I usually have clever, innovative supplements and protocols up my sleeve to add into someone's programme once the basics are in place – but often don't need to use them. It's as if your body is a complex clockwork mechanism, where perhaps one cog is stuck or out of place, or there is a layer of rust in various patches, which means the hands on the clock face aren't turning. Replacing the hands won't fix the clock. If you sort out the cog or clean off the rust, the whole mechanism can start moving again, including the hands.

So this book is largely about what the cogs do and how to keep them moving.

Make it personal

There are also opportunities at the end of each chapter to reflect, as well as practical tips and/or recipes that are relevant to the chapter content. There's no point knowing all the theory if you don't try putting it into practice!

If you are reading this for your own benefit, then I hope these will help support your progress. If you are practising or studying nutrition, then you may find these useful for both your own personal development and to share with your clients.

Reflection time

- **What nourishes you?**
  Write a list of everything that makes you feel truly, deeply nourished
  How often do you experience the things on your list?

- **What is your aim with nutrition?**
  Write a list – however short or long – of what motivates you, and any issues you would like to address or prevent.

Action plan

- **Practise being present**
  - *At least once a day, take time to feel your feet on the ground, the temperature of your skin, the sights and smells around you, the taste in your mouth, the feeling in your belly.*
  - *Try to avoid judging sensations as "good" or "bad". Instead savour every sensation as if it were a new and curious experience.*
  - *Then let it all go and get on with your day.*

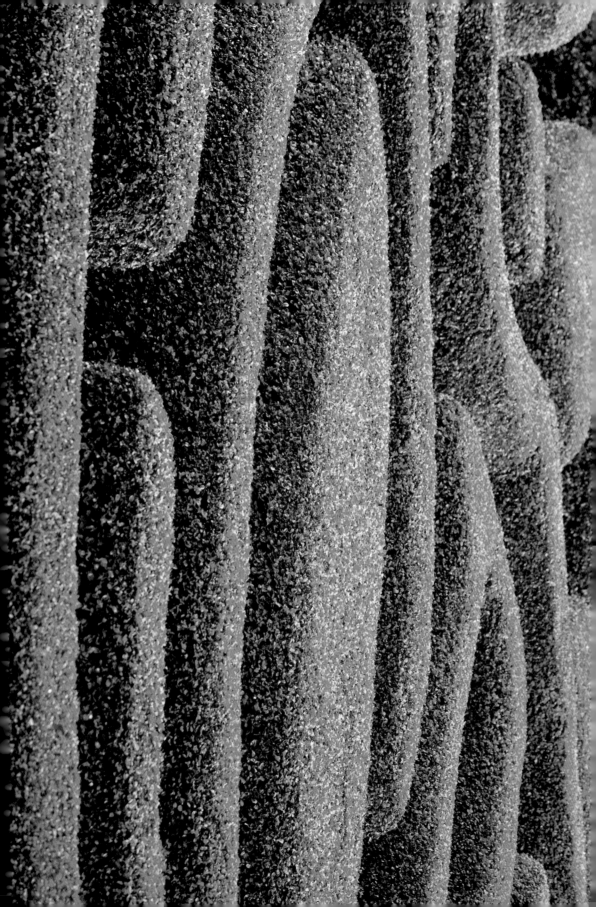

Chapter 2

Digestion
~ a brief look inside ~

To understand how to nourish yourself effectively with food, you need to understand how your digestive system works. After all, there's no point spending time, effort and money putting together an amazingly nutritious meal if you're then not going to digest and absorb its nutrients very well. Being fully present when you eat is one aspect of this, as I'll explain.

This is a brief introduction to your digestive system – there will be a more detailed one in chapter 6. What I first want to make clear is that, if you pulled this system out of your body and fed it some food, it wouldn't work. It relies on your heart to pump blood around and help clear toxicity, your kidneys to help regulate your blood's contents, your lungs to breathe in oxygen to help you make the energy you need for digestion, your hormonal system to send out the right triggers and messages at the right times, your nervous system to do the same, as well as to monitor what is required and act on new information, your limbs to hunt/gather/buy/prepare your food and so on. Everything within you is interrelated, and it all works together like a complex and magical piece of superintelligent machinery.

As we take a quick tour through your digestive system, bear in mind at all times that it is connected to, relies on and is relied upon by many other aspects of you.

Your brain
Most people wouldn't consider their brain to be part of the digestive system, and yet most anatomy and physiology text books will mention the cephalic phase of digestion – cephalic meaning related to the head. Thinking about, seeing and smelling your food will alert your brain to what you are about to eat, and your brain will tell the rest of your digestive system to make ready.[1]

Your mouth (aka oral cavity)
Your teeth rip and grind the food, and together with your saliva, break it down into a paste (if you are chewing well enough!). Saliva is released from three sets of glands in your mouth – the average person produces about 1.5 litres of saliva a day! Two of those glands – the parotid and submandibular glands – also release enzymes that start to break down carbohydrates. Your tongue is there to help shape the chewed up food and direct it towards your throat to be swallowed.

Your oesophagus (aka esophagus)
This is the foodpipe that directs your food towards your stomach. There are sphincters at the top and bottom, and it also has to pass through your diaphragm, so it's a little more controlled than a drainpipe.

Your stomach
Your stomach is higher up in your body than what you might think of as your tummy. It is the most acidic part of your digestive tract – and body – and it's where proteins start to be broken down.

Your small intestine (aka small bowel)
There are three parts to your small intestine: the duodenum, jejunum and ileum. This is where most of the breaking down (digesting) and absorption of nutrients takes place.

Your pancreas
Some of the enzymes involved in digestion in your small intestine are produced in your intestinal wall, but many of them are produced by the pancreas, and released when the time is right.

As your stomach releases food into your small intestine, your pancreas squirts out a fountain of enzymes plus alkalising juices. If your pancreas didn't do this, the acid from your stomach would burn a hole in your small intestine, and you wouldn't have enough enzymes to fully digest your dinner.

Your liver
Whatever gets absorbed into your bloodstream is now carried to your liver to be processed and sent to where it needs to go.

Your liver also produces bile, which is stored and then released by your gallbladder when you eat something fatty. Both the pancreas and the liver make use of the common bile duct to release their substances into the small intestine.

Your large intestine (aka colon or large bowel)
What hasn't been absorbed generally ends up here, to be further processed and excreted as faeces (aka poo). Some water and water soluble nutrients are absorbed here.

This is also where the majority of your bowel flora resides (aka gut bacteria, aka microbiota). And you have an appendix there too, which many people have found they can live without. However, it's not the useless dangly thing medical professionals once believed it to be. We now know it is an important part of your immune system, and possibly also a kind of seed bank for beneficial bacteria.

Your GI tract

The route from mouth to anus is known as the gastrointestinal tract, or GI tract for short. Like a tunnel, it has walls, known as the gastrointestinal wall. This wall is mostly made of four layers:

1. Adventitia – the outermost layer, sometimes in a slightly different form called serosa

2. Muscular layer – the next layer in, largely muscle as the name suggests

3. Submucosa – just underneath the mucosa, contains lots of blood and lymph vessels and nerves

4. Mucosa (aka mucous membrane) – innermost layer, often contains an extra layer of muscle

The mucosa contains lots of mucus secreting cells called goblet cells, to keep itself moist and protected from damage.

In the small intestine, much of the mucosa has a brush-like surface to help you absorb more nutrients.

The muscles are there to contract and pulse, to gently drive its contents along. This motion is called peristalsis, and is the same kind of movement you might see when watching a snake consume a mouse, for example.

In fact, all of your organs are in a continual state of motion. They're not just hanging there inside of you, but are busy all day and all night long. Every time you breathe out and in, your diaphragm, a kind of elastic sheet cutting across your middle, rises and falls, massaging and kneading your lungs above it and your stomach, liver, pancreas, kidneys and so on below it. Your heart is continually pumping and your arteries pulsing, your blood and lymph flowing, urine gathering, sweat and mucus seeping, body hair twitching with temperature changes, neurotransmitters jumping from nerve to nerve and lighting them up like Christmas.

All of this takes an enormous amount of energy, before you even think about walking down the street, let alone going to the gym. Fortunately, it is also the very process (or at least one of them) that supplies you with energy. Much of what you absorb in the small intestine can potentially be converted into energy. Let's have a look at how you do this.

Reflection time

- *Just take a few moments here to send some appreciation to your digestive system! We'll look at it in more detail in chapter 6.*

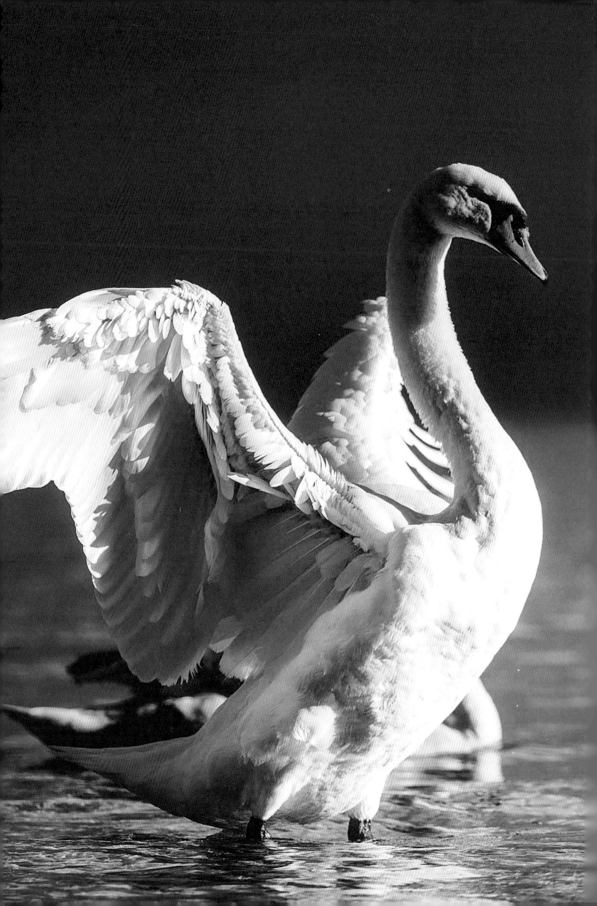

Chapter 3

Vitality
~ harnessing nature's energy ~

Energy is the power to do things and drive processes; it's the force that creates movement; it's the vibration of light waves and the subatomic particles that make up our universe – including us.

We often think of food purely as fuel – or calorific intake – so that we can keep going without flagging. To a certain extent that's true, but it's a very superficial view of something really quite magical.

It also gives us a very bland view of food as just calories: it doesn't matter what we eat, as long as we eat the same amount of calories as we burn. This notion of food is not just dull, it's incorrect.

For a start, we have a continual turnover of cells, so we need a daily source of raw materials to make them. So as well as providing fuel, the proteins, carbohydrates and fats (lipids) that make up the food we eat are broken down and restructured to make parts of us: our organs, limbs, nerves, flesh and blood. We can also use them to make enzymes, hormones and other substances we use in our bodies to perform specific tasks.

There are also vitamins, minerals and other nutrients in food that we need as sort of factory workers for energy production, body part production, enzyme and hormone production, nerve cell activity, tissue health and protection and much more.

Proteins, carbohydrates and lipids are called macronutrients, while vitamins, minerals and other smaller nutrients are called micronutrients.

Meet your macronutrients

Proteins are made up of chains of different kinds of amino acids. When we digest proteins, we break them down into these individual amino acids, often called the building blocks of life. They are used to make various structures in your cells and cell membranes, and so are essential for all the different kinds of tissue that make up your body (not just muscles!). They are also used to make enzymes, some hormones, antibodies and more. In some instances they can be burnt for fuel, and therefore represent a source of energy.

Food sources: most foods contain some kind of protein, but the most protein-dense sources include meat, fish, eggs, dairy, pulses, nuts, seeds and spirulina.

NB: "Complete proteins" contain all the amino acids you need to obtain from your diet, and include all the animal protein sources plus soya products, quinoa and amaranth. Certain combinations of other vegetarian protein sources can make up a complete protein: generally speaking a pulse plus either a nut, a seed or a grain, but this may not be necessary in the same meal.

Carbohydrates are made up of chains of sugars; longer chains are called complex carbohydrates, and solo sugars or chains of just two together are called simple carbohydrates or sugars. We think of them as being just a source of energy, but actually they provide a lot of structure too, for example in cell membranes, mucus and some hormones. We can also store them as fat if we have too many in our diet.

Food sources: whole grains (e.g. whole wheat, brown rice, oats) and starchy vegetables (e.g. potatoes, sweet potatoes) contain complex carbohydrates; refined carbohydrates (e.g. white flour, white pasta, white rice) contain complex carbohydrates stripped down without the fibre and nutrients to help us digest them; fruit and honey contain simple carbohydrates (sugars); refined sugars, such as white cane sugar and some syrups, contain simple sugars without the fibre and nutrients we need to process them healthily.

Lipids are fats and oils, and are made up of different kinds of fatty acids. We can use them for energy or for structure. Most fats and oils, including butter, olive oil, sunflower oil and coconut oil, contain a range of different fatty acids. People generally like to divide them into "good" and "bad" fats, but it truly isn't that simple.
     Some are saturated: i.e. made stable by being completely covered with hydrogen ions. Others are unsaturated: i.e. mostly covered with hydrogen ions except for one or more small areas – which means they sometimes have more exciting roles in the body, but also that they can oxidise and go rancid quickly, especially in the presence of heat and light. That's one reason why oils that are rich in unsaturated fatty acids, such as sunflower, olive, flax, hemp and fish oil are not considered safe to heat. Heating them also produces carcinogenic substances. Fats that contain mostly saturated fatty acids, such as coconut oil and animal fats, are much safer to heat. You may not want to eat huge amounts of these, however, depending on your lifestyle.
     Some unsaturated fatty acids are referred to as omega 3, 6 or 9 fatty acids, which describes their structure. Modern diets tend to be over heavy on the omega 6s, which may contribute to chronic inflammation.

Food sources: fish, algae, flax seeds, chia seeds (omega 3); nuts, seeds (omega 6); olives (omega 9); animal fats, coconut oil, palm oil (saturated fatty acids).

NB: There are also different kinds of each omega fatty acid. e.g. omega 3 fatty acids appear as ALA in flax and chia seeds, and the longer EPA and DHA in fish oil and algae. We can convert ALA to EPA and DHA, but not very efficiently. EPA and DHA are needed to help counter inflammation and make healthy tissue, especially in the brain.

Solar powered people

The energy that you get from food, be it from the carbohydrates, proteins or lipids, originally comes from the sun.

The sun is a massive ball of gases that shoots out energy, and we feel it warming our faces, bathing our whole bodies sometimes, as golden sunshine, bringing light and heat into our day. Sunshine can be measured as waves or as tiny, highly energised particles called photons – whichever way you choose to measure them, they oscillate their way down through space and the earth's atmosphere, to eventually shine upon and be absorbed by plants and other living beings.

We are very familiar with the way that plants capture the energy from photons and use that to grow – we call this photosynthesis. Then you eat the plant, or an animal that has eaten the plant, and your body has very specific ways it extracts the energy that the photons brought from the sun.

So you may not think beyond the concept of getting energy from the food you eat, but actually you're getting it from the sun. The energy you get from your food is the solar power that has travelled down with the sun's rays.

In very brief terms, you break foods down to their simplest forms, and some of these then have the energy extracted from them. Carbohydrates, for example, may be broken down to glucose, a rich store of calories, or solar power. To get at that energy, you have to put it through a multi-staged process called cellular respiration. The final stages take part in tiny structures in your cells called mitochondria. Because you need so much energy to drive so many processes every second of your lives, your cells contain hundreds and sometimes thousands of mitochondria.

The energy harnessing process gets to a point where you have released a whole bunch of highly charged subatomic particles from your food called electrons and protons, but you have to be careful you don't just let them bounce around causing havoc like a herd of miniature bulls in a china shop – or indeed your mitochondria. Mitochondrial damage has been linked to many serious diseases, including cancer, Alzheimer's disease and Parkinson's disease.[2] So the mitochondria have a kind of dam set up that forces these tiny particles through in single file, like a hydrodam harnessing the power of a river. At the end of the dam, the energy is stored neatly in molecules called ATP, which I like to think of as minuscule batteries. When your body needs some energy – perhaps to recall a memory, or to contract or relax a muscle – it pops in one of these batteries and uses it for power.

Ketone bodies

Although we mainly think of sugars and carbohydrates as providing energy, you can also harness solar power from fats and proteins. You can slot fats and proteins into the same ATP production process, and if you were starving, your body would eventually start to break down the protein in your muscles for energy. Alternatively, you can convert fat into ketone bodies, which are then easily convertible into ATP.

Your body will seek to make ketone bodies from stored and consumed fats before it starts to break down proteins from muscle tissue. Just to feed your brain, your body would need to be breaking down nearly a kilo of muscle tissue a day.[3] So fats are definitely a more preferred option.

The ketogenic diet – a diet high in fats and low in both carbohydrates and proteins – works with the body's ability to convert fat into ketone bodies. Brain cells are especially good at harnessing energy from ketones. The blood-brain barrier conspires with this by supplying specific transporters for ketone bodies into the brain when carbohydrate intake is very low and during starvation.

The ketogenic diet was originally used for people with epilepsy. In many ways it mimics fasting, which had been observed to reduce seizures. The processes involved in restricting carbohydrates and producing ketones seem to have specific anti-seizure mechanisms.[4]

Scientists have now realised that some cancer cells aren't so good at making energy from ketones, so ketogenic diets have also become an interesting area of research, particularly with certain brain tumours.[5] The premise is that a ketogenic diet will starve at least some kinds of cancer cells that are reliant on glucose for ATP production, while supplying healthy cells with all the energy they need.[6]

Take a walk on the wild side

Some scientists would also argue that we have our own version of photosynthesis – that electrons clustering around each of our cells can absorb the energy from photons directly. As light photons (from sunshine, for example) come into your body and shine upon your cells' outer walls, electrons there start to vibrate at a faster frequency. They become energised directly by the sun. That is now stored energy that your body can use.[7]

The electrons are in the unsaturated fatty acids that the outer walls of your cells contain. Note that the lipids with the highest number of electrons are EPA and DHA, the omega 3 fatty acids found in fish oil and algae, and AA, an omega 6 oil found largely in animal, fish and dairy fats.

It seems you can also conduct electrons directly from the earth into your body.[8] These electrons carry stored solar energy too. Walking barefoot, getting your hands in the soil, really having physical contact with the earth can not only feel very grounding, but can also energise you and form part of a health restoring process.

So in many respects we can equate electrons with a potential for vitality, and therefore a well-functioning, healthy body. We can also perhaps more confidently include spending time outdoors in nature and in gentle sunshine in our list of things that nourish us.

Co-factor support

Your energy processing systems need teams of little helpers every step of the way, and this is where many of the vitamins, minerals and other nutrients we consume come into play. We call any substances that are needed to carry out a process a co-factor, and the list of co-factors for ATP production includes magnesium, B vitamins, antioxidants, amino acids (proteins) and much more.

My generation has been brought up to believe you need carbohydrates (such as sugar, starchy vegetables and grains) for energy, and the more active you are, the more carbohydrates you need. So there seems to be a general belief out there that you need to eat more pasta, potatoes, bread, cakes and sweets when you play sports, go running or go to the gym. We can already start to see, however, that it's not that simple. Apart from also being able to produce energy from fats and proteins, we also need a vast array of vitamins, minerals and other nutrients from a variety of food sources to carry out the processes of harnessing the solar energy from foods and storing it as ATP. We need still more to then access and release that energy. We need vegetables, fruit, good quality oils, good levels of hydration, fresh air, mindful exercise, effective stress management... the list goes on!

Paradoxically, we have also been brought up with an obsession for calories. Just like the carbohydrate-energy myth, we have been taught that to lose weight we need to restrict calories, to gain weight or to support higher levels of exercise, we need more calories. As there are more calories, gram per gram, in fats than in carbohydrates, this has led to a diet industry that focuses on low fat. So at the same time as promoting the belief that you need high levels of carbohydrates for energy, food companies are also selling you low fat, high carb "diet" foods to help you lose weight. No wonder we're all so confused about food! And on top of that, no mention of any of the vitamins, minerals, amino acids or other co-factors you need to successfully and efficiently make ATP molecules.

Main co-factors for ATP production:

Magnesium *Food sources: green leafy vegetables, seeds, nuts*	Alpha-lipoic acid *Food sources: spinach, broccoli, organ meats*
Vitamin B1 (thiamin) *Food sources: sunflower seeds, peas, beans*	Coenzyme Q10 *Food sources: meat, fish, nuts*
Vitamin B2 (riboflavin) *Food sources: spinach, yoghurt, eggs*	L-carnitine *Food sources: meat, fish, dairy, asparagus*
Vitamin B3 (niacin) *Food sources: oily fish, meat, brown rice, avocados*	Other amino acids *Food sources: meat, fish, eggs, nuts, seeds, pulses*
Vitamin B5 (pantothenic acid) *Food sources: shiitake mushrooms, avocado, sweet potato*	D-ribose (a sugar that is actually part of the structure of ATP) *Your body can make this from riboflavin (see vitamin B2 above)*

Energy boosting meal ideas:

- Poached salmon with a salad of babyleaf spinach, rocket, avocado, toasted pumpkin and sunflower seeds
- Brown rice salad with asparagus, peas, wilted spinach, avocado and chopped hazelnuts
- Slow-baked sweet potato with houmous, spinach and walnuts
- Shiitake and asparagus stir fry with chard and black beans served with brown rice

The air that you breathe

In order for the mitochondria in your cells to harness energy from food as efficiently as possible, they need oxygen. Every time you breathe, you bring oxygen into your body. Your tree-like lungs expand, you breathe in life-giving air, the capillaries in your delicate lung tissue exchange oxygen for some carbon dioxide your blood needs to get rid of. Most of that oxygen is transported by your red blood cells: oxygen attached to iron embedded in your haemoglobin, which is a protein-based molecule that makes those blood cells red. To manufacture red blood cells, you need some B vitamins, including B2, B6, B12 and folate, plus vitamin A and copper. Oxygen can then diffuse from the blood into the rest of your cells like flavour moving from a teabag into a cup of hot water.

There are various factors that may affect how much oxygen is taken up by the cells for use by its mitochondria, including glucose levels, glutamine levels and how much oxygen is there already, as well as how much oxygen is circulating in your blood. If your red blood cell count is low, or blood vessels are constricted (for example due to stress or inflammation) or blocked (for example in heart attacks and strokes), then there will be less circulating oxygen, either in a specific area or generally in your body. Or perhaps you have been exercising so vigorously that you are unable to breathe in enough oxygen to help fuel your activity.

If your cells have access to plenty of oxygen, then normal ATP production can continue. This is called aerobic respiration. If oxygen levels are low due to high bursts of physical activity, then all is not lost: your muscle cells can revert to anaerobic respiration, the process of making ATP without oxygen. This is much less efficient: for every molecule of glucose you can make two energy batteries of ATP, compared to about 32 with aerobic respiration. Plus there's the interesting by-product of lactic acid with anaerobic respiration, the same lactic acid produced when making yoghurt, sauerkraut and other fermented foods. That's why anaerobic respiration is also called fermentation.

This works well for muscles, but other healthy cells, such as brain cells, cannot survive without oxygen. Brain cell death will occur rapidly once any oxygen supply is cut off.

Tumour cells, however, seem to have the ability to switch to anaerobic respiration, and there is evidence to suggest that hypoxia (low oxygen levels) and the resulting acidity (from the lactic acid) may help tumours to survive and spread.[9]

Nobel Award winning Otto Warburg was the first to notice how much glucose cancer cells generally consume, and how much lactic acid they produce, both in conditions of hypoxia and where there is plenty of oxygen present. This focus on glucose metabolism in cancer research fell out of favour for a long time, but scientists have started to pick up on it again, to see how it ties in with all the other complexities of cancer behaviour we have noted over the years, but still cannot pull together cohesively enough to fully understand.[10]

A simplistic response to Warburg's observations has been to shout from the rooftops that "sugar feeds cancer" and so sugar should be avoided. Oncologists and cancer nurses are fond of pointing out that the body can break down most foods to sugar, and in progressive stages, will even start to break itself down, seemingly to feed the cancer. They are right to point this out, but I still do not believe this justifies the frequent advice to cancer patients to eat vast quantities of cakes, biscuits, chocolate bars, fast food and so on to "build up". Such a diet will still have adverse effects on insulin pathways and inflammatory processes that seem to me a priority to avoid, as we shall see. Sadly, most orthodox consultants, doctors, nurses and dieticians seem to focus more on calorie intake than the many other impacts of high levels of sugar and refined carbohydrates.

How much do calories count?

The traditional standpoint is that we count the energy provided by each foodstuff in calories, and it doesn't matter which foods those calories are from, it's just the number of calories that counts. So eating 1000 calories in roast chicken will have the same effect as eating 1000 calories in doughnuts: the same amount of energy will be released either to burn for fuel or turn into fat. And so a whole industry of calorie-obsessed diets was born, where the calorie count is deemed to be the only nutritional factor that makes a difference to weight loss.

As there are more than twice as many calories per gram in fats than in carbohydrates (approx. nine compared to approx. four), fats have been demonised by the diet industry: you eat fat, you get fat, we are told. With that reasoning, a few generations have now been brainwashed to believe that fatty foods, including nuts, seeds and avocados, are fattening and therefore to be avoided, and substituted for low fat fruit yoghurts and rice cakes if you want to stay trim.

Meanwhile, there has been growing dissent from those of us who believe the body and its relationship to food is more complex and dynamic than that.

I mentioned the ketogenic diet with regard to energy production, and indeed we can make more energy from fat, gram per gram, than from sugar and other carbohydrates. However, that does not mean eating fat makes us fatter compared to eating carbohydrates. In fact, Dr. Atkins raised the profile of using a ketogenic diet for weight *loss* in the 1970s. His version was high in both dairy fat and animal protein. The Dukan diet, Paleo diets and others also promote weight loss through carbohydrate reduction. Contemporary versions of the ketogenic diet are more focused on restricting proteins as well as carbohydrates, and keeping fat levels high, particularly levels of Medium Chain Triglycerides (MCTs). MCTs convert rapidly to ketone bodies, and are only minimally stored as body fat, while increasing how much other fat you burn generally through the day.[11] Yes, you read that correctly: eating higher levels of fats called MCTs helps you to burn fat and lose weight.

The increasingly popular coconut oil is relatively rich in MCTs. Coconut oil has been measured to have 8.62[12] calories per 100g, which is about par for the course for fats and oils: butter has 7.17, lard has 8.98, olive oil has 8.84. Compare that to a stick of Brighton rock, which is 100% sugar and has 4.29 calories per gram. You'd think that eating coconut oil would lead to putting on twice as much weight as sucking on seaside rock, as that's what the calorie counting industry would have you believe. Instead, coconut oil can help you burn calories, lose weight and be healthier as a result. It seems not all calories are created equal after all, and we have known this for some time.

A study carried out over 30 years ago compared an intake of 2tbsp coconut oil daily with the same intake of soybean oil (7.63 calories per gram). The participants were women who were otherwise on a low calorie diet and went for daily walks. The women in both groups lost about 2lb by the end of 28 days, but *the women in the coconut group lost belly fat, while the soybean oil group gained belly fat.*[13] So even where overall weight loss was comparable, the effects on health and wellbeing may be markedly different.

Belly fat, also known as visceral adiposity, has been linked to a whole range of cardiovascular health risks, some cancers, diabetes and impaired blood sugar mechanisms, including glucose intolerance, increased levels of insulin and insulin resistance in the liver. People who are more prone to store their fat below the belly – sometimes described as more pear-shaped than apple-shaped – are less likely to die from these kinds of diseases.[14, 15] Belly fat tissue releases pro-inflammatory cytokines and is associated with inflammation in the liver, and in later chapters we shall see how inflammation underpins all chronic illness.[16]

On the other end of the scale, cancer patients with cachexia, a concerning degree of fat and muscle loss, are often encouraged to "build up" by eating high fat dairy products and fried foods. The aim is to increase calorie intake, with little or no regard for the differing effects of different types of foods on metabolism and general health. Quite a number of cancer patients have reported to me that they've been told by their nurses and dieticians to eat McDonalds and other takeaway foods, cream cakes, ice cream and milk chocolate bars, all to put on weight. Weight gain through increased calories is seen as a priority above all factors, despite increasing evidence that cachexia is a complex condition strongly related to inflammation, hormonal changes related to long term stress responses, insulin resistance and a number of additional complex factors.[17] Many of these factors are worsened, not helped, by the kind of gut irritating, nutrient-depleting diet often advised. In fact, we have just seen how some kinds of fat – in the above example, omega-6 rich soya bean oil – may contribute to pro-inflammatory belly fat, and there is a big health difference between this kind of weight gain, and more general fat and muscle development. In addition, the processed meals and snacks often included or even relied upon may contain a hornet's nest of sugars, additives, damaged fats and other toxic and/or pro-inflammatory factors.

Cachexia is a more extreme example, but actually a similar range of complex factors determines everyone's ability to gain or lose weight, to make enough energy for all our bodily processes, to keep our cells and tissue healthy and generally to keep illness at bay. The next chapter looks at one of these in more detail: your insulin pathways.

Reflection time

- *Have you ever counted calories?* How did it make you feel? On what levels did it seem to work for you / not work for you?*

* Counting calories is where you add up the calories in each meal to make sure it contains a particular amount. This is usually done either by weighing foods and working out the calories of the proteins, carbohydrates and fats they contain, or by taking the information from labels in processed foods.

Recipes

It's not just carbs that you need to feel energised. These recipes contain nutrients and co-factors that you need to make the ATP "batteries" of energy that drive most of your body's activities.

- ***Energising salad*** *– p.264*
- ***Nutty asparagus and brown rice salad*** *– p.264*
- ***Rousing risotto*** *– p.252*

A little note about science

The views I express and activities I describe have been informed by reading hundreds of scientific documents, including research papers, reviews, books and more – as well as by working with many hundreds of individuals, and my own experience. I am completely open to revising my opinions at any point as and when new information and insights come about. So the information in this book is not set in stone, but the best I can offer at the time of writing. I have spent well over a decade researching scientific studies relating to nutrition and health, and it's true that much of it is problematic. It's hard to carry out a double blind placebo test on eating carrots, for example, because both the carrot-eating group and the control group are going to know if they've been eating carrots or not. There is no suitable placebo I can think of for a carrot.

Many studies involve asking people what they eat or drink and then either monitoring or asking about their health status. Some such projects involve thousands of people over many years, and so seem to offer a wealth of data. However, we also need to remember the data that will be missing: both false reporting of what people actually eat, as well as answers to questions that might not have been asked (e.g. how the carrot was cooked). In addition to that, data can be interpreted in different ways, and there is often disagreement as to what the results actually mean.

To give a very basic example, you could ask 200,000 people how many apples they eat each day for 20 years, and then also how often they visit a doctor. You could then take the results of that research to answer the question, "Does an apple a day keep the doctor away?" For a number of reasons, some of the people you ask will lie, even if it is an anonymous questionnaire. In addition, whether an apple a day is useful for keeping the doctor away may depend on a number of factors, such as:

- Is the apple raw or cooked? If cooked, how is it cooked?
- What else did you eat with the apple? What time of day was it eaten? Were you stressed or distracted when you ate it?
- Where was the apple grown, and what were the soil conditions like? Was there much sun/rainfall that year?
- How fresh was the apple and how had it been stored?
- What variety of apple is it?
- Do people that eat a daily apple also tend to eat or do other things that might be contributing to good health, such as exercising more?
- What is your access to GP services like?
- Are you the kind of person that calls the doctor for any old thing, or who avoids calling the doctor unless absolutely necessary?

You may have the foresight to ask some of these questions, but there may be other factors that you might never even consider asking about.

The human body is too complex for us to perhaps ever fully understand. In addition, your body has a lifetime of unique interactions with your environment, lifestyle choices and other influences that impact how you will respond, for example, to eating an apple a day. Scientists talk about the need for approaches to health to be "evidence-based", which means they are supported by tests and observation – but there will always be new tests, new observations, new insights and new information that come along and change what we thought we knew. So while I support an evidence-based approach, it is with eyes wide open that the current evidence base is, and will continue to be, limited. Note this is not just true of nutritional research. There are limitations to all kinds of scientific research, and a study is only ever as good as the questions it asks.

In my opinion, anyone who insists that something has been proven to be true beyond doubt, doesn't really understand science. Equally, anyone who insists that something is definitely not true because there is no evidence, is blinkered and doesn't really understand science. There is always room for doubt, and there is always room for further possibilities. To my mind, a true scientist is open to any and every possibility, and questions everything!

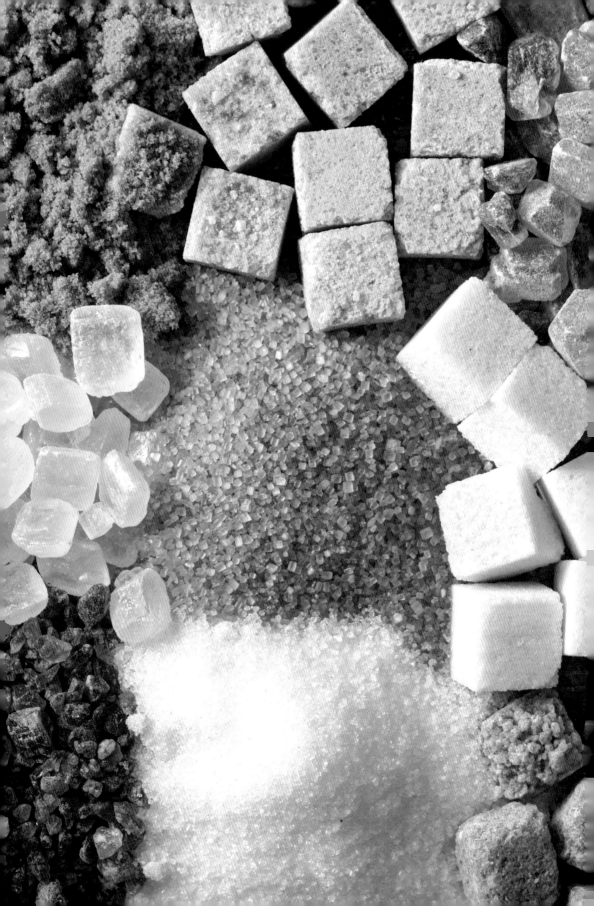

Chapter 4

Sugar
~ the highs and the lowdown ~

When life is sweet, I don't seem to crave so much sugar. I may enjoy sweet foods from time to time, but I don't actively seek it out. When my mood or zest for life drop, when I feel let down, or when I feel like the ground has fallen away beneath me, my thoughts turn to sugar. It's a pattern I learnt when I was very small, and reinforced with abandon as I grew up. It's one I now smile at like an old friend I have drifted away from. We sometimes hang out for a brief while, but I spend more time with my other friends these days. They don't challenge my insulin pathways so much.

Insulin and glucagon – balancing blood sugar

When you eat, your pancreas releases hormones that directly affect your energy pathways and fat levels. Remember that your pancreas sits near your stomach, and most of it is busy producing digestive juices to squirt into your small intestine. A small section of it, however, has a specialist role in balancing blood sugar.

About 2-3% of your pancreas, an exotic resort called the Islets of Langerhans, releases blood sugar regulating hormones called insulin and glucagon, plus a moderating hormone called somatostatin. These hormones then course through your bloodstream, with instructions for what to do with glucose, the sugar released from your latest meal or snack:

- *When you have high levels of glucose in your blood:*
    - insulin can trigger some of it to be sent into your cells to make ATP "energy batteries";
    - any excess will be converted to a substance called glycogen in your liver, where you can keep a store cupboard of about a day's supply;
    - if there's still more glucose left over, insulin will turn it into fats, which are then sent to your fat cells (aka adipose cells) for more long-term storage – this is how sugar can make you fat.

- *If your blood sugar is too low:*
    - glucagon will tell your liver to release some of its short-term storage.

In this way, you should always have enough fuel for your cells to carry out their day-to-day and moment-to-moment functions, and the delicate balance of your blood is never overloaded or damaged by an excess of glucose. Simple, clever, effective.

Insulin resistance

That is, as long as your insulin receptors keep working. Insulin receptors are like very selective doormen on the surface of your cells: they'll shake hands with insulin, listen to its message and pass it on, but completely ignore everyone else. In this case, the message is: "Open the glucose gate and let some sugar in."

They can get overwhelmed, however, if there is too much insulin trying to be heard too much of the time – perhaps due to a high sugar diet – and start ignoring the insulin as well. We call this insulin resistance, and it's bad news on a number of levels. In simple terms, we end up with high levels of circulating insulin (not being listened to), and long term high blood sugar levels, which can eventually cause damage to your blood vessels, nerves and kidneys.

Insulin resistance is an integral feature of obesity, hypertension, diabetes, heart disease and cancer,[18, 19] as well as Alzheimer's disease.[20]

To begin with, the pancreas's Islets of Langerhans will continue to produce more and more insulin, to try and get its message heard, but eventually they will become worn out. In the meantime, the liver keeps releasing more glucose from its personal energy stores, which drives blood sugar levels even higher; but it still responds to the high blood sugar situation by producing more fats from glucose.[21] So you end up with more fats floating around in your liver, your blood and your fatty tissue.

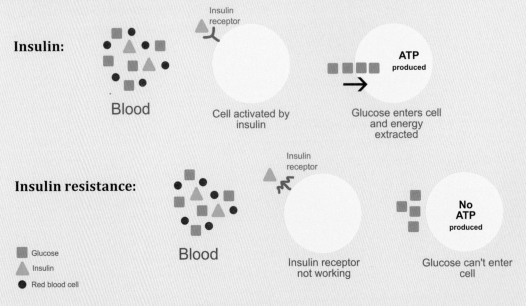

Insulin:

Insulin receptor

Blood

Cell activated by insulin

ATP produced

Glucose enters cell and energy extracted

Insulin resistance:

Insulin receptor

Blood

Insulin receptor not working

No ATP produced

Glucose can't enter cell

Glucose
Insulin
Red blood cell

The impact of diet on insulin resistance

In recent years, we've started to look at how we might resolve insulin resistance. A 2013 study compared the effects of three different types of diet on 164 participants all in the early stages of hypertension (high blood pressure) but without diabetes. Each person had six weeks on each of the following: a) a high-carbohydrate diet similar to one often recommended for hypertension, b) a diet focused on plant-based proteins and c) a diet rich in monounsaturated fats, like olive oil and avocados, for example. The conclusion: "A diet that partially replaces carbohydrate with unsaturated fat may improve insulin sensitivity in a population at risk for cardiovascular disease."[22] So once again, carbohydrates are shown to contribute to a problem where certain kinds of fats may be beneficial.

Monounsaturated fatty acids (MUFAs) such as those found in olive oil and avocadoes are known to have a heart protective effect.[23] This more recent study suggests that lowering our carbohydrate intake may add to these benefits. In fact the evidence is steadily growing that high carbohydrate diets are a much greater health hazard, as well as more fattening, than diets high in certain kinds of fat.

Taking that a step further, a 2015 study of children on a high sugar diet showed that replacing almost 2/3 of their sugar with starch – a different kind of carbohydrate – also had a beneficial effect on insulin sensitivity.[24] So there are further nuances within the effects of too much carbohydrate that I'll come back to shortly.

Nutrition for healthy insulin pathways

Specific nutrients have been identified that support various aspects of how well your insulin pathways work.

Zinc is involved in both insulin production as well as the way that insulin binds to receptors, and opens the gates that take sugar out of the blood and into the cells to make energy. You can find zinc in pumpkin seeds, chickpeas, nuts, seeds and shellfish, for example.

Chromium also helps insulin bind to insulin receptors on your cell membranes, and additionally helps you make more receptors. Broccoli, barley and oats are all good sources of chromium.

Magnesium helps prevent insulin resistance, and is found in green leafy vegetables, nuts, seeds, blackstrap molasses and green powders such as chlorella and spirulina.

Manganese is needed to make the actual insulin itself, and helps insulin receptors to work properly. You can find manganese in oats, rice, spinach, pumpkin seeds and blackstrap molasses.

A while ago I developed a snack recipe, a variation on a flapjack, for those with a sweet tooth. Spiced fig and apple flapjacks are as mouthwatering as they sound, and include impressive levels of all these nutrients. You can find how to make them on page 284, in the Recipes section of this book.

Fat cells, leptins and insulin resistance

Adipose cells – the technical name for your fat cells – also play an important role in sugar metabolism. They produce proteins called leptins that help to regulate how much glucose you burn and how much of it you store, whether as glycogen or as fat. It's another beautifully simple system that complements your insulin and glucagon activity:

- If you have a lot of fat stores, you produce more leptins. These leptins send a signal to the hypothalamus in your brain to reduce your hunger pangs as well as your reward system – the feel-good factor your body produces when you eat sugar-dense food such as fruit (in the wild), or fast food, cakes and chocolate (in modern lifestyles). The fatter you are, the less you want to eat.

- Equally, if you have low reserves of fat, then your adipose cells produce fewer leptin proteins, so your hunger and reward systems are given free rein, and you are encouraged to eat more. So essentially, your fat levels should be self-regulating.

However, just like the insulin receptors, your hypothalamus seems to stick its fingers in its ears if it's being bothered by too much leptin, coming from an excessive amount of fat tissue, and keeps sending out hunger signals even when you have plenty of fat already there. At the same time, it will downgrade any non-essential activity that needs a lot of energy, such as laying down new bone tissue and reproduction – so leptin resistance can have a direct impact on your fertility and bone density.

Leptin resistance and insulin resistance seem to accompany each other, but there is debate as to what comes first and why. We spend a lot of time trying to figure out a linear timeline of events with disease, so we can figure out a single point in time where we can intervene and fix everything. Sometimes that may be possible, but for the most part I suspect it is an inevitably frustrating approach. Often what becomes increasingly apparent is that most things have many factors, often happening simultaneously, and with varying results, dependent upon other factors.

One area of research into leptins of particular interest to me however, is connected with a type of sugar called fructose.

As sweet as sugar candy

Just as not all calories are created equal, the same can be said of carbohydrates and sugars.

Carbohydrates are chemical structures that include carbon, hydrogen and oxygen, and include both starches and sugars. Starches are complex (long chain) carbohydrates found in potatoes, unripe bananas, wholegrain products such as wholegrain bread and pasta, quinoa and brown rice, and pulses such as peas, beans and lentils. They are long chains of sugars joined together to form a molecule that takes more effort to break down when we eat them.

Simple carbohydrates are made of just one or two sugars, and can be found in fruit, white sugar, brown sugar, treacle, molasses, honey and all the different syrups you can now find in your local shops. Most complex carbohydrates are ultimately broken down to simple sugars in the gut. That doesn't mean they all have the same end result, however.

For a start, there are different types of simple sugars, including glucose, fructose and sucrose. Different foods contain varying selections and ratios of these, or of starches that break down to them. So, for example, white sugar is predominantly sucrose, a compound that's 50% glucose and 50% fructose. Honey also has the same ratio, but there is a world of difference between eating refined white sugar, which has had most of its nutrients removed, and raw honey, which is richly nourishing and so more likely to support your body and keep it more balanced while it deals with the sugar rush. Blackstrap molasses is what's taken out of sugar when it's refined, so the sweetness comes from a similar make-up to both white sugar and honey, but it's also rich in manganese, calcium, iron and many other nutrients.

There has been a lot of press condemning high fructose corn syrup (aka glucose-fructose corn syrup or just corn syrup) in many processed foods and drinks. This is a manufactured sweetener that takes glucose rich corn syrup and adds fructose, so that it ends up being 55% fructose – probably because fructose has a sweeter flavour. Before we look at why this is an issue, it's worth noting that agave syrup and agave nectar contain an even greater ratio of fructose to glucose, as much as 75%. Agave syrup has been an impressive marketing success sweeping health food shops, supermarkets, the raw food movement and the more general world of nutrition and healthy cooking. I stopped using it a long time ago, and when I want to use a sweetener, I generally opt for raw honey, molasses or whole fruit.

Higher levels of fructose can be problematic for two main reasons. Firstly because a lot of people struggle to absorb fructose in the small intestine, and so it can end up hanging around in the gut creating bloating and inflammation, thus affecting digestive health and immune function. Glucose helps with fructose transport from your small intestine into your blood, so sugars with equal amounts of glucose and fructose are often easier on your digestive and immune system.

Secondly, and more importantly, excessive fructose is increasingly being recognised as one of the major health hazards of modern day living, and so deserves a section all to itself.

The fructose factor

The thing about fructose is that you process it in your body differently to how you process other sugars. To begin with, it's absorbed differently in the small intestine. Then much of it is carried to the liver where most of it seems to join a factory production line for triglycerides, i.e. fat.

Triglycerides are made up of three strands of fatty acids (broken down fats) on a kind of coat hanger made of glycerol, and fructose is rapidly converted to glycerol for this purpose.[25] These triglycerides are then put into a little carrier and are transported in the blood as VLDL (Very Low Density Lipoprotein). VLDL has been associated with increased levels of inflammation in the blood vessels, which means a greater risk of cardiovascular disease.[26]

While all this is going on, fewer leptins are triggered, and more ghrelin, a major appetite stimulator, so you're more likely to want to keep on eating beyond what you actually need, or is healthy.[27]

As the liver busily turns fructose into triglycerides, it produces uric acid as a side effect, and deactivates nitric oxide.[28] Uric acid build up can be bad news, eventually leading to painful conditions such as gout and kidney stones, as well as chronic kidney disease. High uric acid levels are also associated with... yes, you guessed it, diabetes and heart disease.[29] Nitric oxide, on the other hand, is something we want to have in store as much as possible, not least for keeping our blood vessels healthy and so avoiding high blood pressure, stroke and other features of cardiovascular disease.

As with everything, scientists are still debating and researching the precise effects of fructose metabolism, but a large number of studies have connected high fructose levels with higher levels of obesity, insulin resistance, high blood pressure and other markers clustered into what's now known as "metabolic syndrome", a group of risk factors for cardiovascular disease.

A recent study, mentioned above, took 17 children on a high sugar diet, all between the ages of 8-18, and modified their food intake so that sugar was reduced from 28% to 10% of their diet, and replaced instead with complex carbohydrates. Although it was not measured, we can reasonably assume that the sugar in their diets had been fructose heavy. After just nine days, triglycerides were reduced, insulin sensitivity improved and blood pressure came down as well.[30] Calorie intake didn't change, just the quality of the carbohydrates.

In a laboratory study on rats (please note I do not condone animal experiments in any way), scientists tried to induce metabolic syndrome through diet. There were four groups of rats, each fed either wholewheat flour or refined flour. In two groups, 60% of the flour was replaced with fructose. In both fructose groups, metabolic syndrome markers were apparent within four weeks, and in the refined flour group, the rats had higher blood pressure, blood sugar, insulin levels and blood triglycerides at eight weeks. The fructose clearly had a devastating effect, but this was accelerated when the rest of the diet was essentially white flour, and slowed down with the help of the additional nutrients and fibre in wholewheat flour. So again, the quality of carbohydrates does seem to make a difference.

It has been suggested that the research carried out to date, although increasingly extensive, is still limited in its ability to single out fructose as a culprit.[31] This would be tricky, as fructose, once ingested, becomes part of an intricate cascade of effects. Varying levels of fructose and glucose can affect each other's metabolism, suggesting that the ratio of these sugars may be an important health factor – and perhaps another argument in favour of using raw honey and molasses instead of high fructose corn syrup and agave syrup. Fructose may also have a more damaging effect when the diet is high in carbohydrates generally.[32] With the current information available, I would suggest keeping a lid on total carbohydrates and an even tighter lid on fructose.

But isn't fructose a healthy fruit sugar?

Fructose is indeed the sugar you find in fruit, alongside glucose and sucrose. When you eat an apple or some berries, you are consuming fructose together with a spectrum of vitamins, minerals and phytonutrients that support your digestion, metabolism and overall health – plus fibre, which seems to reduce the impact too.

We've known for years that fruit juice usually spikes insulin more than the whole fruit, and blood sugar drops less after absorption. Appetite is satisfied for longer with whole fruit too.[33] When you drink fruit juice, you are denying yourself the benefit of that all important fibre; when you consume food or drink with a high fructose sweetener, you generally lack both the fibre and the wealth of nutrients provided in whole, real food.

Recent research has also been looking at a type of fibre called Resistant Starch Type 3. This is a type of indigestible fibre that can be created by cooking and then cooling or freezing carbohydrates like potatoes and pasta – and its presence also seems to help prevent insulin spikes.[34]

Back to fruit, an interesting and more recent study sought to find out how much of the benefit of the whole fruit is down to the fibre, and how much is down to antioxidant polyphenols, protective pigments found in plant-based foods. It's sadly more laboratory research on rats, this time feeding them either standard rat chow or a high fructose diet, then adding in either an unprocessed blackcurrant pomace rich in polyphenols (pomace is what's left after the juice has been squeezed out), or blackcurrant pomace processed to make it low in polyphenols. Both pomaces had beneficial effects on the rats that enjoyed them, but the greatest fructose-protective effects were experienced by the rats that ate the polyphenol-rich blackcurrant pomaces.[35] So it's not just the fibre that's helping. It's most likely a combination of benefits, which makes total sense as that's how most things seem to work. Our bodies have evolved to work with fruit, vegetables and other natural foods that contain a kaleidoscope of vitamins, minerals, phytonutrients, proteins, lipids, carbohydrates, fibre and fluids – and are delicately balanced to interact with these as a group rather than with any in isolation.

Quantity is key too. Once upon a time, the fructose in our diet would have been limited to a small amount of seasonal fruit (note that seasonal means none in the winter in the UK, although we may have had some dried fruit), and occasional foraged honey. After the tight rationing of World War II was over, Cinderella went to the ball, the sugar market exploded and the way we eat started to change dramatically. We wanted sweets, cakes, chocolates and soft drinks, and as our collective sweet tooth developed, we became hooked, with the food industry our increasingly savvy dealer.

Whether this story ends happily ever after really depends on your definition of happiness...

Reflection time

- *Have a think about the quality of carbohydrates in your diet:*
  - *How many of them are whole grains, such as brown rice, millet, whole wheat or rye bread, whole grain or brown rice pasta and noodles?*
  - *Does eating whole grains make you feel more satisfied? More energised for longer? Do you find them easier or more difficult to digest?*
  - *How much of your diet includes refined carbohydrates, such as white bread, white pasta and noodles, white pastry, biscuits, cakes and sweets?*
  - *How do refined carbohydrates affect your energy (immediately and later in the day)? Mood? Digestion?*
  - *How much fruit juice, squash or other sugary drinks do you have?*

Action plan

- *Add more whole grains to your shopping list:*
    - *Try replacing white rice with brown rice*
    - *Try replacing white pasta with whole wheat pasta or brown rice pasta*
    - *Try replacing white noodles with brown rice or buckwheat noodles*
    - *Try replacing white bread with whole wheat or rye bread*

- *Try eating smaller portions of carbohydrates, or having very low carbohydrate meals such as fish with broccoli, cauliflower and steamed greens*

- *Try replacing fruit juice, squash and sugary drinks with water or refreshing infusions – see below for recipes*

Recipes

Snack times are where the sugar and refined carbs often creep in. My delicious spiced fig and apple flapjack recipe gives you more flavour and yet less sugar than standard flapjacks and cakes, while satisfying that desire for something sweet. It's also richer in protein to help keep blood sugar levels more stable, together with nutrients that help your insulin pathways to work better. One of these squares is great as a snack, a quick breakfast or a lunchbox treat.

My Superberry chia pot recipe is a great way to combine nutrient-dense chia seeds with just a few berries to provide a delicious, blood sugar balancing snack or breakfast.

Then instead of a fizzy drink or fruit juice, make up a refreshing infusion to keep in the fridge or put in with your packed lunch – or have freshly made and warm in the colder months.

- **Spiced fig and apple flapjacks** – p.284

- **Superberry chia pot** – p.287

- **Refreshing infusions and soft drinks** – p.294

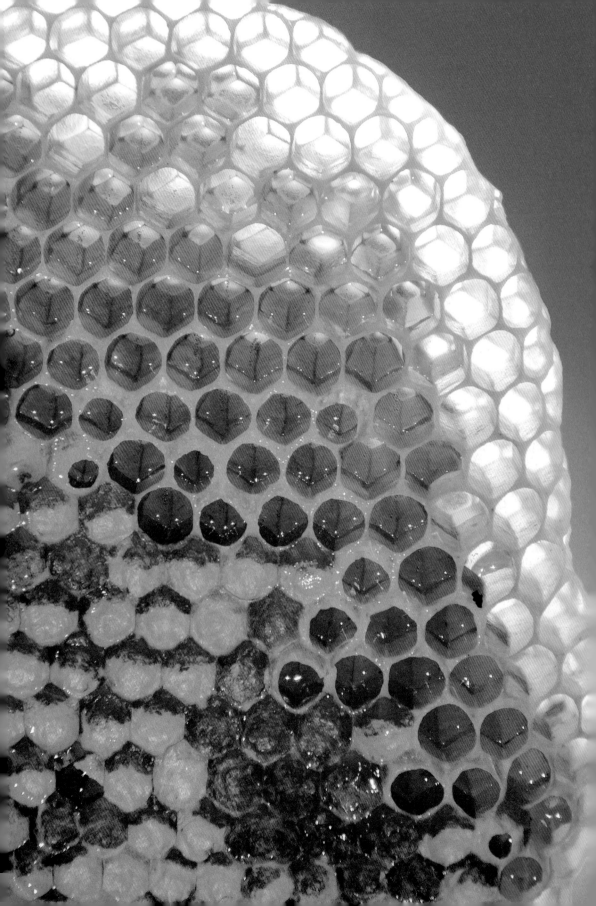

Chapter 5

Sugar pt.2
~ life is sweet ~

The bliss point

The bliss point is a term used to describe the moment when we are most satisfied by something: less of the substance wouldn't achieve euphoria, more would miss the mark and become unenjoyable. It's a term used in economics – at which point does the excitement and pleasure of shopping become a concern that you've overspent, for example? And it's a concept explored thoroughly by American food industry consultant Howard Moskowitz from the 1970s onwards.

Moskowitz has worked on optimising soups, spaghetti, fizzy drinks, army rations and more. He and fellow researchers compared consumers' reactions and feedback to many different combinations of flavours, texture and colours to find the perfect recipe that would hook the greatest amount of people into that product. Rather than being concerned with nutrient content and physical requirement, these scientists were measuring pleasure: the brain's endorphin rush. Moskowitz realised that there was a certain range of sugar intake that would trigger such a bliss response. This head rush of bliss that we can experience from food is addictive, in that the brain will seek to replicate the thrill. Which turns his goldilocks concept of "not too much, not too little, but just right" into a goldmine for the food industry.

The addictive nature of sugar has been measured in terms of brain chemistry, and seems chillingly similar to how we become addicted to heroin, cocaine, alcohol and other drugs, including how we crave them, how we build a tolerance to them and what happens during withdrawal. In fact, one study has noted how people with drug and/or alcohol dependency issues also have a very sweet tooth, as do children of alcoholic parents, particularly alcoholic fathers.[36] In my own practice as a nutritional therapist, I have witnessed such patterns, and have frequently worked with people who have managed to withdraw from drug and alcohol addictions but then struggled to deal with food addiction and binge eating. In such cases a lot of work needs to be done to keep blood sugar in balance, as well as to reduce inflammation and support optimal function both in the gut and at brain/nervous system level.

A bliss point has also been measured for salt and for fat – although it's interesting to note that the bliss range for fat has no upper level. So there's a point at which a food can be too salty or too sweet to enjoy, but not too fatty. The snack foods, biscuits, cakes, ready meals, breakfast cereals, cereal bars, salad dressings and other processed foods that fill the supermarket and even health food shop shelves are largely formulated these days to provide a heady combination of sugar and salt, sugar and fat, salt and fat – or all three – that will just hit the bliss point. That's why low fat foods are often higher in sugar and/or salt, for example.

It may not surprise you that one of the most perfectly bliss-balanced foods is the potato crisp – or potato chip as researchers called them in a 2011 American study. The researchers had monitored the diet, activity and smoking habits of 120,877 women and men over 25 years. All the participants were health professionals, and so likely to be more conscious about their exercise and nutrition – but even so, over the years, they tended to exercise less, watch more TV and put on an average of 3.35lb every four years. When the researchers analysed their diets, they found that one food item was by far the most responsible for weight gain: crisps. As Michael Moss explains in his article "The extraordinary science of addictive junk food":

"The coating of salt, the fat content that rewards the brain with instant feelings of pleasure, the sugar that exists not as an additive but in the starch of the potato itself – all of this combines to make it the perfect addictive food."[37]

Sensory specific satiety

Sensory specific satiety refers to how satisfied you feel after different kinds of flavours. Complex and intense flavours will generally go beyond the bliss point, so that your brain will feel overwhelmed and dull your desire for more. On the other hand, foods and snacks that are enjoyable and hit the bliss point, but are often relatively bland will be "moreish" – you'll just keep wanting more of them. So one aspect of the ready meal and snack industry is to create crisps, crackers, dips, sauces etc. that are tasty, but not *too* tasty.

The food industry has known about this concept for a long time, but we can make use of this knowledge too. If you find yourself munching your way through whole packets of snack foods, one of the things you can do to help is to create your own deluxe snacks with intense or complex flavours. Make some houmous with fresh coriander leaves, tangy lemon juice and extra garlic. Or instead of milk chocolate coated nuts and raisins, dip brazil nuts in the darkest, richest chocolate you can find, perhaps laced with orange oil, cardamom or ginger.

Let the flavours linger on your taste buds with every bite, so that your brain can fully take on board the intensity. You may find that you are less quick to finish the batch than before.

Protein-rich breakfasts and snacks

Nutritional therapists such as myself have found for years that most people find a protein-rich breakfast more likely to sustain them, and also to prevent symptoms associated with blood sugar crashes – such as headaches, dizziness, and problems with memory, concentration and mood swings. In recent years, countless studies have confirmed this to be the case.

Such studies show that the more protein you have at breakfast, the more likely you are to feel full and satisfied throughout the morning and even eat less for lunch,[38] and that animal protein may keep your blood sugar stable more reliably than plant-based proteins.[39] We'll explore proteins in more detail in a later chapter.

A study of teenage boys with ADHD is quite enlightening here.[40] The boys were given a sucrose drink at various stages through the day to measure the impact on their ADHD symptoms, such as mood, hyperactivity and cognitive skills. Those who had eaten just carbohydrates for breakfast found that the sucrose drink spiked their symptoms alongside their blood sugar. Those who had eaten protein for breakfast found that the sucrose drink had no such effect, and may even alleviate their ADHD symptoms.

Before you start reaching for the grill pan and heading for the butcher, take a moment to check in. You may find that too much animal protein feels too heavy for you right now, in which case you may want to include just a little, or stick to plant-based proteins for now. Obviously, if you are vegan then focus on nuts, seeds and pulses to provide additional protein in the morning. Vegetarians might like to experiment with eggs and yoghurt too. Or it may be that your body is crying out for some substantial animal protein first thing, and you feel amazing for it. Always listen to your body first, as it knows better than any book, article or nutritional therapist.

How much sugar is ok?

Whatever kind of sugar your diet contains, it would be fair to say you don't want too much of it. WHO (World Health Organisation) guidelines released in March 2015 recommend that no one should have a daily intake of free sugars higher than 10%, and that a further reduction to 5% a day, which equates to about 25g (or 6 teaspoons), would provide "additional health benefits".[41]

By free sugars they mean any simple sugars (e.g. glucose, fructose, sucrose) added to food and drink for example in the form of cane sugar, corn syrup, hydrolysed starch, dextrose etc. – plus sugars naturally present in fruit juice, fruit juice concentrates, syrups and sweeteners. The natural sugars present in fresh fruit, vegetables and milk, however, are not included in this. The current UK intake is about 16-17%, the equivalent to a whopping 80-85g or 20-21tsp sugar a day. Actually, considering that's the amount of free sugar in a single can of sugar sweetened soft drink, you can see how that's not hard to achieve.

Sugar coating the health industry

I often discuss the importance of reading labels. I have mostly got this down to a fine art now, scanning quickly for red flags (various added sugars and flavourings, for example), and largely buying ingredients that I cook from scratch. But I understand that for a lot of people label reading is too much of a drain on their time and energy. People are too busy trying to juggle work, family, bills and other daily concerns without wanting to vet everything their local shop sells them. They want to be able to trust shops, supermarkets and the food industry to get it right in the first place, and create food that is nutritious and healthy. Most people are well aware that cakes, sweets and ice cream are full of sugar, but if the packaging of a meal or snack gives the impression of goodness, nature and health, then surely that's what you're being sold? Disappointingly not. For the most part, the food industry often seems more motivated to invest in how well the packaging fools you than in your health.

And if the product is specifically marketed as a healthy option, are you safe to add it to your basket without checking the label? Sadly, even the health food industry often seems to fall foul. If health food shops, and the healthy option sections of supermarkets, were to remove from their shelves anything with added sugars, most would probably be surprised at the resulting expanse of empty shelf space.

One of the most common cereal bars I see in health food shops contains 8.8g sugar – that's more than 2tsp of mostly sugar and glucose syrup. I've seen the same amount of sugar in a supermarket cheese ploughman's sandwich and about 20g in a small (200ml) bottle of fruit juice. So what would constitute many people's idea of a healthy lunchbox would actually take you to the limit of what the WHO recommends for your entire day's intake. Add in a low fat fruit yoghurt (15g sugar) when your energy levels dip an hour or two later, plus breakfast and dinner, and you're in the dangerous zone without even looking at a doughnut, fizzy drink or chocolate bar. Damon Gameau did just that in his experiment in "That Sugar Film": he raised his own sugar intake to health endangering levels purely by eating in a way that most people consider to be healthy – and actually within his government's guidelines.

A glance at the ingredients list of more artisan and specialist looking snacks and treats in your local health food shop still often causes me to raise an eyebrow. They may be free of refined cane sugar, but the first – and therefore weightiest – ingredients in the list are frequently agave syrup and various type of rice syrup. Agave syrup was popularised in the 2000s and particularly championed by the raw food movement. It then transpired that agave syrup (or agave nectar) is generally highly boiled and processed so that it becomes high fructose syrup of questionable benefit. Rice syrup, while largely glucose rather than fructose, usually has most of its nutrients processed out of it so that it, too, could arguably be described as a refined sugar. The quantity of these sugars in such snacks is also quite alarming – in some cases 20-25%.

Actually, it's very easy to make many of these in your own kitchen, with no added refined sugars or sweeteners – see my Recipes section for ideas. You can buy energy balls and bars with very simple ingredients – largely dried fruit, nuts and seeds – but the largest ingredient is still dried fruit, which is very concentrated in fructose. You can very easily make the same energy balls changing the ratio so that there are much smaller amounts of dried fruit, and they will still taste great. (See page 277 for some recipe suggestions.)

Sugar alcohols: sorbitol, xylitol and other –ols

Sorbitol has been around for a while now, once popular as a sweetener for diabetic chocolates and mints and now as a more general sweetener. Xylitol and erythritol are newer kids on the block, and have been creating a buzz the last couple of years as something that sweetens without giving you too much of an, err, buzz. More cutting edge dentists have been recommending xylitol[42] and erythritol[43] as sweeteners that rebalance bacteria in the mouth and so protect the teeth and gums, rather than the tooth decay usually associated with too many sweets.[44]

Sweeteners that end in –ol are technically sugar alcohols. This doesn't mean they'll get you drunk, it just refers to their chemical structure. They are naturally occurring in fruit and vegetables, although the ones used to sweeten your "healthy" chocolate bar are probably industrially synthesised. Their structure means that they activate your taste buds to create that sweet sensation, but with far fewer calories and without spiking your blood sugar or affecting your insulin pathways (except for maltitol). Most have a laxative effect in high doses, however – with the exception of erythritol – and some people find that they are intolerant to sugar alcohols in that they cause digestive problems and bloating. Please also be aware that xylitol is highly toxic to dogs, so do not share your xylitol-sweetened treats with them.

Don't forget the honey!

Honey has been getting a bad rap lately, but it's still one of my favourite sweeteners and contains a wealth of minerals, antioxidants, polyphenols and other nutrients. But preferably raw, i.e. unpasteurised honey – there's a world of difference between this and the highly processed honeys that dominate today's market. This doesn't mean you have to pay a fortune for high quality honey that has racked up thousands of air miles. There are small commercial hives in both urban and countryside communities up and down the land, and you just need to ask them if they pasteurise their honey.

The pasteurisation process for honey is just a matter of heating it. Honey doesn't have to be heated for very long to be pasteurised, but honey producers are prone to heating the honey for much longer to reduce the water content. The aim is to keep the honey liquid – i.e. prevent it crystallising and setting – and to give it a longer shelf life. Unfortunately, this is at the expense of quality. A recent study of Malaysian honeys showed that heat treatment substantially reduced the levels of vitamins B2, B3, B5 and C, as well as proteins and enzymes. At the same time, the carbohydrate and calorie content increased.[45]

Heat treating may also kill the beneficial bacteria found in honey that probably contribute to honey's renowned healing properties. Scientists have found six species of lactobacilli and four species of bifidobacteria, all beneficial for the gut and immune health, depending from which flowers the bees have been foraging. Honey from winter bees fed with sucrose was lacking in lactobacilli.[46] These "beneficial" bacteria are not the only therapeutic agents in honey, however.

Local honey and manuka honey – even when heat treated – are both therapeutically effective even in small amounts against a wide spectrum of bacteria, fungi, as well as biofilm-producing organisms and resistant organisms.[47] This is much more impressive than it may sound. Some very serious chronic illnesses are characterised – or at least accompanied – by a high level of fungal and biofilm (a kind of slime that bacteria and mould use to colonise and spread) activity and bacterial imbalance, including cancer, ME, Lyme's disease and AIDS.

And as we are becoming increasingly aware, bacteria are very good at adapting to antibiotics, so that there are many more resistant varieties – or "superbugs" – around that are difficult to treat. Bacteria can be prompted to become drug resistant or virulent, or to create an overgrowth of biofilm, by a process called quorum sensing, which can tell how big the bacterial population is. As the population grows, quorum sensing will trigger increasing genetic activity to do all of the above – honey can interrupt this process and help to keep bacterial levels manageable. This has been shown to work for E. coli and salmonella enteric bacteria, as well as biofilm producing Pseudomonas aeruginosa, among others.[48]

Honey is already recognised for its antimicrobial and wound healing properties when applied to cuts and other injuries, and not just in complementary healthcare. Some time ago I cut the end of my finger quite deeply, and after sewing it up, the NHS dressed it with honey and silver. Honey can actually help new tissue cells to grow when you need to heal a wound.[49] Silver also has antibacterial and tissue regeneration properties.[50]

The other interesting thing about honey is that it seems to be tolerated better than sucrose or glucose alone, even by diabetics (both mild and severe), and may actually improve blood sugar control and insulin sensitivity.[51] In addition, we tend to use less of it, as it's sweeter.

Honey is often described as being "as bad as white sugar" because they both contain sucrose and glucose – but it's worth noting that there are some major chemical differences between the two. For a start, the glucose and sucrose in sugar is bound together, while in honey they are independent from each other. Honey also contains a wealth of nutrients and enzymes that sugar does not.

I'm also partial to using molasses from time to time, for its remarkable nutrient content. Molasses contains all the nutrients that are taken out of sugar when it's refined to white sugar. It's particularly rich in magnesium, calcium, manganese, and potassium. This makes it excellent for bone strength, as well as providing electrolytes necessary to keep fluids flowing around the body, and in and out of each cell. Magnesium is super important for ATP production, and a mineral I have found most people I work with to be deficient in.

Molasses also contains impressive amounts of vitamin B6, which is needed for red blood cells, detoxification processes and methylation (an important process that triggers fundamental biochemical activity in your body) and improves the bioavailability of magnesium (how well we absorb and use it). It's also rich in iron and copper, which together with magnesium and manganese make up many of your detoxification enzymes, and selenium, a powerful protective antioxidant. Molasses has a strong treacly flavor, which means you won't want to eat too much of it; just as well as it's about 75% sugar (mostly sucrose, also glucose and fructose), but I like to use it when I make flapjack type snacks and occasionally in my porridge.

Comfort eating

Sugar and simple or refined carbohydrates are often the central theme of our comfort food – be it toast and marmalade, sweets and chocolate, chips and crisps, ice cream, jam doughnuts or endless packets of dried fruit. For many, comfort food might be stodgy meals with pasta or mashed potato, or sugary takeaway curry or stir-fry with piles of white rice, or just a mound of bread or toast. When we are down, we reach for something that's going to bring us up. Snacks rich in sugar and simple carbohydrates have an additional stimulant factor, provide a thrilling energy rush (usually followed by a crash riddled with self-recrimination) and reach the bliss point with ease.

In Chinese Five Element theory, the sweet taste is related to the Earth Element. The Earth Element relates to everything that nurtures and supports you. Imagine yourself in a warm meadow, resting against a beautiful tree, feeling connected, centred, at one and at peace with your environment, and fully content. Imagine that your roots run deep and wide, intermingling with those of the tree, being nourished by the same mineral rich soil and energised by the same gentle sunbeams from above. Perhaps a ripe apple or juicy peach falls softly into your lap from the tree's branches and you take a fresh, invigorating and deeply satisfying bite of gentle sweetness. Wouldn't it be amazing to feel this nourished and cradled every step of our journey through life?

Every now and then, however, something pulls the rug out from under your feet. It may be a sudden trauma or shock that sends you into freefall; or it may be insidious, niggling stress factors that inch the rug away tug by tug. Either way, that sustaining Earth connection feels lost, and without it you may feel vulnerable. There may be a sense of loneliness, worry, panic or disconnection; or a sense of distractedness, lack of focus, floatiness or dizziness. Have you ever felt like your head was floating in the air? Or that you were stuck in your head, with thoughts short-circuiting round and round?

In such moments, what you really need is to ground: re-establish that connection, earth those short-circuiting worries and images, and regain access to the sustenance your environment naturally provides.

In reality, you might find yourself reaching for comfort foods instead. The sweetness they provide – either directly to the tastebuds, or a little further down as they quickly break down to sugars – attempts to make up for that disconnection from the Earth Element. The rapid blood sugar rush is a tangible sensation that may mimic (or mock) the contentedness of before – but this is often empty and short lived. And far from helping you to feel present in your own body again, comfort eating is often an absent activity, a way to put up barriers rather than to reconnect, a way to disappear into a strange fog rather than face reality.

Over time, your body may also start to crave sugar to feed bacterial imbalance in your gut, which annoyingly, can make it all the harder to change your eating patterns. You may recognise you need to slow down on the sugar and comfort food, but the physical and mental cravings can be strong. Many scientists have compared the brain chemicals and responses in drug addiction to those evident in sugar addiction;[52, 53] if you try and "battle" this with willpower alone, you will more than likely end up feeling tense, irritable, and perhaps even failure and desperation. If that's the case for you, then it's time to give your willpower a rest, and find a gentler path back to balance.

How to feel grounded and nurtured again

Rather than create a battleground for yourself, remember that this is about finding true comfort to replace deceptive and empty habits. Feeling the rug beneath your feet again and knowing you are home: feeling safe and held.

Being in nature can be invaluable here. Walking in the woods, hills or by the sea; or sitting in your garden or in the park, wriggling your toes or running your fingers through the grass; or digging the soil, planting seeds and harvesting your vegetables, fruits and flowers.

All of these activities can feel deeply connecting and satisfying on a soul as well as a physical level, and literally bring us back down to earth again. If none of that is feasible, then imagine yourself there, imagine the smells and sensations, how it all looks, sounds and feels.

Chinese Five Element theory also teaches us to seek out the gentler sweetness in vegetables such as carrots and parsnips, pumpkins and squash. These are all grown close to the ground, and glow with the Earth Element colours yellow and orange. You can also include orange lentils, yellow split peas, golden turmeric and cantaloupe melons in your weekly menu. Enjoy the dandelions brightening up your garden and the buttercups in the lawn, and maybe add splashes of yellow to your home and accessories. If you find yourself filling your world entirely with these colours, then that would suggest the imbalance is still there, however, so avoid getting carried away!

Whatever you're eating, find pleasure in it. Savour every mouthful and allow the nourishment in. Remember this is about nurturing – how well do you actually nurture yourself, and let yourself be nurtured by others and your environment? Are you too busy trying to look after other people? Or do you struggle to even do that?

Wherever you're at, it all begins and ends with your own self-nourishment. Which is essentially about self-love. This is an unconditional sense of love and acceptance of yourself for who you are – not *despite* aspects of you or things you do or have done that you feel uneasy with, but *including* all that, alongside the rest of the miraculous, amazing you.

When you can sit fully in your own skin and feel comfortable and happy there, then you are in the perfect place to plug into the universe and let everything flow.

Getting to that place is a daily commitment of small steps and kindness. You can gently shift the way you eat to help you along, using the wisdom of Five Element theory and nutritional support for blood sugar balance and ATP production.

You can use mindfulness practices to help keep you present in your body, and nature to help keep you grounded.

Reflection time

- *How much sugar – of any kind – is in your regular, daily diet?*
  - *Include sweets, biscuits, cakes, drinks, fruit juice and fruit as well as hidden sugars in sauces, soups, takeaways and processed foods.*

- *Do you use sugar **regularly** to keep your energy up? Or to focus your concentration? Or as an emotional prop, to help you deal with difficult emotions, as a comfort food etc?*

Action plan

- *Read the labels on foods and snacks you commonly buy.*
  - *Do any contain unnecessary added sugars?*
  - *Can you find or make tasty alternatives?*

- *Try introducing more protein at breakfast time – perhaps with eggs, nuts and seeds, plain organic yoghurt or even meat or fish.*

- *As odd as it may sound to many of us, a bowl of soup is a very common start to the day in parts of the world, and makes perfect sense. It's hydrating, warming, soothing, gently nourishing and, providing there's some protein in there (e.g. lentils, beans, meat, fish), beautifully sustaining.*

- *Note any changes – positive or otherwise – to how you feel as a result.*

Recipes

What people most frequently struggle with are breakfasts and snacks. So here are a few recipes to start you off on the right foot, and then make sure you have something healthy to hand during the day for those moments when you need a little something extra. These recipes are designed to be delicious, simple and quick to make. They also contain as many ingredients as possible that you need to make ATP really efficiently (see chapter 4) and keep your blood sugar and metabolism steady.

- ***Soft egg omelette** – p.249*
  This is a kind of coddled eggs recipe. Coddled eggs are traditionally steamed in little ceramic pots, but in this method I use a few stir fried greens to nest the eggs in. You can also think of them as a soft-yolk version of an omelette.

The longer you cook eggs, the more copper, iron and manganese you lose, as well as choline and B12. So don't overcook them! Choline and B12 are great for your brain and nerves and are essential for the healthy function of every cell in your body. B12 and iron are particularly important for making your red blood cells, which carry oxygen to your cells to help you make ATP molecules of energy. And of course eggs are a fabulous source of protein, which is why they usually keep you going for so long.

- **Avocado smoothie** – *p.291*
  This is my favourite breakfast in the summer. It also makes a really tasty and filling snack that you can either keep in the fridge or take with you anywhere in an airtight container. Avocados are a great source of the B vitamins you need to make ATP, as well as easily absorbed antioxidants that help protect the mitochondria that make the ATP, and your whole body.

- **Energy balls** – *p.277*
  These are a perfect alternative to the sugar dense snack bars and energy balls you can buy in the shops, as you get to control how much fruit and other sweeteners go in them. They refrigerate and freeze well, and you can really get creative with different flavour combinations.

- **Guacamole** – *p.279*
  Savoury snacks are often the way to go – help your brain forget that sugary sweetness ever existed! Guacamole is super easy to make and a light, creamy dip with an optional added kick for oat cakes, celery and cucumber/ courgette/carrot sticks.

- **Stewed apple pancakes** – *p.289*
  These are my favourite comfort food, but nowhere near as sweet as a bought cake or dessert.

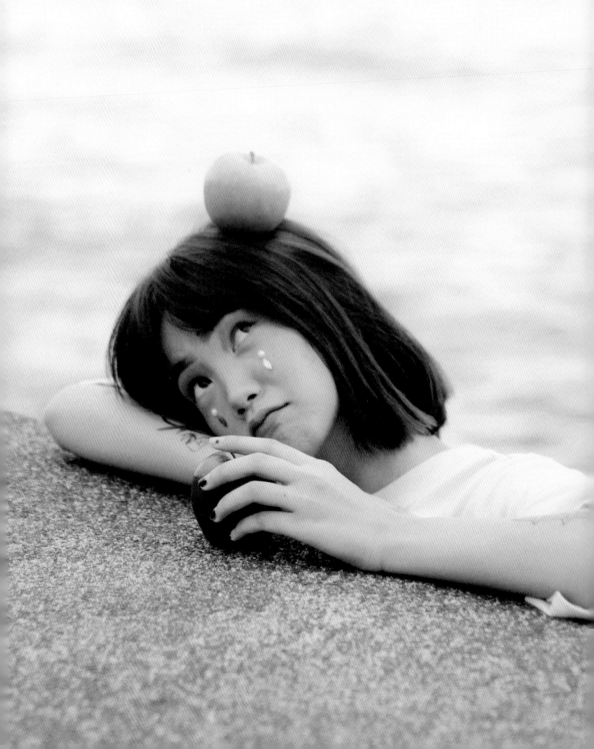

Chapter 6

Digestion, absorption and mindful mouthfuls

Nutrition and diet specialists traditionally concentrate on the balance of foods on the plate. Indeed it is important to ensure that your body has access to an appropriate range of macronutrients (proteins, carbohydrates, fats and oils) and micronutrients (vitamins, minerals and phytonutrients) for your current needs. Before we delve deeper into all of this, however, I want to emphasise that *nutrition is not just about what's on your plate* or indeed in your smoothie bowl. What you should also be paying attention to is how well you are actually digesting the food you eat. You could pride yourself on having "the perfect diet", and yet still be deficient due to poor digestion, absorption and metabolism of your food.

So you can understand this fully, let's revisit and take a little trip through the digestive system.

It's all in your imagination

Your digestive system actually starts in your mind. As soon as you start to think about what you're having for dinner, your brain starts gathering information. Perhaps you're picturing a Thai curry: a few brightly coloured vegetables with succulent chunks of tofu or chicken simmering in a pan of creamy coconut milk. You may already be imagining the warm smell of the spices, the sensation of that first delicious mouthful… and as you do so, your brain begins to send messages to your digestive system so that it can wake up and get ready.

Fluids will be sent to various aspects of your digestive system to make sure it has enough to make all the different digestive juices. Your cells will arrange to manufacture some more hydrochloric acid for your stomach, so it can break down the proteins in the tofu or chicken more effectively. Minerals, vitamins and previously digested proteins will be gathered to make the digestive enzymes you need for that particular meal. You may even start salivating at the thought of such a welcome meal, as your mouth readies itself to chew everything up and start to process the carbohydrates in the rice, sauce and vegetables. Your digestive system has gone from *standby* mode to *at the ready*.

Flooding your senses

If all that happens when you're just thinking about food, imagine how your digestive system can be set into action once dinner actually arrives. You can now see the reds, oranges, greens and creamy whites; you can smell the fragrant yet pungent aroma filling your nostrils. As you dip your fork in, your proprioception picks up clues about the density, the weight, the texture of your curry, and as the food enters your mouth, thousands of nerve endings confirm and more deeply probe the textures and landscapes of that forkful. Your 10,000 taste buds are now party to an explosion of flavours: the sweetness of the coconut, rice and peppers, the sourness of the lime, the saltiness and deep "umami" flavour of the chicken and seasoning, the pungency of the garlic and spices; the bitterness of the coriander and spinach. Your brain is working hard to process all of this information and send it down to where it is needed. There can now be no doubt that there is Thai curry on its way in, and your digestive system can switch from *at the ready* to *all systems go*.

Give yourself a heads up

This is all called the *cephalic phase of digestion*. "Cephalic" means that it involves your brain. I believe it is one of the most crucial stages of digestion.

What this means is that if you are mindfully engaged with your food, you will be able to switch on your digestive processes nice and early. This will maximise your chances of absorbing all the nutrients you need from it, while avoiding indigestion, bloating, inflammation and some of the root causes of chronic illness.

On the other hand, if you don't pay much attention to your food, perhaps grab something quickly from a shop or the freezer, and wolf it down mindlessly while watching TV or working at your desk, then when that food hits your stomach it's going to come as quite a surprise. There may have been a few indications, but it's not going to be nearly as well prepared as it perhaps might like. As we shall see below, that can have a knock on effect through your whole system.

So the sensible thing would be to give your digestive tract a heads up. The more information you can send its way, the better. There's a little ritual you can practise for the first few mouthfuls of each meal or snack that I call "Three Mindful Mouthfuls". Like any habit, the more you do this, the more engrained it becomes, until it becomes a natural part of how you eat.

Every now and then you might enjoy an eating meditation where you do this for the entire meal or snack, but in general I recommend this for the *first three mouthfuls*. That gives you enough of a chance to engage fully with your meal, and send as much information as you can to your gut about what's on its way.

Three Mindful Mouthfuls

Setting the scene:
- Even if you won't be doing the cooking, take an active role in deciding what you're going to eat. To help you make this decision, tune into what your body feels it might want – or not want – to eat today.
- When it gets nearer to mealtimes, remind yourself of what you're going to have, envision it, and get a sense of what it's going to taste and feel like.
- Just before you eat, imagine a bubble of calm around you, a space that stretches out timelessly in all directions. Even if – in fact especially if – you are surrounded by chaos and noise.

Mindful mouthfuls:
1. When the food is in front of you, have a good look at it. Enjoy it like a work of art, or a beautiful view.
2. Lean in and inhale the amazing smell of your meal.
3. Allow and encourage a deep sense of gratitude and joy. Gratitude has an uncanny way of opening us up to receive things.
4. Slowly savour the taste and sensations of your first mouthful, the temperature and textures, as you chew your food thoroughly.
5. Pause to gather some more food onto your spoon or fork, and repeat the process for at least 2 more mouthfuls.

Perfect posture:
Sit up straight as you swallow, and throughout and after your meal. This will help the mechanics of digestion, ensuring the food can travel easily through the plumbing of your digestive system, and that the sphincters at each gateway can fully operate.

Then you may want to check in with a mindful mouthful sporadically through your meal, to keep the connection in place, and to listen for any cues that what you are eating is still appropriate or that perhaps you have had enough.

Note that this is a practice, which means there's no pressure to be good at it! If you find it hard to be present, then try and enjoy the process of practising, and let go of any attachment to "success" or "doing it right." Also note that if any mindfulness practice, including this one, brings up feelings of trauma, then you may need professional support before being able to work in this way.

Stress and digestion – how the Three Mindful Mouthfuls practice works

Taking Three Mindful Mouthfuls will trigger your cephalic phase of digestion, which will optimize how much physical nourishment you will glean from that particular meal. At the same time, this is a bite-sized mindfulness practice that will directly impact how you process and respond to stress.

Your natural stress response downgrades your digestive processes. This is a sensible move: faced with a problem or threat to overcome, you need to focus as much energy as possible resolving or getting away from the situation. Then you can get back to digesting your food. (The same can be true for your reproductive processes, so this is also pertinent for anyone trying to have a baby or with any kind of menstrual problems.) At the same time, stress can actively increase inflammation in your digestive tract, affecting how you absorb nutrients into your body, as well as impacting your immune system and nervous system. This is how stress can make you feel run down, strung out and depleted.

Stress can come in many forms: work-related, relationship issues, financial worries, anxiety about your health or the health of a loved one, lists of things to do building up... In addition you may still be holding stress patterns from unresolved physical or emotional trauma, sometimes from many years ago. Added to all that, your body may be working hard to cope with modern excesses of pollution, pesticides and electromagnetic stress. Or to deal with foods that it struggles to digest. All of this can keep you in a continual state of heightened anxiety that may affect your mental, emotional and physical health.

This is where the bubble of calm comes in. Your imagination is a powerful tool, and your digestive system will listen to it, as we have already seen with the cephalic phase of digestion. Take a few deep breaths, and settle into that perfectly calm space: where there's nothing to do, nothing to think, no demands, nothing pressing, just time and space stretching out eternally. The stresses in life may not go away, but your shift in focus away from worrying about them may allow your body to downgrade its stress responses enough for you to digest your meal more effectively.

Then in that beautifully clear space you can begin what is essentially a mindfulness practice. You focus first on the food – something physical in your immediate environment – with all your senses. This helps to anchor you to the present moment. Then as you bring that food into your body, still focusing with all your senses, you will be able to become more fully present in your body. As you chew, taste, feel, swallow and maintain a gentle awareness of your posture, you practise staying fully present in your body, in the here and now.

There are countless studies showing how being present in the here and now switches your central nervous system from high alert back to a calmer, more fluid state.

Remember this is a *practice*. This isn't something to be perfect at, or to score or judge yourself on. In fact, this is a place where you can practise letting go of judgements, criticisms, and anxieties. Just as you would in a mindfulness meditation,[54] when these or any kind of thoughts appear, smile at them and let them float away, as you bring your awareness back to eating. If you need to do this a lot – i.e. there are a lot of thoughts, anxieties or judgements distracting you – then be grateful that you have a lot of opportunities to practise letting them go! If you find the practice itself stressful, then trust that it won't always be that way, and giggle to yourself at the irony. Humour is one of the most helpful stress-relievers I know.

Eventually – or even sooner than you think – you may find yourself naturally enjoying this practice every time you eat or drink. It becomes as effortless as pausing to savour the first few mouthfuls of each meal. The effects of something so simple can be profound, however, and we'll explore that more in the next chapter on Mindfulness and Your Health.

Chew your food!

For some, the mouth is a convenient funnel to shovel food into before gulping it down. This is a bit like throwing whole eggs into a cake tin with handfuls of flour and sugar and a packet of butter, with no mixing, beating or blending, and expecting it to come out as a cake. Your teeth, tongue and salivary glands are there for a reason, and you would be well advised to use them.

Chewing your food helps grind it down so that digestive enzymes can get to work on it more easily. Plus, of course, chewing feeds back more information about what you're eating to help trigger digestive processes throughout your digestive system. As with many practical tasks, the secret is in the preparation: if you do a good job here, then everything will be easier further down the line.

It also stimulates the release of saliva from various sets of glands in your mouth. The saliva is an important ingredient in your "cake mix" to help moisturise it and ease its journey when you finally swallow. Some of it also contains an enzyme called ptyalin that specifically breaks down complex, starchy carbohydrates, such as bread, rice and potatoes. The longer you chew and savour the food in your mouth, the more chance the ptyalin will have to do its job. The ptyalin gets deactivated in the stomach, so make the most of it while you can.

Another handy feature of chewing is that it stimulates the regular pulsing contractions that move substances down your oesophagus (foodpipe) into your stomach, then through your intestines and finally out of your anus. This movement is called peristalsis, and is essential for a healthy digestive system. If you're constipated or feeling congested, try chewing your food more.

Sit up straight!

Remember being told to sit up straight at the table and chew your food? Well, I used to understand why I should chew my food, but I thought that being told to sit up straight was just an etiquette thing. It turns out that your posture is important for your health too.

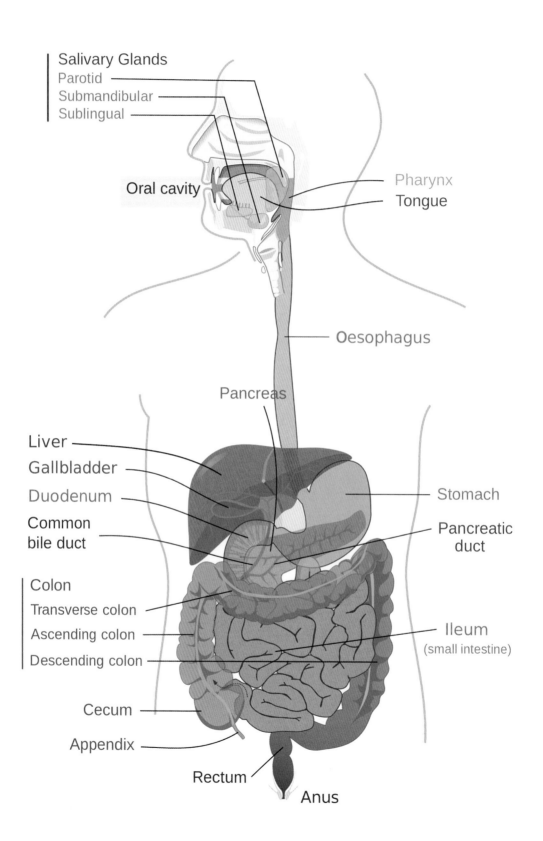

Salivary Glands
Parotid
Submandibular
Sublingual

Oral cavity

Pharynx
Tongue

Oesophagus

Pancreas

Liver
Gallbladder
Duodenum
Common
bile duct

Stomach

Pancreatic
duct

Colon
Transverse colon
Ascending colon
Descending colon

Ileum
(small intestine)

Cecum
Appendix

Rectum
Anus

Your oesophagus (or esophagus – pronounced a-*soff*-a-gus) is the 8-inch food pipe that channels what you swallow down into your stomach. The tissue cells lining it can take quite a battering – especially if you haven't chewed your food very well! As a result, the inner lining – the mucosa – of the oesophagus is continually shedding and growing new cells.

The oesophagus doesn't just dump the food you swallow into your stomach like a rubbish chute. There is a sphincter towards the top that you can consciously activate by burping, and another sphincter further down between the oesophagus and the stomach. This lower sphincter acts as a kind of lid that stops your highly acidic stomach contents spilling back up and damaging the tissue in your food pipe. If the lid doesn't seal properly, you can end up with acid reflux.

Your posture can be really important here. If you sit up straight during and after a meal, and in fact are generally aware of your posture, this helps the sphincters to seal properly. The seal is relaxed and the lid allowed to open in response to swallowing – and also in response to the stomach stretching, which is what creates a belch from your stomach to let gas out and up. Because this lid is on the upper right side of your stomach, lying on your left side can help to release any trapped wind, or alleviate reflux.[55]

Your oesophagus passes through your diaphragm, a dome-shaped sheet of muscle that stretches across the inside of your chest just above your stomach. When your diaphragm contracts and moves down, air rushes in to fill your lungs and you inhale, and when it expands and moves up, it squeezes air out and you exhale. This movement massages the organs below the diaphragm, and helps the flow of fluids through your veins and lymphatic system. Contraction of the diaphragm also acts as an additional sphincter to help prevent reflux of stomach acid and contents.[56]

A hiatus hernia is when the upper part of the stomach gets squeezed up through the hole in the diaphragm that's there for the oesophagus, and then gets stuck. So there's a bit of squashed stomach that's also pressing on the diaphragm, the oesophagus and the vagus nerve (more on that later), and this can create breathing problems, chest pains and even heart palpitations alongside indigestion. Or sometimes there can be no symptoms that you can feel.

Your stomach: your very own protein processing plant

Your stomach is slightly on the left hand side of your lower chest, and its contents are always acidic. Most of the time, your stomach contains fluids that are moderately acidic, but if your brain has told it that proteins are on their way, then your pH can shoot down to around 1.5, which is extremely acidic (the lower the number, the more acidic it is – you don't get much more acidic than 1). So as you can imagine, your stomach has a thicker and more protected lining than the rest of your digestive tract, including a thick layer of mucus excreted by specialist cells called goblet cells.

Fluids with a pH higher than 4 can probe their way into this mucus, but the hydrochloric acid in your stomach is usually too acidic for this. It's a surprising situation where strong acids just can't get through or erode the mucous, while weaker acids can.

To produce enough stomach acid to digest the proteins in your diet, you need:
- to be hydrated (gastric juices are fluids, after all)
- to have enough zinc available
- to have triggered its production by thinking about/smelling/tasting etc. your food
- to be in a relatively calm place.

Think about that for a moment, and ask yourself: *how efficient do you think your stomach acid production is right now?* The answer to this question has ramifications that may impact your health in a number of ways.

Your stomach acid is actually hydrochloric acid (remember that from the chemistry lab at school?) and is released via cells in your stomach wall called parietal cells. At the same time they deploy a substance called intrinsic factor, which protects acid-sensitive vitamin B12 from acidity. If your stomach isn't producing sufficient levels of hydrochloric acid, then you may not release enough intrinsic factor. However, the B12 will still be destroyed by the weaker acids, resulting in B12 deficiency. This can result in a type of anaemia called pernicious anaemia, as B12 is crucial for blood building. And that's just the tip of the iceberg, as you also need B12 for your nerves, your brain, energy production, plus an important chemical process called methylation. This is why many practitioners recommend sublingual B12 tablets, which dissolve under your tongue straight into your bloodstream, or patches that send B12 through your skin, and it's why GPs are able to offer B12 injections into the bloodstream.

Hydrochloric acid also has the important job of killing of as many pathogens as it can so that you don't get ill from your food or water. Pathogens are bacteria, viruses and other tiny organisms that can cause disease. Your gastric juices need to have a pH of about 1-2 to do this job well, so this is another situation where your stomach acid production can directly impact your health. Some scientists have expressed concern that people taking frequent antacids for indigestion and stomach ulcers are leaving themselves vulnerable to food- and water-borne disease.[57]

Finally, you also have chief cells in your stomach lining that release pepsinogen during what we call the *gastric phase of digestion*. The hydrochloric acid released at mealtimes unlocks the pepsinogen and converts it into pepsin, an enzyme that breaks down the proteins. Proteins are long chains of chemical structures called amino acids, found in most foods, and in particularly high amounts in meat, fish, eggs, mushrooms, nuts, seeds and pulses. Pepsin will break these down into much shorter chains called peptides. Your stomach will churn your food up like a blender to continue the job your teeth started, and so that as much pepsin as possible can get to the proteins. The resulting "smoothie" is called chyme, and when your stomach registers a change in pressure and a high peptide content, a sphincter at the lower end of your stomach will open and allow the chyme to flow into your small intestine and the next stage of digestion begins.

Note: if your stomach acid production doesn't cut the mustard, then this trigger may be delayed. The contents of your stomach may then have to swill around in there for a while, perhaps feeling uncomfortable and giving you symptoms of indigestion.

Your pancreas: fire department and enzyme factory

The chyme travels next into your small intestine, for the *intestinal phase of digestion*, but this couldn't happen without the interception of your pancreas. We mostly tend to think of our pancreas as something to do with blood sugar and diabetes, but as we have seen, only 2-3% of its cells are involved in this (the Islets of Langerhans). A large proportion of your pancreas is concerned with the safety and effectiveness of your small intestine.

The chyme is still highly acidic, and left untreated, would burn a hole straight through your duodenum (the first part of your small intestine). Fortunately, the pancreas is at the ready, dousing it with alkalising juices via a hose system called the common bile duct. The alkalinity is provided by bicarbonate ions, which are made in the same bit of biochemistry that produces the hydrochloric acid for your stomach. I love how cleverly efficient the human body can be.

At the same time, if you have made good use of your cephalic phase of digestion, your pancreatic juices will be packed full of all the enzymes you need to break down everything into its smallest component part: the carbohydrates that have been partially broken down in your mouth can now be broken down into the simplest sugars; the peptides from your stomach can be split into amino acids; and the fats and oils will also have their enzymes, but they still have a little way to go yet.

Small intestine

Your small intestine is also an enzyme factory, and so all the enzymes get to meet up and have a feeding frenzy here. Peptides (partially broken down proteins) are converted into amino acids, while carbohydrates and sugars are broken down to their simplest forms, glucose, fructose and galactose. Lipids (fats and oils) are also broken down here, as we shall see below.

Your small intestine is considered to have three sections: the duodenum, the jejunum and the ileum. Most of the activity happens in the jejunum. The brilliant thing about the small intestine is its inner wall. Instead of being smooth like the inner tube of a bicycle wheel, it is rough with thousands of tiny little projections, like a lawn. And each blade of grass in that lawn is covered with a miniature lawn of its own. This is called a brush border, and it's where the extra enzymes are produced. It's also where most of the absorption of nutrients into the body takes place. (Although you may think your food is already in your body, your digestive tract is actually more like the hole in a doughnut – so anything here is still technically outside of the doughnut.)

So imagine you are an ant, walking the length of your small intestine but having to do so by walking over each individual minuscule blade of mini-grass on each individual tiny blade of grass – and you get some idea of how this clever design increases the surface area of the intestinal wall. Which means loads more capacity for absorbing stuff.

Amino acids and sugars can pass through the cells that make up the blades of mini-grass into your bloodstream, and then make their way to your liver. A lot of other nutrients are absorbed here too. Water soluble nutrients (e.g. B vitamins, vitamin C, minerals and some phytonutrients) can be absorbed throughout much of the digestive tract, while fat-soluble nutrients (e.g. vitamins A, D, E and K and other phytonutrients) need to be absorbed with the lipids here in the small intestine.

Lipids (fats and oils) like to be different. They don't mix well with water, which is what most of you and your internal fluids are made up of, so they're a little harder to break up and transport around. They need a little help from bile acids, which are produced largely by your liver and are made from cholesterol (one of the many reasons you need good amounts of cholesterol in your body). Your gallbladder, a small organ next to your liver, acts as a storage container for bile, and releases it whenever appropriate into the common bile duct – the same pipework used to secrete pancreatic juices. If you don't have a gallbladder anymore, then your liver will need to take on this role – and how well it manages seems to vary from person to person.

The bile salts break up the fats and oils into droplets and create little clusters called micelles that can now travel happily through the watery intestinal fluids to the brush border. The micelles allow lipases – enzymes that break down lipids – greater access to these fat droplets, so they are broken down into smaller fatty structures.

In technical speak, they are converted from triglycerides (glycerol-based structures that contain three lipids, or fatty acids) into monoglycerides (glycerol structures that contain one fatty acid) plus free fatty acids (i.e. single fatty acids that aren't attached to glycerol). Fatty acids are to fats what amino acids are to proteins, i.e. their most basic building block. Just as there are many different kinds of amino acid, there are also many different kinds of fatty acid, and we'll explore them more in a later chapter.

Fatty acids are transported through the brush border, but often in a different way to amino acids and sugars. Instead of being passed through into blood vessels, fatty acids and monoglycerides are packaged into another form of transport called a chylomicron, and then absorbed into a lymph vessel. The lymphatic system runs alongside the blood vessels in your body; in the area above your heart, they drip into your blood, so the lipids can finally make their way to your liver.

Liver

Your liver is a phenomenal workhorse, and its role as an accessory organ to the digestive system is just one of many. We have already seen how the liver produces the bile salts that help you digest and absorb lipids. We have also traced the path of digested nutrients through the wall of the small intestine into the blood (via the lymphatic system in the case of some lipids), and from there to the liver. It's now the liver's job to decide what happens to them.

Your liver may put some of them together to form new substances, such as cholesterol (to make bile, for healthy cell membranes, for vitamin D production in the skin and for the production of many of your hormones). It may send some of them to various parts of the body to where they are needed right now, or to be stored for later use. It may use or store some of the nutrients itself. Before it does any of that, it may convert some of them to slightly different substances.

For example, if your blood and liver register a great deal of sugar that is surplus to current requirements, your liver can arrange for much of it to be stored. It can either convert it to fatty acids and triglycerides and send it to fat cells for storage (which it can also do with excess proteins), or convert it to glycogen and store it in its own cells. This activity, as we know, is triggered by the hormone insulin.

Your liver is also a storage site for iron, copper, vitamins A, D and K and vitamin B12.

Large intestine

Meanwhile, back in the doughnut hole, not everything has been absorbed. If your digestive tract is in a good healthy state, any proteins that haven't been fully broken down to amino acids will be strictly prevented from entering. This includes harmful pathogens and allergens that have made it through your stomach acid, as well as carbohydrates that haven't been broken down to the smallest sugars, either due to poor digestion or because they were never supposed to break down, as in the case of dietary fibre.

Dietary fibre can be either soluble or insoluble. Soluble fibre dissolves in water and forms a gel that can slow down your absorption of some nutrients, including sugars – which is why it's important to eat whole fruit and not just drink fruit juice. The juice doesn't contain the fibre you need. The gel formed may also be soothing to your digestive tract, which may in turn calm down the nerves there and help prevent spasms (e.g. in IBS, irritable bowel syndrome). Calming down the nervous system in the gut may also have a soothing effect for the rest of your nervous system, and so your whole body. Chia seeds, psyllium husk, oats, barley, peas and beans are all good sources of soluble fibre – but note that you also need water for them to dissolve in to form the necessary gel. If you've ever soaked chia seeds, you'll know exactly what I mean.

Insoluble fibre won't dissolve in water, but instead absorbs it and puffs up like a sponge. It can then act as a sweep through your digestive tract, and so be helpful for constipation and for clearing stagnation. Too much insoluble fibre can also be highly irritating, however, especially where there isn't enough hydration. Insoluble fibre is found in nuts and seeds, the bran portion of whole grains and in the skin of fruit, such as apple peel.

Although fibre is often recommended for digestive health, in practice, blanket advice to increase dietary fibre is misleading. With people whose diet is low in dietary fibre, an increase alongside improved hydration may be helpful in many cases. In a few of those cases, and with people who already have a good intake, increasing fibre can either show little benefit or may even worsen symptoms.[58]

In any case, the leftovers from digestion and absorption in your small intestine will form an unappetising soup of dietary fibre and other undigested substances, and then make their way out through a valve into your large intestine.

You large intestine – or colon – is actually much shorter than your small intestine, but is substantially wider. Like the rest of your digestive tract, it gradually squeezes its contents through its plumbing system, which in this case goes up the right side of your abdomen, across the top, down the left side, and then wiggles its way to your rectum and anus. Along the way, as much water is absorbed as possible (together with any remaining water soluble nutrients), and the rest is compressed with masses of gut bacteria into packages of faeces/stools/poo. The main bulk of your stools are, in fact, bacteria, but that is not the only role of gut bacteria, as we shall soon explore.

It's also worth noting at this point that your liver and colon have an additional role: that of detoxification and elimination. Your liver contains several different kinds of detoxification enzymes that process toxins delivered to it from throughout your body (via your blood and lymphatic system). These include carcinogens, environmental toxins, drugs and their metabolites. It can send the end results to your intestines along with the bile it releases, and then your intestines have the opportunity to eliminate it all when you empty your bowels.[59]

So how well you can let go here is important not just for your colon health, but also to help rid your whole body of any toxic load it may be carrying. We'll look at this in more detail in chapters 7 and 18.

Poor digestion and malabsorption

There is even more to the digestive system than this, and there are separate chapters devoted to the gut bacteria (also known as bowel flora or microbiota), the vagus nerve and your gut's relationship to your brain.

However you can already see how easy it is to disrupt your digestive processes. Stress, overeating, eating too late, eating inappropriate quantities or ratios of foods and nutrients, eating poor quality foods (especially processed and refined foods with reduced nutrient value), eating too quickly and/or mindlessly, poor hydration and even posture can all contribute to poor digestion and absorption.

If you're not digesting and absorbing foods efficiently, you will end up with higher amounts of undigested or partially digested nutrients in your small intestine. Some of these may contribute to bloating, discomfort, pain, cramps, constipation, loose stools, and general inflammation throughout the gut. Inflammation will then set the scene for the paradox of poor absorption alongside leaky gut.

Leaky gut is where irritants and pathogens can sneak through the gut lining into the bloodstream, and potentially cause havoc throughout the body. So the paradox is that you end up absorbing things you don't want in your body, and unable to absorb much of what you need.

Poor absorption of nutrients, whether because they haven't been fully digested or because the brush border is too inflamed to do its job properly, means that you will be depleted in the proteins, lipids, carbohydrates, vitamins, minerals, other nutrients and energy you need to function on both fundamental levels – i.e. those needed to avoid illness and death – and on higher levels, including memory, speech, intelligence and emotional wellbeing.

Hydration

Crucial to all of this is hydration. You need to be well hydrated to make all of your digestive juices, from the saliva in your mouth, to the secretions in your stomach and intestines, and the juices released by your pancreas and gallbladder. Your enzymes break down foods through a process called "hydrolysis", which means that water needs to be present for that to work. The tissue that makes up your digestive tract is largely made of water. The mucous coating that lines and protects that tissue is predominantly water. Then you need your blood, lymph and tissue to be well hydrated for all the digested and absorbed nutrients to be able to travel to where they are needed.

Some people find drinking a lot of water with a meal gives them indigestion, so you might want to try drinking water between meals, so it is already in the wings waiting to be used.

We breathe, sweat and wee out approximately four litres of water a day. We can recoup much of that through a hydrating diet, which means one that is rich in vegetables and salad, soups and casseroles and other water-rich foods. The rest we can get from our fluid intake. I have found over the years that 1.5-2 litres seems to be a helpful quantity for most people – but not all in one go. It can be dangerous to drink too much water, especially in one sitting. After particularly strenuous exercise or sweating lots in a hot environment, you may need to increase your water intake, but again, not all at once. Some people prefer to continuously sip water; I prefer to drink a large, warm glass on waking and then at intervals through the day. If you regularly find yourself wanting excessive amounts of water, you should probably ask your doctor if you need a diabetes test.

The quality of your fluid intake is key, however. Many common drinks are diuretics, which mean they make you wee more, so you may need to drink more plain water as a result. Diuretics include coffee, tea, fizzy drinks and many herbal teas.

Plain water is often the best option for hydration. For the most part, room temperature or warm water seems easier for the body to comfortably assimilate. A lot of people don't like the taste of water, and so prefer to add ice, lemon or squash. I suspect the underlying issue in most cases is poor water quality. Good quality water tastes better, and commonly it feels easier to drink more of it, too.

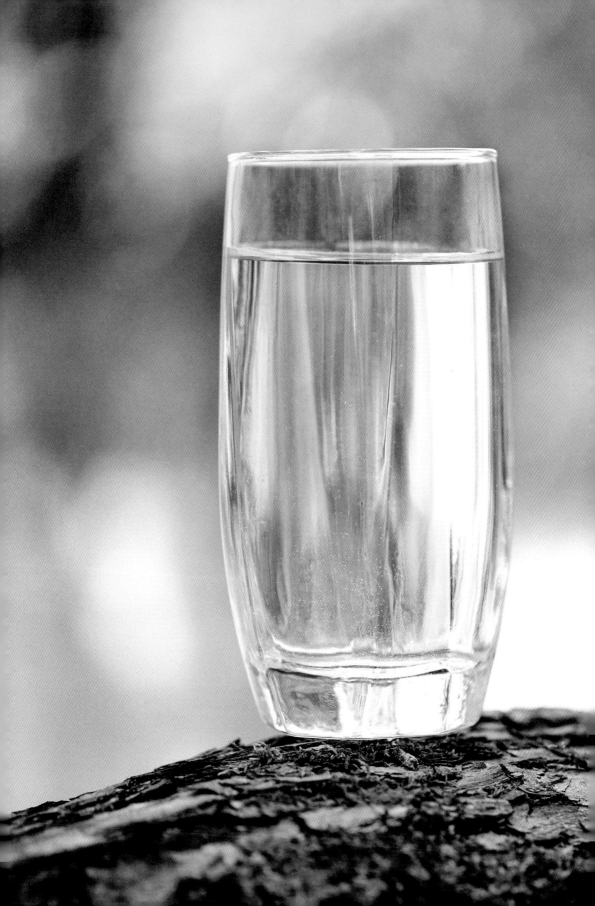

Water quality

So where can you get good quality water? Well, my ideal would be fresh spring water from pure glacial mountains in a pollution-free environment. That's something I don't have access to, however, so I do my best to get as close to that as I can. Sometimes, that will mean buying reputable mineral water, preferably in a glass bottle (by reputable, I mean not bottled tap water, but actual spring or well water). Other times it will mean tap water, because that's the best on offer and I'm grateful that I have access to water at all. When I'm at home, this currently means reverse osmosis filtered water that has been remineralised and reoxygenated! A system I am very fortunate to have, but that still isn't anything like fresh, unpolluted, mountain spring water.

There are many filter systems out there, and each has its own pros and cons. I've chosen this one because I like the fact that reverse osmosis (or RO) takes pretty much everything out, including hormone disrupting chemicals, something that most other systems aren't capable of. What you're left with, however, is empty of minerals and vitality. Spring water has been whorled and eddied through stones that add minerals, electrons and oxygen; I have remineralising and oxygenating add-ons instead. A poor substitute, perhaps, but one I am grateful for. RO filters are notoriously wasteful, so I also have a pump that recycles waste water, for the benefit of the environment and my water bill. I am aware that there are many other systems out there with various benefits, and you will need to find your own preference within your budget and kitchen cupboard space.

Linseed tea

Linseed tea is a wonderfully hydrating drink that you can make with just golden linseeds and water. The recipe is simple and I have included it in the recipes section. The end result is a slightly thickened, golden elixir that soothes your digestive tract, deeply hydrates, and seems to fill your body with calming light.

Most people seem to really enjoy linseed tea. Some have unfortunately been put off because the linseed tea they have made is far too gloopy. It doesn't need to be excessively thick, and can even get quite unpleasantly snotty when over-reduced. So remember to simmer the tea very gently indeed and with the lid on.

I prefer my linseed tea simple and warm. Some like to add cinnamon for flavour. I have also successfully made cool mint linseed tea for hot days and extra digestive support. However I have my linseed tea, my body, particularly my digestive tract, is always very grateful!

Reflection time

- *How do your current eating patterns serve you?*

- *Do you have any signs of poor digestion or absorption?*
    - *If so, how long have they been there?*
    - *How often do you notice them?*
    - *Are there any obvious triggers?*
    - *Have you noticed anything that usually helps?*

- *What do you do that you know really helps you to digest and absorb your food?*

- *How often do you manage to do this?*

- *What habits and patterns would you like to let go of, or introduce?*

Action plan

- *Practise the Three Mindful Mouthfuls eating meditation*
    - *Remember to avoid judging sensations as "good" or "bad".*
    - *Instead savour every sensation as if it were a new and curious experience.*
    - *Then let it all go and get on with your day.*

Recipes

- ***Linseed tea*** *– p.293*
  This feels so good to drink! It's a slightly thick, golden elixir that soothes, hydrates, and seems to fill your body with calming light.

- ***Golden milk*** *– p.292*
  Again, soothing, hydrating and calming, with anti-inflammatory and antioxidant spices that make this the perfect comfort drink.

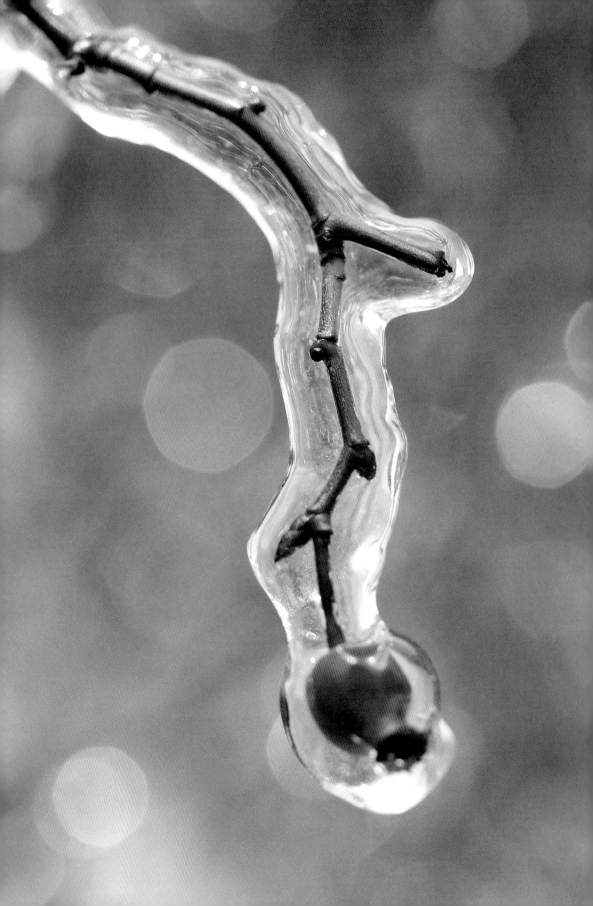

Chapter 7

Melting the freeze response and letting go

It's all about the flow

I am fond of saying that hydration is not just about how much water you drink, but about how well that water is flowing around your body. Putting a bucket of water in the garden won't water the plants: you need to stand there with a hose or have a sprinkler system, to allow the water to reach each and every plant, and you need to make sure the taps are open and that no one is standing on the hose.

Similarly, you might be putting a good amount of water into your body each day, but how well is it actually hydrating you? Is it effectively helping to create the gel-like and fluid structures that make up your body? Is it usefully helping you to transport nutrients, hormones and enzymes around your body to where they need to go? Is it perfectly helping to flush waste material and toxins out of your cells?

There are so many things that can get in the way of water doing the jobs it needs to do, but I believe one of the biggest ones is stress. Your natural trauma and stress response involves the kind of physical tension that can stop fluids flowing around your body. Your immediate response to stress and trauma is to contract. You are like a runner in a starting block, but can all too easily get stuck there, in a kind of holding place. Waiting, holding on, your muscles and connective tissue tense.

That tension restricts the flow of fluids. The big muscles we usually think of, as well as the ones that wrap around your blood and lymph vessels, may both respond to a surge in adrenal fight/flight/freeze hormones by contracting.[60, 61]

So the amount of water you are drinking may not be not the whole story in how hydrated you actually are. To be fully hydrated, and so able to digest your food properly, and in fact function better on every level, you may need to look a lot deeper.

Fight, flight or freeze

When something stressful or traumatic happens, you go into a response that is often referred to as "fight or flight". Your body prepares to either fight off or run away from a threat. It does this by:

- speeding up your heart rate and breathing;
- activating the ancient part of your brain that triggers action without thinking;
- downgrading non-essential activities (such as digestion and reproduction);
- energising and tensing the muscles in your arms and legs so that you are coiled, ready to spring into action.

Fighting and running in that moment releases that coil and expends the excess energy. Sometimes, however, no physical action is necessary: perhaps the threat was a wild animal in a jungle that has been distracted, or a mugger that has been intercepted, or an argument, or financial stress, or grief.

In such a case you need to do something else to release the tension and help energy to flow back to your other organs and systems. Otherwise you might get stuck in this response: at least partially frozen in position, wound up, tense, digesting poorly, struggling to think rationally, with a general lack of flow through your organs and tissue – meaning that fluids, nutrients, waste materials hormones and other substances can't efficiently get to where they need to go.

You have a natural mechanism to avoid this scenario: you can literally shake it off. Have you ever found yourself trembling after a scary or traumatic event? Perhaps shaking with nervous or hysterical laughter? Or uncontrollably sobbing? It's a very neat way of getting things moving again, while grounding yourself back into your physical body.

Peter Levine in his book "Waking the Tiger" talks about an aspect of the fight or flight response that involves deliberate freezing. He describes a gazelle being chased and then caught by a cheetah. In that moment, the gazelle collapses, going into a state of numbness to avoid feeling the full pain of being eaten alive. This may also fool the big cat into a false sense of security, so it relaxes its immediate grip and potentially allows an opportunity for escape. In this particular scenario, the gazelle does indeed get free, and then shakes to bring itself out of its freeze response.

Possums are particularly good at "playing dead", their version of the freeze response when they are caught. Predators often aren't hungry when they come across prey, and so will stash them in a secret food store rather than eat them straight away. If they seem dead already, then there's no need to kill them, so the predators just hide them. Once stashed, the possum comes to and steals away before their predator returns. So freezing or fainting is a very clever self-protective response. It offers either survival or numbness from pain.

We also seem to have the ability to downgrade our consciousness in some way, so that we at least partially numb the pain of the threatened trauma. We freeze emotionally as well as physically. If we don't manage to escape or resolve the threat, and then shake off our physical response to it, then we can get stuck in that frozen place.

In the short term, this freeze response can be life saving. Over time, however, it can have quite a detrimental effect. The drain on resources and prevention of full activity in your body sets the scene for stagnation, exhaustion, inflammation, depression and illness. When you start to become more present in your body, you become more aware of this, which may feel painful or uncomfortable on physical and/or emotional levels. You might therefore find it difficult to settle into yourself and really feel what's going on within you.

Becoming more present may therefore initially be very difficult, as it's going directly against an important self-protective mechanism. In some cases, we will do anything to avoid that – even behaviour that seems quite irrational and destructive.

One such behaviour might be binge eating. A classic binge session will often take place almost in a trance, where the person is shovelling down food without even registering what it tastes like. It's almost a pushing down of feeling, a filling up of a place that has started to register distress, so it can't be heard anymore. Rationality and mindfulness is absent, it can feel purely animalistic, even a struggle for survival. The feelings that are bubbling up are far too painful to address, so it is easier to distract and absent oneself – whether that be with cramming down food, self-harming in other ways, drinking, taking drugs, excessive exercise or losing yourself in your work. Binge eating is rarely about being greedy, and more commonly about pain avoidance, a self-protection mechanism against ongoing or unresolved trauma.

These seem like extreme responses, but you may be surprised at how common such behaviours are. You may even recognize one or more of them in yourself, to a greater or lesser degree. Thankfully, there are tools that wise and insightful people have developed over thousands of years which can help guide you through and out of any stress response you might be stuck in. One of those is mindfulness, which I have already touched on and will explore further in the next chapter. Another, also from the Orient, is an understanding of the Chinese Five Elements.

Dissolving stress with the Chinese Five Elements

Chinese Five Element Theory has a lot to contribute to this discussion, but I'll try and keep it relatively brief here. If you – like me – are intrigued by what I share here, then I encourage you to explore further, whether through further reading,[62] through finding a good qi gong class, or studying something like shiatsu or Five Element acupuncture.

It's described as a theory, but I think of it as a way of viewing the world, and seeing all the patterns, connections, how things move and how things get stuck.

It's a particular perspective, and has a lot in common with, as well as differences from, the Ayurvedic viewpoint, ancient European approaches, Native American perspectives... we're all exploring and describing the same world, just from a slightly different angle. They are all insightful and inspiring, and Five Element Theory in particular has intrigued me since I started practising qi gong 20 years ago.

Imagine the universe is a tapestry made up of five different coloured threads. The tapestry's pictures are multi-dimensional and moving, an ever shifting story. Each thread represents a different element: the green thread represents the Wood Element, the red one is Fire Element, the yellow one Earth Element (I have described this a little already), the white one Metal Element, and there is a blueish black one that represents Water Element. Everything in the universe is made up of a combination of these threads, each combination telling a different story, and shifting as the story unfolds. You are part of this universe, so you are also made up of your own unique and evolving pattern of colours.

Even a fairly superficial understanding of your current make-up and that of the tapestry around you can bring incredibly useful insights. If you choose to delve deeper then there are layers and layers of understanding to explore.

The Water Element is connected to winter time, when we can be still, reflect on what has gone before and prepare for the year ahead. The Wood Element has the energy of springtime, where our plans are pushing upwards into action. The Fire Element is midsummer, where we are active, creative and full of joy. Earth Element is the fruit-bearing time of late summer, while Metal Element represents letting go of excess fruits in autumn, letting them fall to the ground and nourish the soil. And so we are now empty and ready for the stillness and contemplation of winter again.

For the time being I'd like to focus in on the Water, Metal and Earth elements.

Water Element

Picture a scene of snow covered stillness on a wintry evening in the countryside. There is complete calm. The trees are bare and the lake is frozen over. There is life, but it is mostly at or below the surface: the tree's roots are active deep in the earth; the lake's deeper waters still flow and are rich with living creatures – and if you look closely, there are creatures sleeping beneath and scurrying around the earth. The essence of Water Element is flow, calm and, of course, hydration.

The emotion associated with the Water Element is fear. Fear can be a lifesaver: it keeps you on your toes, looking out for threats, helping you respond to danger by either fighting, fleeing or freezing. If you get stuck in fear, however, it's as if the lake has frozen too deep, and the ecosystem below starts to suffocate. Five Element Theory teaches that emotions such as fear are neither good nor bad; instead they are useful as long as you can feel them when appropriate, and then move through and beyond them when they are no longer appropriate. It's the fluidity of your emotions that's important.

Perhaps unsurprisingly, the Water Element has a strong connection to your internal waterworks: your kidneys and bladder. Fear is considered to be held in those organs. It's interesting to note that your adrenals, which send out the hormones that trigger your fight/flight/freeze response, sit on top of your kidneys. Your brain tissue and bones are also coloured with this thread, as well as your hair, your knees and your ears/hearing. In some people where the Water Element is either dominant, struggling or stuck, you might observe traits or symptoms that relate to a few of these organs and tissues.

Jing energy

Your kidneys are considered to house your Jing. Jing is described as ancestral energy, and it's the level of vitality you inherit from your parents when you are born. Some people are born with nearly a full glass of Jing, as it were, while others are born with much smaller amounts. As you go through life, you will use up increasing amounts of that Jing energy. When it runs out, your time here is up.

However, you can prolong and brighten your experience on this planet by nourishing yourself with a different kind of energy, called Chi or Qi. Wholesome food, reviving water, energising breathing, being in nature and sunshine and certain movement practices (such as qi gong, t'ai chi, yoga) can provide Qi energy to top up your Jing, so that your glass (or kidneys) takes much longer to run out – and in the meantime you have much more energy to enjoy life.

Stress, burning the candle at both ends, poor eating habits, dehydration and living a life disconnected from nature and its cyclical rhythms can all deplete your Jing energy. In the West we might call this "living on your adrenals". At some point, you are bound to collapse.

Re-establishing balance, flow, peace and inner reflection will help to steady this trend. Imagine sending your own roots deep into the earth, and feeling the calm and sustained support it provides.

Bring awareness to your own physical body, and imagine a relaxed and fluid state, as if you embody the stillness of a lake with steady deeper currents and life. From that place, a sense of trust can start to melt the frozen effects of fear, and things can start to flow again.

Water Element foods

There are certain foods and ways of eating that are considered to support this process. Many of them are dark in colour like the deep blue-black of the Water Element; some have a natural sea salty nature, such as seaweed and fish; others are hydrating and nourishing in other ways. If you ate just these kinds of foods and nothing else, you might drown out some of the other elements you want to

> **Some water element foods:**
> Kale, asparagus, leeks, aduki beans, black beans, black lentils, seaweed, chestnuts, walnuts, dates, raspberries, blackberries, blueberries, watermelon, black sesame seeds, fish, buckwheat, barley, miso, tamari

keep in balance. So perhaps include them little and often at times when you feel your Water Element needs more support, or during the winter time.

Earth, Metal, Water

The Earth Element is largely about feeling grounded and nurtured; the Metal Element is primarily about letting go. They are both precursors to the Water Element (Earth = late summer, Metal = Autumn, Water = Winter), and so are important for setting the scene.

If your Earth Element is *well nourished*, you feel supported and safe enough to *let go* of anything you no longer need. This might include blockages, toxins, insecurities, fears and any crutches you are gripping onto that no longer serve you. In this way, tending to your Earth Element will pave the way for a balanced Metal Element. With well supported Earth and Metal Elements, you feel safe and now also clear enough to allow things to flow and be healthy again – a prerequisite for a balanced Water Element.

So to allow your Water Element to fully flow, you need to make sure there is sufficient support for the Earth and Metal Elements that precede it.

Earth Element

The Earth Element is represented by late summer, the time when you are reaping the harvest of your creative activity. It's a very physical time, where you have put your plans into action, added your own creative fire, and can now see and feel the results, as a mother can see her babies. It's a time of fullness, and a deep connection to the earth, which nourishes you just as it feeds the apple trees and squash plants around you. You can feel satisfied here, deeply content.

That sense of connection to everything around you brings with it an ability to empathise with all those around you, to feel a shared experience.

If you remember, an imbalance in the Earth Element might be experienced as feeling disconnected – from the people around you, from earth beneath your feet and even from your own body. From that disconnection might come an inability to feel empathy or that the universe is nourishing you, alongside a sense of ungroundedness and perhaps anxiety or worry.

There may have been a trauma that has pulled the rug out from under your feet. It may be a series of events or an ongoing situation that has built up an increasing sense of instability and isolation. Or it may be that you have always felt this way, as long as you can remember. Either way, it's difficult to achieve the inner calm and flow of the Water Element when you feel disconnected from the Earth.

Eating for the Earth Element

The Earth Element relates to the stomach, spleen and tongue – all aspects of how you take in – or reject – nourishment. Its colours are the golden yellows and oranges of harvest time, and its taste is sweet, like carrots, squash and pumpkins, apples and nectarines. We looked at this a little in chapter 5 too.

Too many raw and cold foods can be problematic when the Earth Element is struggling. You might experience this through indigestion or loose stools, or just a sense that you don't want too much cold or raw

> **Some earth element foods:**
> Carrots, squash, parsnips, sweet potato, orange and yellow melons, nectarines, apples, yellow split peas, orange lentils, quinoa, millet, yellow and orange edible flowers

right now. Warm and gently slow-cooked foods are often much easier for and more nourishing to a system that is lacking digestive strength. Soups, casseroles, stewed rather than raw fruits (or sometimes avoiding fruit completely), and using cinnamon, ginger, turmeric and other spices to add some warmth.

Sugar addiction and self-deprivation

When you feel in a state of disconnection, you might desperately seek out sugars and carbohydrates, grasping at sweets, cakes, biscuits and sugary drinks. Or perhaps you overload with bread, pasta and potatoes – or even with excessive amounts of fresh or dried fruit. Such foods will give you a similar kind of dopamine hit to recreational drugs and alcohol. The potentially addictive qualities of such foods can be enhanced by a sense of isolation, of not being nourished or supported. Or you might be flung in another direction, where you dislike or deprive yourself of anything sweet.

Human beings are great at tying ourselves up in knots with this. Feeling malnourished on any level can equate to feeling neglected and rejected. We often take this a step further by rejecting nourishment and care in an effort to protect ourselves from feeling let down.

It's easy to see this play out emotionally, but it also seems to play out physically. I have already mentioned how I see it in people who are seemingly doing all the "right" things with diet, exercise and self-care, but little of it seems to be getting in and having the desired effect. The freeze response seems to create a barrier to self-nourishment, not least through creating inflammation in the part of your digestive tract that absorbs nutrients, and through downgrading your digestive processes in general.

Digestive and eating disorders

Sometimes we take this to an extreme of rejection, as a way – consciously or not – of trying to exert control over an unstable or unpalatable situation. We may lose our appetite for sweet things, lose our appetite entirely, experience indigestion when we eat or vomit up our food, sometimes with conscious effort. Or food may just pass through poorly digested and barely absorbed.

This may be tied in with complicated emotions and responses around self-love, self-care, relationships, and feeling ungrounded and out of control, sometimes due to trauma. This sets the perfect scene for eating disorders, such as anorexia nervosa and bulimia. In anorexia nervosa, food is rejected before it enters the mouth. There are usually psychological factors that play out, but there is also usually a very physical block to digestion in the background. It may be that stress and trauma has told the digestive system to pretty much switch off, or it may be that there is so much discomfort in the digestive tract it is sending signals to the brain to avoid putting more food in that might add to the problem.

With bulimia, the combination of indigestion and microbial imbalance in the gut provides the perfect backdrop to bingeing: the body and the gut microbes both crave simple carbohydrates, the psyche craves nourishment, and both body and psyche seek a numbing of the discomfort, as well as a filling of a bottomless void and a solid anchor to hold onto.

The result of such a binge will, unfortunately, be further discomfort, both physical and mental/emotional. The physical discomfort of indigestion interwoven with feelings such as self-loathing, disappointment and despair can lead quickly to a rejection of what has been binged upon, usually through either vomiting or laxatives. Which might then perpetuate self-critical feelings and keep the person in an ongoing state of stress, disconnection and freeze response.

Obviously this is a very simplified sketch, and for each individual experiencing eating disorders there will be a unique set of circumstances, influences and response patterns. My main point here is that addressing the person's digestive health alongside work to melt the freeze response can for many be an integral part of the therapeutic process.

Disconnection and reconnecting

There are other ways in which an Earth Element imbalance can play out. Perhaps trying to attain fulfillment with material possessions, or needing approval through popularity or public recognition, or chasing extreme sensations to make up for a sense of disconnection or frozen numbness. Or alternatively, through an active rejection of nourishment by depriving oneself of material possessions, relationships or experiences, or with various kinds of self-destructive behaviour. All of this may be experienced in subtle or more obvious ways, but in every case can be linked to being somehow un-earthed.

This state of disconnection is related to the disembodiment we have explored with relation to our stress responses. Part of the freeze response is to remove conscious awareness from the physical body in case the pain and trauma is too much to bear. Reconnecting with the Earth Element helps you to settle back into your physical body, and to establish that, even though there may be discomfort, it's safe and bearable enough to feel again. To open up and allow things in again – be it nutrients, breath or love. It's a physical step in the direction of good health.

One of the most useful ways I have found to do this is with the Three Mindful Mouthfuls described above. When you focus on the food you are about to eat, you are placing your awareness there. As you bring that food into your mouth, and then swallow it deeper into your body, you are by default bring your awareness and consciousness back into your body again. You are using the gifts of your tongue and stomach (aspects of the Earth Element) to help you reconnect with your physical body, and with your physical environment. In doing so, you encourage your fight/flight/freeze response to melt a little, and you start to be able to allow yourself be more fully nourished. If this practice is too overwhelming, then start with one Mindful Mouthful, or seek professional support to help get you to that stage.

From there, you can begin to explore the kinds of foods that bring you true nourishment. Does the way you are currently eating feel fulfilling? If not, which foods feel more satisfying? What quantities, which mealtimes?

Feel your way through it. The minute you start to judge the foods you are eating as "good" or "bad", you start to also judge yourself as "good" or "bad", and the stress starts to clam you up again. Trying to figure things out too much in your head will also encourage that disconnection from what your body is trying to tell you. Treat this as a fun exploration where there are no rules, just a gentle guidance to keep feeling, keep connecting inwards and to the earth, and to keep things flowing.

Metal Element

The Metal Element is that important phase in the cycle where you feel safe enough to let go of anything that is holding you back. Emotions, patterns, habits, beliefs – anything that is no longer appropriate or nourishing to you.

The fruits that have adorned you in the late summer of the Earth Element are now overripe and ready to fall. You can let them go now to decompose into the soil and provide rich minerals to feed next year's harvest. You can trust the soil to transmute even things that are rotten into something precious and life giving.

For this reason, the Metal Element, and autumn time, are about letting go, separation, sadness and grief. Grief and sadness are by no means pleasant emotions, but it is necessary to feel them and go through them as part of the process of moving on and letting go. Whether we are saying goodbye to people, places, habits or beliefs. The Earth Element can help us feel held while we do this.

On a physical level, it should be no surprise that the organs connected to the Metal Element are those connected with elimination. The large intestine, where we make and let go of faeces, the lungs where we breathe and sigh out air, and the skin that we sweat through. We can use all of these as routes out for toxins and waste, in a process of letting go that leaves us purified. This creates an environment where our Water Element can then flow unhindered by rubbish or stagnation.

Constipation, irritable bowel syndrome, shallow breathing and skin complaints are all potential signs that you might be holding on rather than letting go. If your body feels it has the energy and space to do so, it might produce a fever or rash, a mucousy cold, or a bout of diarrhoea to blast toxins out and shift any stagnation. Otherwise things might build up and, over time, your whole system can become sluggish.

Metal Element foods

The foods that encourage us to sweat more and generally eliminate are the pungent ones: spices, such as ginger, cinnamon, cumin, turmeric and pepper, alongside garlic, leeks and onions. This pungent flavour is unsurprisingly related to the Metal Element. The colour associated with the Metal Element is white, to reflect its yearning for purity. So we can add in white foods, such as garlic, onions, turnips, coconut, cauliflower, butter beans and rice.

Note that brown rice, especially when well soaked and cooked, will aid the colon in letting go, while white rice is stripped of much of its fibre and nutrient content. I have heard some say that only white rice relates to the Metal Element, but I believe that to be a misunderstanding. Short grain brown rice, properly prepared, will look white enough in any case, and help to gently sweep through the lower bowel.

> **Some metal element foods:**
> Onions, leeks, garlic, cauliflower, cabbage, celery, turnips, coconut, butter beans, rice, mustard, ginger, pepper, turmeric, cinnamon, cumin, coriander seed, horseradish

I'm also a fan of a well-placed, gentle enema to help remind our bodies about the process of letting go. In the UK in particular, we can be so good at holding on, with our stiff upper lips and anally retentive nature, so sometimes we need a helping hand!

Essentially, the aim here is to find that place of calm where you can reside in peace, knowing that there is a steady flow of nutrient-rich fluids around your body, and that you have the freedom to move forward in your life in whichever direction you now choose.

Less is more

The approach I find most useful with any health picture is one of gentleness and kindness. A soft nudge here and a gentle reminder there can be so much more powerful and helpful than an extreme approach. So if you feel your Metal Element needs support, for example, you may feel tempted to surround yourself only with white ornaments, flowers and foods, to wear only white, to lace everything with generous amounts of spices and garlic, and perhaps even to do enemas several times a day. This may well throw your Metal Element even more out of balance. It may just require little hints of white, some small additions of pungent flavours, and perhaps just an occasional enema, or just more time to relax on the toilet.

This approach is much more likely to move things forward and support not just your Metal Element, but also your Water Element, so that things really feel like they're flowing and calm again.

Reflection time

- *How grounded and safe do you feel?*
  - *Do you feel completely relaxed most of the time?*
  - *Do you feel that your feet are well connected to the ground, and your head well anchored to the rest of your body?*
  - *Do you ever feel stuck in your head, or slightly floaty or disembodied?*
- *How much are you holding onto that you don't need any more?*
  - *Old resentments, pain, grief, desires, judgements?*
  - *Material possessions, habits, relationships?*
- *How fluid do you feel?*
  - *Do you feel stuck or stagnant on any level?*
  - *Does your body feel stiff or clogged up?*
  - *Do you feel dehydrated, regardless of how much water you drink?*

Action plan

- *Allow time to just relax and breathe*
- *Spend time in nature*
- *Spend time with family and friends*

Recipes

- **Earth Element soup** *– p.245*
  Deeply satisfying for any meal, this soup nods to the principles of the Chinese Earth Element to help ease you warmly back into your body and ground you.

- **Millet slice** *– p.254*
  Another versatile recipe for batch cooking, this Earth Element nourishing dish can be used as a snack, with a light salad or as part of a hearty, warm meal.

- **Cruciferous curry** *– p.257*
  One of my favourites. It includes pungent and white Metal Element foods and spices to help you release toxins and anything you are ready to let go of – plus helps you to make detoxification enzymes, as described in chapter 18.

- **Black bean and seaweed stew** *– p.253*
  Beautifully nourishing for the Water Element, this soup provides nutrients for bone and kidney health, and helps to keep everything flowing and calm.

- **Kombu & ginger tea** *– p.293*
  A feisty Water Element drink providing minerals and anti-inflammatories.

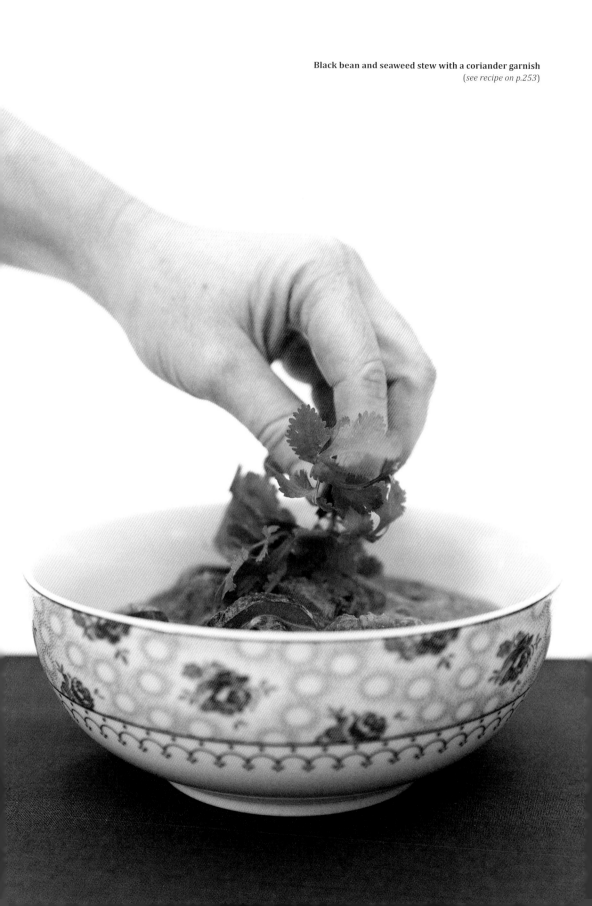

Black bean and seaweed stew with a coriander garnish
(*see recipe on p.253*)

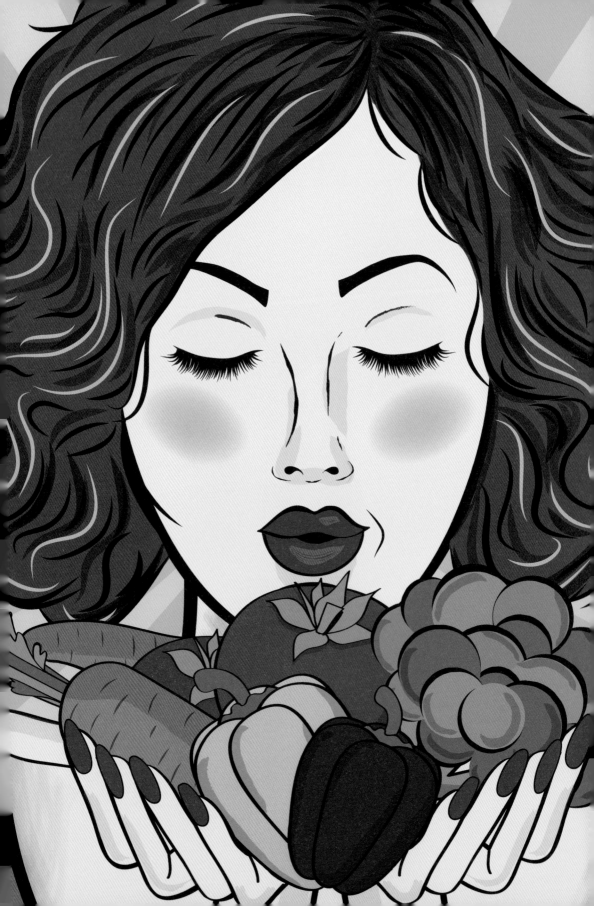

Chapter 8

Mindful eating and your health

"Suffering is not abstract or conceptual. It's *embodied*: you feel it in your body, and it proceeds through bodily mechanisms."[63] Neurologists and other scientists have known for a long time that your mind and your physical body are connected, and how you can influence their behaviour. Aspects of how they connect are well established, and new research is increasing our understanding all the time.

When you experience stress or trauma, hormones and nerve signals ripple out from your brain to alert different aspects of your body to what's just happened, and alter how your body is behaving to better match the situation. You may need to put up a fight or quickly run away, so you need to activate whatever is useful to this, and downgrade anything that isn't.

Electrical nerve signals shoot through your sympathetic nervous system (SNS), which may then increase your heart rate, raise your blood pressure and reduce your digestive juices. At the same time, a part of your brain called the limbic system intensifies your emotions, in particular fear and anger.

Meanwhile, *hormones* (chemical messengers) are sent out from your pituitary gland in your head to your adrenal glands above your kidneys, which then trigger stress hormones that similarly affect heart rate, blood pressure and breathing patterns. Adrenal hormones also release a surge of blood sugar in case you need extra energy to fight or run away, and ensure energy and resources are diverted away from digestive, reproductive and immune functions and towards the large muscle groups.

At the head of all this (quite literally) is the hypothalamus in your brain, an area that is part nervous system and part hormonal, and fires both communication networks up at the same time so that your body can put itself on physical, mental and emotional red alert.

Just to reiterate, in this state you downgrade digestion, reproduction and immune function. These are not priorities when you are on red alert. So your saliva, stomach juices and intestinal juices may dry up, making it difficult to digest and absorb nutrients. This is manageable in the short term, but when stress is long term, this may lead to a state of malnutrition, where you don't have the nutrients or energy you need to keep physically or mentally healthy. Some of the neural and hormonal cascades can affect your memory and how you make new memories, as well as concentration, mood and behaviour. Your fertility or menstrual cycles may also be adversely affected. Plus the various processes that help to protect you from and deal with illness and infection may be compromised.

What's more, these processes might be triggered not just by a stressful or traumatic event or situation, but also by your own thoughts. So you could potentially increase the effect of a stressful event on your body by responding to it in a particularly stressful way. In fact, you might even trigger a stress response by anticipating a stress that may never even happen (worrying about something that may or may not occur in the future) or by dwelling on something that is long gone. Such is the power of your mind, that you can experience the same physical outcome from replaying or imagining a stress or trauma as from the actual trauma itself.[64]

That is not to say that you should be suppressing your responses, or burying your head in the sand. That's just another form of stress, simmering away below the surface.

What is needed is a whole system of stress management that:
- Calms down the sympathetic nervous system and adrenal response
- Allows normal bodily functions to resume
- Replenishes the nutrients and energy depleted by being on red alert – sometimes for many years
- Enables the repair of any damage done to the body in the process

Mindfulness meditation is an exceptionally good start, due to its known effect on soothing your nervous and adrenal systems. Meditation has been well researched, and we now know of a number of specific ways in which it can switch off the high alert sympathetic nervous system (SNS), and instead activate its soothing and calming opposite, the parasympathetic nervous system (PNS).

Meditation is also known to downgrade adrenal activity and strengthen the immune system. As a result, meditation has been shown to help a variety of medical and psychological conditions, including cardiovascular disease, type 2 diabetes, asthma, chronic pain, PMS, insomnia, anxiety, phobias and eating disorders.[65]

Eating mindfully, like meditation, helps us stay in the here and now, be fully present in this moment.

Mindful eating has also been researched, largely for its impressively beneficial effect on weight loss,[66, 67] diabetes management[68] and a whole range of eating disorders,[69, 70] including decreasing binge episodes, improving one's sense of self-control with regard to eating, and diminishing depressive symptoms in binge eating.[71]

A unique study in this area taught mindful eating to overweight and obese women, not specifically to help them lose weight, but primarily in order to measure its effect on their cortisol levels – i.e. their adrenal/stress response processes, and the subsequent benefit to their overall health.

Abdominal fat was used as a way of measuring this. One of the effects of long-term stress is hypersecretion of the adrenal hormone cortisol. Cortisol is known to increase levels of abdominal fat, and indeed higher levels of abdominal fat have been recorded in healthy men and women who have more exaggerated cortisol responses to laboratory stress tasks.

What's significant here is not that stress can contribute to weight gain, but that it can contribute to abdominal fat, the kind that is associated with diabetes and cardiovascular disease. Stress can also trigger emotional eating, particularly of the type of high carbohydrate foods that we have seen can also contribute to abdominal fat and metabolic disease.

In the mindful eating study, the women who were taught the mindfulness practices had a greater reduction in waking cortisol levels than those in the control group, particularly among the obese women. Mindful eating also reduced anxiety levels and emotional eating. Without adding in any kind of dietary restrictions, the women's weight either stabilised or dropped – compared to an average gain of 1.7kg in the control group of obese women who were not eating mindfully.[72]

Mindfulness meditation

Classic mindfulness mediation is an ancient practice whose results have been extensively studied, but we probably still know just a minute fraction of its benefits. It usually involves sitting in a relaxed but upright way, breathing normally, and gently focusing on your breathing. It's a way to help you become present in your physical body and in the moment. Fear and anxiety attach to things in the past or the future, while just being consciously present in this moment now frees you from both.

Sometimes it's taught to begin your mindfulness meditation session with a body scan, where you slowly visit each part of your body, settle into it and get a sense of how it feels. Not to get drawn into any sensation or start thinking about it, judging it or worrying about it, but just to feel it. This is perhaps an opportunity to reconnect with your physical self, and to let your body know you are listening to it – without getting caught up in any habits, patterns or dramas about it.

After the body scan, you can either follow your breathing – perhaps counting your breaths ten at a time – or imagine slowly filling your body up with white light that pours in from above.

Whichever approach you choose to practice, it's important to know how to deal with the thoughts that will pass through your mind and try to distract you.

So many people say, "I can't empty my mind," or "I get distracted by my thoughts" and use that as a reason not to meditate. You may be pleased to hear that even the Dalai Lama reports finding it difficult to empty his mind! And that's not really what it's about. It's about how you respond to the thoughts that pop into your mind, or race around it, or keep prodding at you. So rather than getting caught up in them or frustrated by them, it's about practising just letting them be. It's not about suppressing them or pretending they're not there, it's just about not engaging with them. And it's important to remember that meditation is an opportunity to *practise* this, not a time to beat yourself up about not being perfect at it.

So if you find that you have lots of thoughts distracting you while you meditate, then thank them for giving you something to practise with! And most teachers recommend you consider a regular practice, rather than just meditating every now and then.

If you don't have a class you can go to, then have a look at Andy Puddicombe's Headspace app. I know many people who have found it useful in setting up a regular meditation practice that nourishes them just as surely as a plate of amazing food. It may on some levels feel counterintuitive to use an app to help your mindfulness practice, but if something works for you then don't judge it!

Why mindfulness can be so difficult!

What I struggle with most is keeping up a daily practice of something. I know it's not impossible, though, as there are plenty of things I do every single day, without fail. In fact I clean and floss my teeth at least twice a day, for example. That's a daily habit motivated by the knowledge of what might happen if I don't, and also by how nice it feels when I do. A short meditation, by comparison, should seem just as easy to do, but until it becomes a habit, it's too simple to just keep putting off.

Another layer that can get in the way is the intrinsic nature of our freeze response to stress and trauma. While mindfulness meditation is about being fully present in this moment, and fully conscious in this body, every cell in your body may be screaming: "No! Don't come in here! The pain and horror might be too much to bear!" This seems especially true when there has been unresolved trauma, and the freeze response is deeply set. So the act of meditation might, for some, initially feel like a conflict between opposing impulses. It can take some real patience and commitment, along with some expert support, to work through that.

Bite-sized mindfulness

The Three Mindful Mouthfuls practice can be so useful here. It can be a gentle introduction to bringing awareness inside the body. Once there, your awareness may register that it is, indeed, an uncomfortable place to be, but that it's bearable. Or that it's perfectly comfortable and even pleasant to be reconnecting in this way.

The other great thing is that most of us eat at least a couple of times a day, so the habit is already there. You don't need to make extra time for your mindfulness practice.

An additional and wonderful benefit is that you are now interweaving moments of mindfulness through your day, which means that you become used to slipping into that space in various environments. Sitting silently in mindfulness, perhaps following the breath, for 10-20 minutes a day is undoubtedly a profound and amazing way of transforming your life; but you also need to be able to instantly access that mindfulness wherever you are. Many mindfulness teachers advise doing both: finding time for a daily meditation, and then finding opportunities to practise being mindful in different situations. Perhaps while walking; or, as we have explored, while eating; perhaps by pausing to feel the sun, rain or wind on your face, or to smell what's around you, or to feel the sensation of your feet on the floor.

Benefits of mindfulness

The more you practise, the easier and more natural it will become, so that you might notice your general approach to life being calmer and more considered. Or you might notice that you don't feel so frozen or constricted by an old trauma any more. Or that you don't get caught up and stuck so easily in anxiety, resentment or fear. Or that you feel emotions in a new way, that is very real but also recognises their transient nature.

Meditation is the opposite to numbing and escaping life: it is learning how to fully experience each moment of it, moving fluidly onto each next moment as it unfolds.

At the same time, you may notice physical benefits. Perhaps you experience less pain[73] or your insomnia improves.[74] Or you feel fresher, and have more vitality. Or it's easier to breathe, and you experience asthma[75] with less frequency and intensity. Or your joints are less inflamed,[76] your digestion settles,[77] or your blood pressure is easier to manage.[78] There are so many studies now on the health benefits of mindfulness that its validity is impossible to ignore.

Gratitude and joy

Mindfulness and meditation can sometimes seem like a serious practice, but it really doesn't have to be. In fact, mindfulness meditation can help foster a lightness and cheerfulness, as well as heartfelt gratitude and joy.

Gratitude carries with it an energy that opens you up to receive nourishment on all sorts of levels. When you feel grateful, you are acknowledging that you have something in your life. So it helps to melt any walls you may have built to protect yourself from the possibility that you can't have those things. I believe that gratitude for your food similarly helps switch on your digestive system, lets it know that nourishment is there right now and it's time to interact with it.

And what is the point of anything without joy? We talk about "enjoying good health" for a reason. True joy is an intrinsic measure of how healthy and nourished we are. Healthy living shouldn't be full of "I mustn't have this" and " I can't do that", or having to be serious and dull all the time. Instead, let's opt for, "Wow, life's amazing and fun and breathtakingly beautiful. I can do so much, and the choices I'm making are bringing me so much joy!"

Joy, creativity and fire

Some fire element foods:
Red berries, pomegranate, watermelon, red peppers, red lettuce, kale, cabbage, radishes, red edible flowers, chamomile, chicory, cocoa and cacao powder, dandelion

Joy is literally at the heart of who you are, as Five Element theory shows so clearly in the form of the Fire Element. The Fire Element relates to high summer, and the phase(s) of life where we are at our most expressive and creative. It is the colour red, the heart, the blood and blood vessels, the small intestine, the womb and sexual function – the creative spark that produces new human beings as well as new ideas. It is the seat of your passion and your joy. If your inner fire is steady and strong, then you will take the nutrients offered to you by your small intestine, transmute them into new tissue following the pattern of your own unique DNA, and use their energy to keep burning. This will feed into the Earth Element we explored before, providing the ability to produce fruit with which to nourish yourself.

A weak or scattered fire will struggle to produce such fruit and security, however. You can nurture your Fire Element with the colour red, including red foods such as pomegranate, red peppers, radishes, red lettuces, cabbages and onions, and red nasturtium flowers in your salads. You can gather and strengthen a scattered Fire Element with bitter tasting foods, including dark green leafy vegetables, chicory and chamomile.

I wonder whether many of us are so drawn to the bitter flavour of coffee and chocolate because we are lacking that steady inner flame of joy. Excessive and oversweet coffee and chocolate, however, may hyperstimulate instead – and make it even more difficult to settle into mindfulness, or indeed a solidly happy and creative state. So this is not an excuse to have more coffee and chocolate than your body feels comfortable with in the name of nurturing your Fire Element!

This is an invitation, however, to consider: how readily can you access your creativity and joy? And, of course, a great way to work with that can be with your food. Get creative in the kitchen, engage with your food, delight in the flavour and texture combinations you have produced – all of this feeds right back into the Mindful Mouthfuls practice of easing out your stress response, switching on your digestive system and getting more nourishment from your food.

Reflection time

- *Do you have a regular mindfulness practice?*

- *If not:*
  - *How might be the best way to introduce one?*
  - *Would you find a local class or an app useful? What time of day would this be easiest for you?*
  - *What might be preventing you from having a regular practice?*
  - *Can you / would you like to try changing this?*
  - *Would you benefit from any kind of professional support?*

- *If you do already have a regular practice:*
  - *What benefits have you noticed?*
  - *How do you feel when you maintain your practice?*
  - *How do you feel if it slips?*
  - *Has the quality of your practice changed over time?*

Action plan

- *Interweave moments of mindfulness through your day*
- *Pause to experience the physical sensations of that moment:*
  - *the smells*
  - *the feeling of your feet on the floor or your back against the chair*
  - *the temperature of the air on your skin*
  - *the textures and taste of the food in your mouth*
  - *the light and colours around you*
  - *the sound of your swallowing or your footsteps on the ground*

Recipes

The perfect way to practice mindful, joyful eating is with a decadently bitter chocolate mousse! Here's a classic, creamy vegan version with calming nutrients alongside the cocoa hit.

- ***Avochocolate mousse** – p.288*

Mindful cooking

*As well as suggesting new recipes, in this chapter I want to focus on **how** you prepare food. Bringing mindfulness into the kitchen can have a profound effect on how your meals turn out, how they taste, how you digest them and what you choose to eat.*

So firstly, take a few breaths and become as present in this moment as you can. Then go to your fridge/cupboard/larder and decide what ingredients you want to use. Try to feel rather than think your way through this: which foods are you most drawn to right now, and which foods are you least drawn to? Is there a recipe that springs to mind for these ingredients, or do you need to go and look one up – or get creative and make one up?

Of course, you also need to consider which foods need using up! Let's keep this as practical as possible.

Then, when you are washing your vegetables, slicing/grating/stirring your ingredients, do so carefully and mindfully, as though you are working with precious and amazing beings or works of art (which in many ways you are!). Perhaps you always chop your carrots into discs, but today you get the urge to slice them lengthways.

Have a listening and respectful quality to your food preparation, and at the same time, fill your heart with gratitude and joy: for the food and its gifts, for your ability to enjoy them, for your hands to cook and your tongue to taste, for the people who will share your meal or the space you have to enjoy it by yourself. Kitchens seem to be prime locations for singing, dancing and laughter: so sing, dance and laugh as you cook! Infuse your food with joy, and that joy will nourish everyone who eats it.

Avochocolate mousse with a garnish of raspberries
(see recipe on p.288)

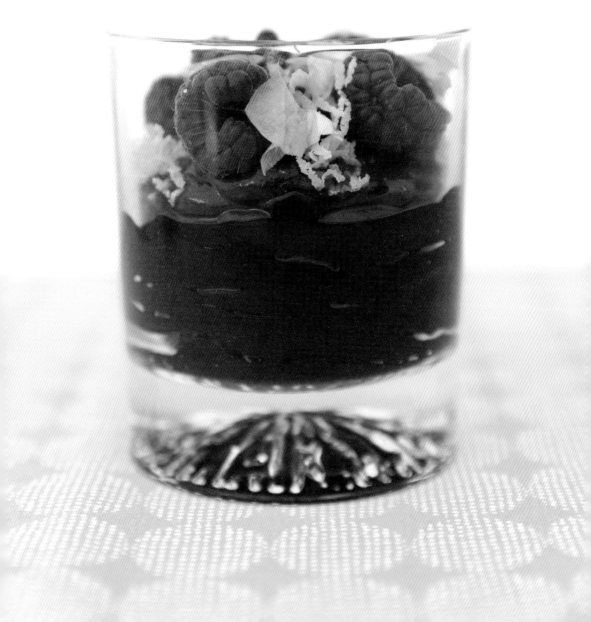

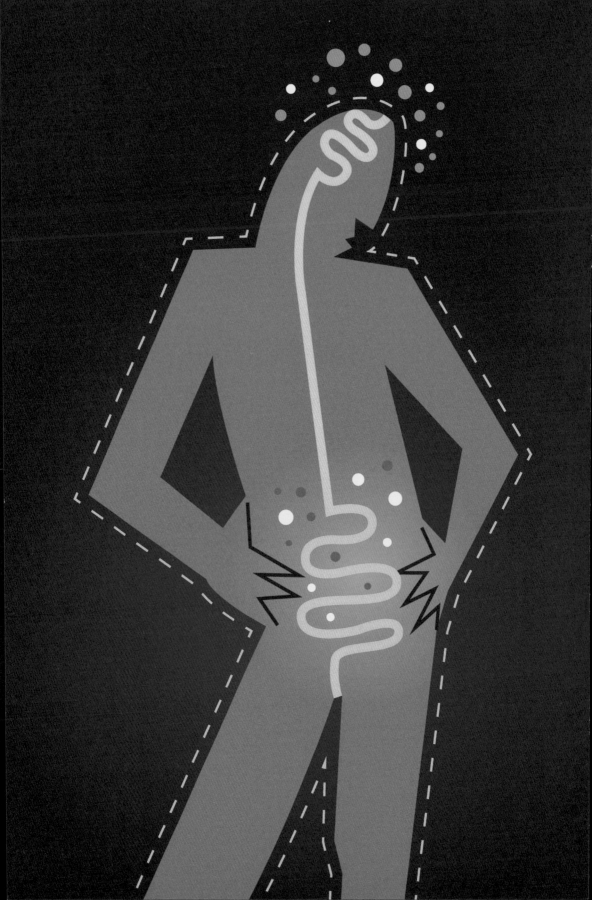

Chapter 9

The gut-brain-adrenal triangle

Much has been written in recent years about the gut-brain connection, how the gut is an integral part of your nervous system and so your stress response, moods and behavior. The next few chapters are about just that and more – and how you can influence all of it with diet.

I find it impossible to talk about the gut-brain relationship without including the involvement of the adrenals, which send out your stress hormones. We have already looked at some of the potential impacts of your adrenals being in stress mode for a long time. Apart from anything else, the continual production of stress hormones will take up lots of energy and resources, which may then lead to energy slumps and/or a continual need for stimulation. Chapter 10 will look at how to replenish and rebalance the adrenals – but first of all I'll describe the gut-brain-adrenal connection. Essentially, this is about how your physical and mental stress responses are driven by 1) your gut, 2) your brain and nervous system, and 3) your adrenal hormones, and how these three aspects influence and trigger each other.

Actually you can't separate out anything in the human body, as it's all connected. No part of us operates in isolation. As you read this paragraph:

- Your eyes are receiving information about the patterns the writing makes;
- nerves are sending that information to parts of your brain to be interpreted into words and concepts;
- to help make this possible, your blood is delivering glucose to your cells to provide the energy required for movement (your eyes tracking the page/screen) and thought, memory and other cognitive processes;
- your cells are busy producing ATP from that glucose;
- hormones from your pancreas are getting involved in keeping the glucose levels in your blood adequate for this;
- your lungs are ensuring there is enough oxygen to make the ATP;
- your heart keeps pumping blood fluidly around your body, delivering the glucose, hormones and oxygen required;
- and also keeping fluid levels in your eyes at the pressure needed to work;
- and to keep your brain hydrated enough to process information efficiently

... and so it goes on.

But for the purposes of the next few chapters, let's focus specifically on the interactions between the gut, the nervous system (including the brain) and the adrenals. First, the gut and the brain:

The enteric nervous system

To begin with, a few brief definitions:

CNS: Your Central Nervous System is your brain and your spinal cord.

PNS: Your Peripheral Nervous System is all the nerves feeding back information from the rest of your body – such as hot, cold and ouch – and receiving orders from your brain – such as sweat, shiver or flinch.

ENS: Your Enteric Nervous System is the realm of nerve activity in your gut. When we talk about the gut, we are usually referring to the digestive tract, and in particular the stomach and intestines. It contains as many nerve endings as your spinal cord. When those nerve endings flutter, you might get butterflies, usually in response to excitement or apprehension. Your enteric nervous system connects to your brain largely via your vagus nerve.

The vagus nerve

The vagus nerve is actually a pair of nerves that connects the brain to most of the internal organs, and has a calming influence on the heart and digestive system. It has been called the superhighway between the brain and the gut, as it sends information in both directions rapidly and directly. Some of these signals affect how well you digest food and how hungry you feel; some communicate important information about the health of your digestive tract.

We used to think the vagus nerve's job was to help your brain tell your gut what to do. We now know, however, that most of information flows in the other direction: from your gut to your brain. So it may be that your gut is more in control of your brain than the other way round.

Acetylcholine messengers on the superhighway

The vagus nerve uses neurotransmitters called acetylcholine as messengers to relay information along its superhighway. So, for example, if there is inflammation in the lining of the intestines, the vagus nerve will tell the brain.

The brain will hopefully register that this is not an ideal long-term situation for the gut: nutrients may not be absorbed so well, and the gut lining may become so damaged that it can no longer efficiently prevent toxins from entering the bloodstream ("leaky gut"). The vagus nerve will hopefully then send acetylcholine with soothing, anti-inflammatory instructions from the brain back to the gut.[79] Meanwhile, the messages from your gut will have had a direct influence on how your brain behaves.

This may partly explain why inflammation and congestion in your digestive tract seems to be able to affect your ability to concentrate, remember and think clearly, as well as your emotional state.[80]

Foods for making acetylcholine

Nutritionally it may be wise to help the work of the vagus nerve by providing foods that contain choline, so that you can make more acetylcholine. Egg yolks are good sources of choline if they are soft – or even better, raw, as you would find, for example, in fresh, homemade mayonnaise. The more you cook egg yolks, the less choline they will contain. Offal is also a good source, such as liver and kidneys. In either case, I would recommend an organic, pasture-fed source for cleanliness and quality. For a vegan option, lecithin granules (usually from soya, occasionally from sunflower seeds) are great to sprinkle onto foods and into smoothies.

You can also ensure an adequate intake of L-acetyl carnitine (in meat), vitamin B5 (in broccoli, chard, squash, sunflower seeds and eggs) and alpha lipoic acid (from red meat, offal or brewers' yeast) to help with acetylcholine production. Vegetarians and those who eat low amounts of meat can synthesise L-acetyl carnitine from two amino acids: lysine and methionine – fish and spirulina may be useful here.

Vagus nerve stimulation

There is a great deal of research on the effects of electrical vagus nerve stimulation in the laboratory and, for example, how that helps to reset fear states,[81] and improve cognitive function such as memory.[82]

Many have additionally suggested stimulating the vagus nerve with gargling, singing, coffee enemas and more. While I haven't seen much evidence for any of this, there are plenty of documented physical and mental health benefits for singing,[83] so I would encourage you to at least sing in the shower every day!

The fearful amygdala in your brain

The amygdala sounds like a kind of dinosaur, and in some ways it is. It's the part of the brain humans have had the longest, and is sometimes referred to as reptilian. It's highly emotional, and is critically associated with fear and anxiety. It takes over at times of stress and trauma so that you are acutely alert to threat, and can react instantaneously without thinking things through. It's helpful if you need to move your hand out of a fire, for example, without having to weigh up the pros and cons of leaving it there. However, if your amygdala is in charge all the time, then just a walk to your local shop will feel like a dangerous mission with potential axe murderers, venomous snakes and sudden sink holes at every moment.

Gut microbes and fear responses

When your amygdala takes over as part of your fight/flight/freeze response to stress or trauma, this will impact your gut activity;[84] including how much saliva, stomach acid and other digestive juices you secrete – and when – along with blood flow, contraction of muscles and stimulation of nerves, your inflammatory responses, and the balance of bacteria and other microbes in your gut. This at least partly explains how stress and nerves contribute to IBS, Crohn's disease, colitis or even just a stomach-wrenching feeling.

What's exciting is the amount of emerging research about how your gut microbes directly affect your amygdala. If you have a microbial imbalance, then your amygdala is more likely to roar and take over. Whereas if you have a healthier balance of gut bugs, you will be less likely to react so strongly, and will be able to calm down your fearful inner dinosaur much more quickly. This means your response to stressful situations – be they flying in an aeroplane, speaking in public, dealing with confrontation or walking down a dark alley at night – may be much calmer and more measured, and/or much easier to calm down from.

In fact, a lot of recent research points to poor gut bacteria in early life as being a predisposition for PTSD – post traumatic stress disorder. This is because the balance and diversity of your gut microbes in the early stages of your life seem to impact how your whole stress response system develops and behaves. The more out of balance, the more likely that a later trauma will result in PTSD. The good news is that it seems that restoring your microbiome in later years is being regarded is a potential treatment.[85]

More on your microbiome shortly. In the meantime, how do the adrenals fit into all of this?

Nerves and hormones

Well, to begin with, your adrenal response directly affects whether your brain and nerve activity are being dominated by your calm, rational frontal lobe or your fear-based amygdala.

Just like your nervous system, your hormonal system is in charge of relaying messages and commands around the body. You could perhaps think of your nerves as emails, instant messages and texts, and your hormones as a letter in the post. They work alongside each other: sometimes backing each other up in the same way you might both e-mail and post your acceptance to an invitation; and sometimes triggering each other, in the way that a letter from your bank might trigger you to e-mail your boss and ask for a pay rise, or a text from your sister might remind you to send your mum a birthday card.

There's actually a physical part of your brain where your nervous system and hormonal system share an office. It's called the hypothalamus, and half of it is nervous tissue, and the other half endocrine tissue (like the endocrine glands in your hormonal system). In times of stress, your hypothalamus, perhaps responding to incoming nerve signals, barks a hormonal command over to your pituitary gland, an endocrine gland nearby in your brain, and your pituitary sends a hormonal order down to your adrenals glands, and then your adrenals respond by releasing their stress hormones.

This chain of command is called the HPA axis: Hypothalamus to Pituitary to Adrenals. It describes one of the many routes via which the nervous system triggers a chain of events in the hormonal system.

You can't really talk about the communication and relationship between your brain and your gut without bringing in your hormonal system – and specifically your adrenals, which are so immediately involved in your fight/flight/freeze response.

Adrenal hormones, stress and inflammation

The adrenal hormone we've all heard of is adrenaline. Except annoyingly it's now mostly called epinephrine. Your adrenals are also responsible for releasing norepinephrine (or noradrenaline), cortisol (and similar hormones in a family called corticosteroids) and DHEA.

Epinephrine and **norepinephrine** can trigger your heart to beat faster and more forcefully, and direct the increased blood flow to the muscles you might need for running or fighting, and to the older part of your brain. (And away from your digestive tract and reproductive system.) They can also influence sugar metabolism to provide instant stimulation.

Cortisol also influences blood pressure and sugar metabolism. Plus it helps process protein and fats, calm inflammation and may decrease bone formation.

DHEA is a precursor to oestrogen and testosterone, and has been linked to longevity and wellness in old age, especially in men. There also seems to be a (limited) protective affect for male smokers.[86] Some studies suggest a role in immune function, and low levels have been linked to cardiovascular diseases, although scientists are not sure whether DHEA reduces the disease or the disease reduces DHEA.[87]

All of these hormones spike in response to stress or trauma. Once things are resolved, their daily ebb and flow goes back to normal. If the stress or trauma is unresolved or ongoing, however, then you move into a more long-term stress response, where DHEA is likely to drop to a low level.

At the same time, you usually end up over producing cortisol. As we have seen, in an ideal world cortisol calms down inflammation. However, when your adrenals have been pumping out cortisol for too long, your body stops listening to it. Just as if you live by a busy road, after a while you stop hearing the drone of traffic.

Which means you are now no good at calming down inflammation. Which means that any inflammation in your digestive system will have a hard time cooling off.

Why is this a problem? Well, remember that your digestive system has been downgraded, so you may not be breaking foods down efficiently. Undigested or partially digested foods may be causing irritation and inflammation in your gut. You may also now be lacking some of the nutrients you need to keep your gut tissue healthy. Plus there may be a number of foods in your regular diet that are adding to that agitation. And now your gut can't hear the message to calm that inflammation down.

Your gut may be getting quite stressed about all this, which will set your nerves further on edge, and keep your adrenals fired up.

And there you have it in the simplest terms: the Gut-Brain-Adrenal Triangle. And we haven't even got to the *really* exciting bit yet!

Your microbiome and your mind

We've known for a long time that your gut bacteria play a pivotal role within your immune system, but what we are now learning about its relationship with your brain is mind-blowing.

Actually, your gut microbes collectively weigh the same as your brain, about 1kg. There are hundreds of different varieties of gut microbes, each with its own roles to play. We call these microbes gut flora, bowel flora or microbiota, and the realm in which they live, the microbiome. The microbiome extends to other parts of your body too, including your skin and mucous membranes (ears, nose, throat, sinuses, airways, mouth, urinary tract, digestive tract, vagina etc.), but the vast majority resides in your colon. Some swim around freely, and some form colonies grown on biofilm, thin sheets of goo that the microbes produce themselves.

The balance and diversity of bacteria in your microbiome is unique to you, and may vary according to what's going on in your life and your gut. They have beautiful, mysterious, mostly Latin names and are grouped into different families (technically called genera), such as Lactobacillus, Bifidobacterium, Enterococcus and Streptococcus. You may have heard of acidophilus – its full name is Lactobacillus acidophilus as it belongs to that genus of bacteria. Your microbiome also includes other microbes, such as yeasts – you have probably heard of Candida and may have come across Saccharomyces. They sound terribly important, and indeed they are.

There are many more bacteria cells than human cells in your body. They are a lot smaller and so you are still more human than bacteria, but never underestimate their influence on your every waking moment. You have a symbiotic relationship with your microbiota, which means that you mutually benefit from your relationship. You nourish each other in many different ways. In fact, scientists suggest that gut microbes have helped human minds to evolve, and may even have encouraged us to form social structures. So let's have a look at the surprisingly close relationship between your microbiome and your brain.

The chemicals of mood, emotion and behaviour

Psychotherapy and modern medicine have narrowed in on a specific group of brain chemicals that directly impact how happy you feel, how well you store and recall memories, how sharply you can focus, how clear your mind feels, how rationally and socially you behave and more. These chemicals are called neurotransmitters, and you may have heard of a couple of them, such as serotonin and dopamine.

Anti-depressant drugs such as Prozac aim to stop levels of serotonin, your happy chemical, dropping too low. Dopamine and serotonin are both of great interest to psychotherapists working in addiction,[88] as where natural levels are low, addictive behaviours such as drinking, drugs, sex, gambling and overeating seem to provide regular stimulation.

The table of "brain chemicals" in your gut, overleaf, briefly describes the main activity of some of the main neurotransmitters and neuromodulators (chemicals that influence brain behaviour).

You will also notice in the same table some extraordinary information that has emerged in recent years: which gut microbes produce each of these. Where once scientists believed that all this activity was firmly confined to the brain, psychotherapists are starting (slowly!) to listen to the mounting evidence that we should be paying more attention to the gut. To maintain your emotional and mental health, you need to be looking after the health of your digestive tract and the balance of bacteria and other microbes there.

A steady wave of nutritional therapists and naturopaths has been working in this way for a long time, so there are already protocols and clinical experience to draw on here. I'll go into this in more detail shortly. First, just take some time to look through the table below and let the implications settle in.

Table of "brain chemicals" in your gut[89, 90]		
Neurotransmitter/ modulator	What it does	Gut Microbes That Produce It
Dopamine	• Associated with: – *pleasurable emotions* – reward centre of brain, and so *addictive behaviour* • Controls voluntary *movement*	**Bacillus, Serratia**
Serotonin	• Affects *emotion, mood, anxiety* and *perception of pain* • Regulates *sleep*, circadian rhythms and *appetite* • Regulates the *digestive and cardiovascular systems*	**Candida, Streptococcus, Escherichia** and **Enterococcus** Also produced in the gut wall In addition, **Bifidobacterium infantis** can influence the production of serotonin from tryptophan (an amino acid found in many protein–rich foods), and has been shown to have antidepressant action in preclinical models of depression
GABA (gamma-aminobutyric acid)	• Prevents nerve cells from getting over excited • *Reduces anxiety* • Involved in *movement* and control of muscles, limbs and *vision*	Some species of **Lactobacillus** and **Bifidobacterium** The GABA produced here influences the brain via the vagus nerve
Acetylcholine	• Activates the vagus nerve and so *calms the nervous system* • Regulates areas of the brain associated with *attention, arousal, learning* and *memory* • Stimulates *muscles*	**Lactobacillus**
Norepinephrine	• Regulates *mood* and physical and mental *arousal* • Can raise both *heart beat* and *blood pressure*	**Escherichia, Bacillus** and **Saccharomyces**

So it looks as though the lactobacillus in yogurt, miso, tempeh and some other fermented foods may help to reduce anxiety, soothe your body and mind's stress responses, improve your focus, memory and other cognitive skills, as well as help with control of your physical movement and eyesight.

Notice that it's not quite as black and white as "good bacteria produce happy chemicals and bad bacteria reduce them." For example, the primary bacteria associated with serotonin production (Streptococcus, Escherichia and Enterococcus) are associated with disease. Candida is a fungus that can be hugely problematic throughout the body when you have an overgrowth of it. And yet it, too, produces serotonin, a happy chemical. This is incredibly clever and sneaky. Candida is essentially saying, "Feed me and I will give you a hit of happiness."

Candida needs and craves sugar, both because its structure is 80% carbohydrate and because sugar helps it transition to the fungal form that spreads through the body. Could this be an additional reason why sugar can be so addictive? Could candida be instructing your brain to give you sugar cravings?

However, if your microbiome is in a healthy state, then candida's demands won't be dominating the show, there will be less inflammation in your intestinal walls and your gut may then be free to make serotonin in other ways.

Your microbiome and the HPA axis

Your balance and diversity of gut microbes, as well as any probiotic supplements you may take, have been shown to have an effect on your HPA axis, the chain of command that kick starts your adrenals into a stress response.[91]

If you get an E. coli infection in your gut, for example, it can activate the HPA axis. A reduction in or lack of microbiota will have a similar effect. Animals raised with bacteria-free guts in laboratories have shown an exaggerated HPA response to psychological stress. This hyper response then normalises once their gut is populated with Bifidobacterium infantis – but there seems to be just a narrow window of time for achieving this.

However, there are further studies showing that probiotic supplements help take the edge off the HPA response to stress in ways that influence anxiety levels and how the brain processes emotions – and not just on lab rats.[92] There is a notable human study where healthy volunteers were given either a probiotic supplement containing Lactobacillus helveticus and Bifidobacterium longum, or a placebo for a month. The study was double-blind and randomised, which means that no one, not even the researchers, knew who was taking what until the results were in. Urine samples then showed that cortisol levels had been reduced in those who had been taking the probiotics, showing a direct impact on the HPA axis and adrenal response. In addition, probiotic use lowered the scores for anxiety, depression and other mental health factors.[93]

Probiotic supplements also seem to be able to help with gut permeability, or leaky gut syndrome. In cases of irritable bowel syndrome (IBS), activation of the HPA axis seems to be increased still further where there is a leaky gut – but this has improved with probiotic use. People with major depression – which interestingly has been linked to inflammation in the brain – have also shown higher levels of HPA activation where there is a leaky gut.[94]

The interrelationship between the gut, the brain and the adrenals seems irrefutable. Which suggests that:

- **If you are working on gut issues, you may need to work on the health of your gut and your microbiome alongside further adrenal and anti-inflammatory support**

- **If you are working on mental health or cognitive issues, you may need to work on the health of your gut and your microbiome alongside further adrenal and anti-inflammatory support**

- **If you are working on adrenal issues, such as anxiety or fatigue, you may need to work on the health of your gut and your microbiome alongside further adrenal and anti-inflammatory support**

What is more, because of the impact of all of this on inflammation throughout the body, and because inflammation underpins all chronic illness:

- **If you are working on any chronic health issue, ranging from eczema to diabetes, asthma to heart disease, arthritis to cancer, you may need to work on the health of your gut and your microbiome alongside further adrenal and anti-inflammatory support**

The next few chapters focus on exactly how to do that.

Reflection time

- *Do you ever feel tension in your throat, chest or abdomen in response to stress or emotions?*
- *Have you ever noticed your bowels responding to stress or emotions, for example with diarrhea or constipation?*

Recipes

These recipes all contain nutrients that help you make acetylcholine and soothe your nervous system and adrenals.

- **Calm bars** – *p.279*
  A snack that soothes as well as keeping hunger at bay.

- **Sun slaw** – *p.269*
  A sunshine-coloured, sunflower seeded coleslaw.

- **Soft egg omelette** – *p.249*
  Also see chapter 5, where this was recommended as a sustaining breakfast option. Keeping blood sugar stable through the day will also help keep your system calm, plus this contains some great nutrients for resetting stress pathways.

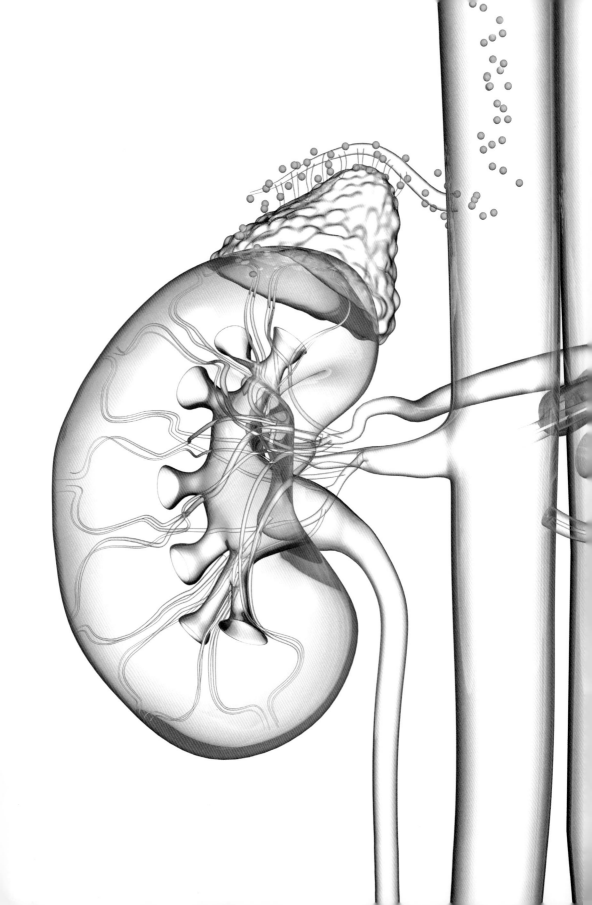

Chapter 10

Specific adrenal support

Adrenal support is essentially all about resetting your stress responses, calming everything down, and getting everything flowing again. Your adrenals are, after all, the glands that send out your stress hormones.

We've already looked at how mindfulness practices, including mindful eating, can be incredibly useful here. Plus we've looked at how your gut health and microbiome balance influence how your adrenals behave. Chapters 11 and 12 will explore your microbiome and how you can nourish it in more detail.

In this chapter, I'd like to address nutrients required specifically for your adrenal activity. These include ingredients and co-factors required for your adrenal responses, and nutrients often depleted by long term or immense stress.

People often express surprise that you can influence your body's hormonal and stress responses so directly with nutrition. And yet when you consider that every single process and activity in your body requires ingredients and helper nutrients (co-factors), nutrition really should be an obvious first port of call.

The building blocks of hormones

In the last chapter we saw how the adrenals release hormones to trigger your response to stress, trauma and threat. Some of these hormones are made primarily from proteins, or amino acids, while some have a ring of cholesterol at their heart. Cholesterol has been given such a bad rap, but this is one example of how you absolutely need adequate levels for health and survival. It is so important, in fact, that if you reduce your dietary cholesterol too much, your body will just make more from ingredients it can find in most different kinds of foods.

Your adrenals have an inner section, called the medulla, and an outer section, called the cortex. In your adrenal medulla, epinephrine (adrenaline) and norepinephrine (noradrenaline) are formed from the amino acid tyrosine, which can be synthesized from another amino acid called phenylalanine.

Phenylalanine and **tyrosine** can be found in good levels in meat, fish, spirulina, dairy and pulses, and there is also some in nuts, seeds and grains.

The cortex is where your corticosteroid hormones are produced, including cortisol, DHEA and aldosterone. These are all cholesterol-based, which means that technically your body can make them from practically any food.

Similar ingredients, plus a host of vitamin and mineral co-factors, are required for many other hormones in your body, including reproductive hormones, thyroid hormones and blood sugar balancing hormones. So you want to make sure you have plenty to go round.

Adrenal co-factors

There are a number of adrenal co-factors that both research and experience have shown to be immensely helpful in mitigating the effects of stress. Many of them seem to act by preventing your adrenal hormones from spiking so readily, or by helping them to recover their balance quickly. Some also help to make the neurotransmitters that your nervous system uses to keep you happy and calm. These co-factor nutrients are not exclusive to your adrenals, but all have additional jobs around your body to help keep you in good health, ranging from detoxification processes to countering inflammation.

Vitamin B5

I first came across vitamin B5 when I was studying for my nutrition exams. I was facing an intensive day of written papers, and had spent weeks revising, developing outlines for any subjects that might come up, and practising essay writing in timed exam conditions. I had learned everything I could about the human body and how it works, the impacts of food and nutrients and so much more. It was at the point when I sat down to learn about B vitamins – why you need them, where you can find them and what happens when you are deficient – that I realised I was at saturation point. I had information overload, study fatigue, a seriously aching writing hand and a continual wired, tense feeling I recognized as stress.

It was just days before my exams, and I felt suddenly blocked. I kept staring at my B vitamin charts, but struggled to focus on what any of it said. I persevered, and eventually, there it was: *vitamin B5 may help support the adrenals and modify the effects of stress*. I bought some as soon as I could (in the form of calcium pantothenate), and the effects seemed almost immediate.

Now, of course, much of this could be attributed to the placebo effect, and at the time I didn't really care – as long as I was calm enough to sit my exams. However, vitamin B5 stuck in my mind. Further research has revealed that B5 deficiency does indeed affect how the adrenals process stress. And vitamin B5 seems to have a very structural involvement in what goes on:

- B5 stimulates your adrenals to produce the cholesterol needed to make corticosteroids, so not enough B5 means not enough hormones
- The structure of the adrenals suffers with B5 deficiency, initially enlarging and then wasting away
- If you catch B5 deficiency in good time, then supplementation can reverse this and improve the adrenals' response to stress[95]

These days, vitamin B5 is often my first port of call when addressing the adrenals. Occasionally it will seem to have the opposite effect, which also makes some scientific sense. As far as I'm aware, there is no effective tool for predicting this, so as with most supplements I would recommend introducing B5 gradually and mindfully.

Food sources of vitamin B5 include avocados, liver, salmon, mushrooms, sunflower seeds and egg yolks (best soft cooked or raw).

Additional B vitamins

Alongside vitamin B5, many practitioners will reach for B6 supplements when wanting to support the adrenals, usually in the form of pyridoxal-5-phosphate (P-5-P). Vitamin B6 is involved as a co-factor in many processes that keep you healthy, happy and alive. It also helps you to convert the amino acid L-tryptophan into 5-HTP, and then 5-HTP into serotonin, your "happy chemical".

You can find B6 naturally in liver, salmon, sweet potatoes, dark green leafy vegetables, garlic and cauliflower, among other foods.

Vitamin B1 helps to rebalance cortisol, and is found in seeds, pulses and grains, in particular sunflower seeds, oats and barley.

Vitamins B3, B5, B6, B12 and folate all play a role in cortisol synthesis. B3 and B12 also help to convert tryptophan to serotonin, and are most easily obtained from meat and fish. Peanuts and mushrooms are perhaps the best vegetarian/vegan source of B3. Adequate B12 levels are difficult to maintain with a vegan diet, and so supplementation is often necessary. Folate, however, has its richest source in green leafy vegetables, lentils, beans and chickpeas.

With all this in mind, many people reach for a high dose vitamin B complex at times of stress. Indeed a 3-month, double-blind, randomised, placebo-controlled trial assessing stress in the workplace gave 30 workers a high dose B complex and 30 workers a placebo. Those who took the B vitamins reported "significantly lower personal strain and a reduction in confusion and depressed/dejected mood after 12 weeks"[96]

However, B vitamins in very high doses do run the risk of side effects, including gut irritation, neuropathy, anxiety and heart issues. In my experience, low to moderate strength B vitamin complexes (usually found as part of general multivitamin formulas) can be just as useful but without such risks.

Whatever the strength, be prepared for bright yellow urine! Your kidneys will assess what you need and want to get rid of, and whatever they discard will make your wee appear almost fluorescent.

Vitamin C

Vitamin C is another common go-to for adrenal support in times of stress, and it does seem to be involved in adrenal activity. Most of the research seems to revolve around keeping cortisol levels balanced during endurance sports such as marathons. However, a 2002 study looked specifically at psychological stress in 120 healthy, young adults. Half were given 3000mg vitamin C daily, and the other half a placebo. Those who took the vitamin C recovered from their cortisol responses to stress faster than those who didn't get extra vitamin C. The vitamin C group also had lower blood pressure responses to stress tests (such as public speaking and mathematics), as well as lower subjective responses to these tests.[97]

Fruit are often considered the best source of vitamin C, especially citrus fruit, but raw herbs, green leafy vegetables and onions are also great sources – it's just the cooking that destroys vitamin C. If you would like to try higher doses, then pure ascorbic acid supplements are always going to be better quality than those with lots of additives and sweeteners, so read the ingredients list carefully. If you find ascorbic acid aggravates your digestion, try mineral ascorbate forms, such as magnesium ascorbate and potassium ascorbate. For a more easily absorbed – but more expensive – supplement, try a good quality liposomal vitamin C.

Magnesium

Claims have been made that magnesium deficiency is related to anxiety, palpitations and panic attacks,[98, 99] as well as a dysregulated HPA axis.[100] So it makes sense to keep magnesium at optimum levels. It's involved in cortisol production as well as the conversion of tryptophan to 5-HTP, and levels inside your cells drop in response to raised stress hormone levels.[101]

Food sources include our old favourites, green leafy vegetables, nuts and seeds. Although I find that mineral depletion in the soil, together with magnesium depletion due to stress hormones, has led to the need for magnesium supplements in most people I have worked with.

Zinc

Zinc has been seen to help cool the adrenal cortisol response to stress,[102] so may also be helpful in taking the edge off. Zinc, like magnesium, is additionally a great anti-inflammatory throughout the body, and needed for enzymes that support detoxification and other processes.

Pumpkin seeds are an excellent source of zinc, alongside most nuts and seeds, chickpeas, chicken, shellfish and lamb.

Fish oil

The omega 3 fatty acids in fish oil, known as EPA and DHA, have been shown to keep cortisol levels calm in the face of stress, as well as reduce subjective feelings of stress.[103] And, like magnesium and zinc, are useful anti-inflammatories to boot. You can convert the omega 3 fatty acids in nuts and seeds (alpha-linolenic acid) to EPA and DHA, but most of us do this inefficiently. So if you don't eat oily fish at least a couple of times a week, then you may want to introduce either a good quality fish oil supplement or a vegan EPA and DHA supplement from marine algae sources.

The smaller oily fish, such as mackerel, herring, anchovies, trout and salmon, are less likely to contain dangerous levels of mercury and other heavy metals than the larger ones, such as tuna, marlin, swordfish and shark.

Phosphatidylserine (PS)

Pronounced fos-fer-tiddle-seer-een, this clever little substance is particularly helpful if you train a lot, whether it's running, cycling, or down the gym. It reduces post exercise cortisol spikes, and so helps your adrenals to recover after you've given them a good work out. PS also helps reduce depression related to overtraining.[104] Yes, you read that correctly: depression related to overtraining. While regular exercise has repeatedly been shown to benefit mental health and mood, there is such a thing as overdoing it.

PS is found in white beans, soya beans, and in extracted soya lecithin, which you can buy in granule form. It is also in organ meats, such as liver and kidneys.

Choline

Choline is another constituent of lecithin, and your body uses at least some of it to make acetylcholine, the neurotransmitter that calms your nervous system. A calm nervous system contributes to soothed adrenals.

So you'll also be able to get choline from lecithin granules and organ meats. Egg yolks are also a good source, but preferably raw or softly cooked. Cooking decreases not only the lecithin content, but also the levels of B5 and B6 in eggs.

Herbal support

There are a great variety of herbs that can be helpful, such as licorice root, Siberian ginseng, bacopa monnieri, chamomile and many more. A herbalist will be able to give more specialised advice on these. Where I have worked with people taking herbs and roots for adrenal support, I have found that some people respond better to different types than others. Note that licorice should be used with caution if you have high blood pressure.

Microbiome support

Your gut bacteria are super important, so the next two chapters are devoted to this.

Who needs adrenal support?

We all do. We all experience stress, so even if we're good at keeping calm, our adrenals are still working hard on a daily basis.

A lot of people need to give their adrenals extra care and attention. How do you know if you are one of these people? Energy levels, sleep patterns and moods can help you to recognise this, as well as other physical conditions. There are many indications, including:

- You have experienced high levels of stress or trauma, or ongoing repeated stresses over a long time
- You find it difficult to get going in the morning, and maybe have better energy in the evening
- Or maybe your energy is flat all the time
- You seem to have lots of energy, but deep down you know this is just you pushing through, perhaps with the help of stimulants, e.g. sugar or coffee
- Or you feel hyperactive a lot of the time
- You experience insomnia, other sleep disturbances, or wake regularly at around 3am
- You have low or irritable moods, or mood swings
- You have other hormonal imbalances, such as menstrual health, fertility issues, blood sugar problems or diabetes, or a thyroid imbalance – your adrenals interact with and provide ground support for all of these systems
- You have any chronic illness or condition, from eczema through to heart disease and cancer – as getting cortisol back into a healthy pattern may help with regulating inflammation and other aspects of disease.

Your adrenals are so tied up with so many of your daily functions, that whatever you want to work on, adrenal support is bound to be part of the solution. Think of it as putting in the fundamental groundwork, some firm ground on which to stand strong.

Reflection time

- *What are your energy patterns like?*
- *How often do you feel wired, frazzled, strung out, tense or unable to sleep?*

Action plan

- *Set up a batch cooking day.*
  - *This is where you cook larger amounts of one or more dishes, then portion up and freeze, or keep in an airtight container in the fridge, as appropriate.*
  - *Then on days where you don't have the time, energy, motivation or headspace to cook, you have something nourishing on hand you can just warm through.*
  - *You can batch cook soups, bakes, nut truffles, pancake mixture...*

- *If batch cooking works for you, you can schedule in a regular day each week or month when you do this. You could even try getting a batch cooking group together, where you meet up with friends and cook together.*

Recipes

- **Mixed bean casserole** *– p.256*
  This recipe includes some fantastic adrenal supportive nutrients, and is great for batch cooking. If you find beans difficult to digest, then make sure you soak and rinse them well, and try cooking them with a couple of bay leaves or a strip of kombu seaweed (both of which can be removed after cooking).

- **Super slaw** *– p.270*
  A true superhero of coleslaw recipes.

- **Warm slaw** *– p.271*
  A warmer, cooked version for colder days, digestive systems that struggle with raw vegetables and thyroids that don't like raw cabbage.*

* Cruciferous vegetables, such as cabbage, kale, cauliflower, broccoli and Brussels sprouts are goitregenic when raw – which means that if your thyroid is underactive, they are best eaten cooked.

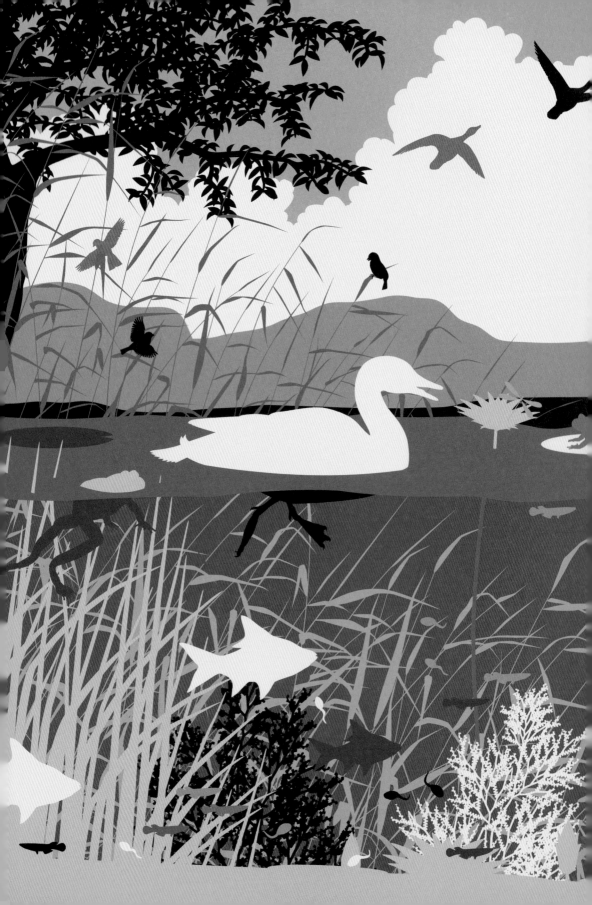

Chapter 11

Your microbiome
~ your inner ecosystem ~

Who's who

Much of your microbiome is made up of different kinds of bacteria. In the realms of microbiology, each species (type) of bacteria is ranked in terms of domains, kingdoms, phyla, classes, orders, families and genera. Within these complex hierarchies, they can also be classified according to whether or not they need oxygen, where they prefer to live, their physical structure, and whether they stain a treated slide purple ("gram positive") or red ("gram negative").

In addition, there are archaea (similar to gram positive bacteria), fungi and viruses, of varying shapes, sizes and activities, and all influencing each other – and you – in different ways.

There is indeed a whole jungle of microorganisms residing among your folds, holes, tunnels, crevices and secret inner spaces.

Most of them live in your colon, the large intestine that is also home to your appendix, which acts as a seed bank for your populations of microbes. Bacteria, yeasts and other microbiota are to be found on all your surfaces, however. The passage that runs from your lips, via your mouth, oesophagus, stomach and intestines, through to your anus, is lined with microbes. Your ears, nose, throat, airways and lungs are similarly inhabited. As are your urethra (where your wee comes out) and vagina (if you have one). Finally your skin, your externally visible surface, is populated with about a thousand different species of bacteria alongside other microorganisms.

In layman's terms, we tend to classify our microbiota into "good bacteria" for a happy tummy, and "bad bacteria" which are associated with bacterial infections, repulsive fungal infections and scary or nasty viruses. This is, of course, both an over simplification and riddled with judgemental emotion. As you may have guessed, the first thing I'd like to do is take at least some of the emotional weight out of the picture, and encourage you to picture instead a richly exotic and beautiful ecosystem of wondrous creatures who have chosen you as their Garden of Eden. But I'd also like to keep things simple, so for now let's think in terms of microbes that are pretty much always beneficial, and microbes that can be pathogenic (disease-causing) when there are too many of them.

Here is a table that lists just a few of these microbes together with some examples of their associations:

Beneficial Microbes	Pathogenic Bacteria	Pathogenic Viruses	Pathogenic Fungi
Lactobacillus acidophilus – digestive and vaginal health – immunity	**Streptococcus pyogenes** – throat infection	**Coxsackie virus** – conjunctivitis – hand, foot and mouth disease – viral meningitis	**Candida albicans** – thrush – oral thrush – other fungal infections
Lactobacillus rhamnosus – anti-diarrhoea and leaky gut – vaginal and urinary health – possibly also protective from eczema, respiratory infections and peanut allergy	**Streptococcus pneumonia** – pneumonia	**Dengue virus** –dengue fever	**Aspergillus flavus** – produces cancer-causing aflatoxin
Lactobacillus plantarum – digestive health	**Staphylococcus aureus** – impetigo – boils – cellulitis	**Ebola virus**	**Aspergillus fumigatus** – causes allergies, respiratory and blood infections
Lactobacillus helveticus – digestion – immunity	**Salmonella** – food poisoning	**Influenza** – flu	**Pneumocystis jirovecii** – pneumocystis pneumonia (PCP)
Bifidobacterium breve – digestive health – immunity – anti-candida	**Shigella** – diarrheoa	**Hepatitis** – liver condition (various types)	**Cryptococcus neoformans** – can affect the lungs and brain
Bifidobacterium longum – digestive health – anti-cancer properties	**Neisseria meningitides** – meningococcal disease	**Herpes simplex** – cold sores – genital herpes	**Blastomyces dermatitidis** – can affect the lungs and skin
Bifidobacterium infantis – digestive health, particularly with IBS – aids serotonin production	**Borrelia burgdorferi** – Lyme disease	**Human papilloma virus** – affects skin and mucous membranes – links to some kinds of cancer	**Tinea corporis** – ringworm
Bifidobacterium bifidum – digestive health, immunity – produces lactase, the enzyme that breaks down lactose in milk	**Chlamydia trachomatis** – chlamydia, a sexually transmitted disease	**Epstein–Barr virus** – glandular fever, also part of the herpes family	**Tinea pedis** – athlete's foot
Saccharomyces boulardii – anti-candida – anti-diarrhoea – norepinephrine production	**Escherichia coli** – abdominal cramps and diarrhoea	**Measles**	**Tinea unguium** – fungal toenails

Pathogenic means disease-causing, but it's useful to remember we all contain many thousands of these within us even when we are perfectly well. We tend to think of pathogens, be they bacteria or viruses, as germs flying through the air with each cough or sneeze, sliming over door handles and lurking in dirty water, and if you don't duck at the right time or keep everything clean, then you'll get ill. But actually, there's a lot more going on than that.

Whether you consider a germ you have "caught" or a pathogen already living within you, the impact of that germ on your health will vary according to the overall balance of microbiota in your gut, and the environmental conditions. A weakened or imbalanced microbiome is known as dysbiosis.

The diversity and balance of wildlife in your inner paradise depends on:

- The microbes passed onto you by your mother in her birth canal during labour, and through breastfeeding;
- the microbes you have been exposed to since birth (and possibly even before then);
- the people you come into close contact with;
- the foods you have eaten and are eating today;
- the pH in your gut;
- the levels of inflammation in your gut;
- the amount of stagnation in your gut;
- the amount and types of antibiotics and other medications you have taken;
- the stresses and traumas in your life and the response of your HPA axis

...and so much more we are yet to understand.

Tribespeople living hunter-gatherer lifestyles have a much richer biodiversity than modern city dwellers. You have an entirely different population of microbiota than me.

It is thought that the microorganisms within us may even encourage us to be sociable, to live in close contact with each other, kiss, hug, hold hands and share germs. This enables their ongoing survival, and provides us with opportunities for enriching our microbiome. We can no longer think of ourselves as independent human beings, but instead as a miraculous and mutually beneficial co-existence of human cells, bacteria cells, virus cells, fungi and more.

When your Garden of Eden is well fed and watered, clear of stagnation and thriving with vitality, then your ecosystem of microbiota finds a balance that enables a number of functions.

Functions of your gut microbes

The roles your gut microbiome play, and their importance to your health and wellbeing, are pretty impressive.

Bifidobacteria, for example, "acidify the large intestine, restricting putrefactive and potentially pathogenic bacteria; produce vitamins and amino acids; stimulate the immune response; repress the conversion of primary bile salts; exert anti-inflammatory activity; and reduce the risk of colon cancer."[105] What a great job description! And we can, of course, now add to that: production of GABA to calm anxiety and the nervous system, and assist physical movement and vision.

If we look at the collective roles of the gut microbiota, we can group these into five main sets of responsibilities:

- Mental health and nervous system activity
- Protection
- Immune function and inflammation
- Nutrient production
- Digestion

Let's look at each of these in a little more detail.

The gut-brain-adrenal connection

We looked at this in the last chapter, so here's a brief review. Your gut wall and microbes between them produce the majority of neurotransmitters (such as serotonin and dopamine) that influence your mood, behaviour and more. They also impact your HPA axis, which governs your stress responses.

As such, your gut microbes and their environment are starting to be taken much more seriously by those working with depression, addiction,[106] anxiety, PTSD (post traumatic stress disorder),[107] Parkinson's disease[108] and other conditions where neurotransmitters and/or triggers to adrenal stress responses play a key role.

Protecting the balance of the ecosystem

The microbes in your gut – and on all the external and hidden surfaces of your body – form part of your protective barrier against the outside world.

Your intestinal wall has its own mechanisms for deciding which particles are food, and so can pass through its cells into your bloodstream (or lymph vessels).

It also contains goblet cells that produce a generally thick and fast-growing mucous barrier that helps prevent large particles (including your gut bacteria) from even reaching your intestinal wall. Your beneficial bacteria are first in line, however, to crowd out and physically prevent toxins and pathogenic bacteria from taking hold before they even get to your mucous barrier.

Many microbes – both beneficial and pathogenic – live in tightly-knit structures called biofilm that adhere to the outer layer of this mucous. Biofilm is an intelligent arrangement that allows microbes not only to survive and grow, but also to communicate and respond en masse to situations. It's when pathogen-dominant biofilm takes hold that we can get into really sticky situations. I'll talk more about biofilms in the next chapter.

Beneficial bacteria can also keep pathogenic microbes at bay by eating all the nutrients available to starve them of food, and by changing the pH and oxygen availability of the immediate environment. Pathogenic bacteria such as E. coli, for example, prefer a neutral or more alkaline environment, while beneficial bacteria usually prefer and are able to create a more acidic environment. (Note that this differs from the pH of your cells and blood, which need to be slightly alkaline.)

Furthermore, bacteria and archaea all emit bacteriocins, some of which seem to be able to kill off pathogens in certain situations. This isn't necessarily a case of "good bacteria" killing "bad bacteria". In fact, E.coli produces bacteriocins that are toxic to E. coli itself. Instead of viewing this as a battleground, we can consider our gut microbiota merely as self-regulating, with the probable aim of maintaining a viable ecosystem where they – and we – can happily reside. Just like a thriving meadow will support a dazzling array of plant, bacteria, fungus and animal life, compared to a less diverse garden lawn, for example.

A communicating community affecting your immunity

As well as being active on the ground, as it were, your gut microbes also communicate directly with systems that assess and respond to substances and conditions, to either allow them or protect you from them. Essentially they have a direct line to your immune system and can trigger or calm inflammation, white blood cell activity and anything else needed to maintain a healthy environment. In the first place, your microbiota are continually sniffing out new arrivals to assess whether or not they belong in that environment. If unsure, they refer the potential toxin to areas in your intestinal wall called Peyer's patches. These are areas of lymphatic tissue containing white blood cells called lymphocytes, which are able to assess the substance. If they are deemed dangerous, a body-wide immune response can be triggered to look out for and disarm any more of these toxins that may be around.

In addition, your gut microbes can signal to your intestinal wall to either tighten or loosen the junctions between its border of cells, and to thicken or thin its protective mucosa. This is one way in which dysbiosis might contribute to leaky gut syndrome, where the intestinal wall has lost its integrity and allows pathogenic substances into the bloodstream. Leaky gut syndrome can lead to the kind of systemic inflammation that has been linked to heart disease and other chronic illnesses.[109]

Inflammation is the starting point for your healing response to pathogens and injury; on the other hand, chronic inflammation provides the backdrop for a long list of illnesses. Either way, inflammation is a critical player in your immune system. Your gut bacteria can influence this directly, for example through triggering cytokines, which are well-studied molecules released throughout your body to regulate inflammation.

What's more, your gut bacteria are able to influence the production of your immune system's white blood cells in your blood, spleen and bone marrow – and so how well your immune system works throughout your body. Laboratory mice grown with germ-free guts were unable to survive a listeria infection – unless their guts were repopulated with bacteria, in which case they were able to produce the white blood cells they needed to recover and survive. In the same study, healthy mice given antibiotics also died from the listeria infection.[110]

Microbiota, inflammation and cancer

There are a number of studies linking gut dysbiosis to colorectal cancer, largely due to the inflammation connection. People with inflammatory bowel disease have an elevated risk of developing colorectal cancer, and a 2009 study demonstrated that bacteria-induced inflammation can be a significant factor here, driving the progression from non-cancerous adenoma to invasive carcinoma.[111]

Further studies have related colorectal cancer to dysbiosis (including higher levels of E. coli)[112] and a reduced diversity of gut bacteria.

There are also strong links between microbial imbalance in the saliva and oral cancer,[113] and bacterial imbalance in the stomach causing inflammatory cascades that increase the risk of stomach cancer.[114]

However, what is perhaps less expected and more interesting is the link that has been established between oral dysbiosis and pancreatic cancer,[115] and also the increasing evidence for a relationship between gut dysbiosis and breast, liver and other cancers.[116] So the inflammatory effects of microbial imbalance are not just local: they can influence tissue health much deeper into the body.

Nutrient production – farming your microbe-rich soil

Your Bifidobacteria are particularly useful for producing some of the *B vitamins* you need for your brain and nervous system, muscles, tissue health and DNA repair, metabolism, reproductive health, detoxification systems and much more. These include thiamine (B1), riboflavin (B2), niacin (B3), folate (B9) and B12. Although studies offer varying data on this, the key bacterial players seem to be B. bifidum and B. infantis. Some lactobacillus bacteria are also involved, in particular L. reuteri and L. acidophilus.

The result is a potentially key boost of B vitamins in the large intestine, where they can easily be absorbed along with water. It would seem, however, that you cannot rely solely on your bacteria for your B vitamins. Perilous levels of vitamin B12 deficiency are still recorded in vegetarians and vegans, for example, where dietary intake is typically low.[117]

Your gut bacteria are also capable of producing *vitamin K2*, a form of vitamin K that seems to be important for bone strength and cardiovascular health. However, the jury seems to be out on how much of this K2 you can absorb, as most of it seems to be produced in the large intestine (colon). As vitamin K is a fat soluble vitamin, it is best absorbed higher up in the small intestine where fats are absorbed.

Amino acids are also synthesized by your gut bacteria, including lysine and threonine. Threonine is needed for your connective tissue, to keep your liver healthy, for aspects of brain function and to help you make antibodies. Lysine is particularly useful for healthy bones and skin and your immune system.

Microbe food: proteins and fibre

Remember that the majority of microbes in your digestive tract are found in your colon (large intestine), which is towards the lower end – which means that they have access to whatever you have eaten *after* it has already passed through your mouth, stomach and small intestine with its various digestive juices and enzymes. So much of what your bacteria gets to work on is what has been either undigested, or digested but not absorbed, further up.

Recent research has highlighted how many amino acids (the building blocks of proteins) make it through to the colon – in addition to the ones your gut bacteria produce themselves. This makes sense, as your microbes need these as much as the human cells in your body to make new parts. Your gut bacteria seem to like the amino acids lysine, arginine, glycine, leucine, valine and isoleucine. The by-products of this feast include a number of fatty acids, including the short chain fatty acids acetate, proprionate and butyrate.[118]

The bacteria in your gut also ferment undigested fibre and carbohydrates from plant foods into the same short chain fatty acids (SCFAs). Incidentally, these particular SCFAs have the capacity to suppress inflammation, and so potentially inflammatory bowel disease and cancer.[119] They also provide your gut wall and bacteria with energy.

If you are lacking non-digestible carbohydrates (i.e. plant fibre) in your diet, then some gut bacteria – feeling hungry – will start to eat mucin sugars from your intestinal mucosal barrier instead. This will bring your gut microbes into closer contact with your gut wall, which means the impact of any imbalance (dysbiosis) will be even greater.[120] And as we shall see below, this thinning of the mucous layer may result in your fat cells being crammed with more fat.

Microbiota and obesity

As the SCFAs (Short Chain Fatty Acids) produced by your microbiota are essentially an additional source of calories – not just for your gut bacteria but for you – it may be tempting to reduce plant fibre as part of a calorie-controlled diet. However, this is a great example of a situation where the environmental impact of a food is more important than its calorie content. Your microbiome affects how much energy you use and how much of it you store.

This is another piece of the puzzle here to add to chapter 3, where I talked about the calorie myth and obesity. Remember that it's not as simple as the old "calories in, calories out" model, where you are overweight if you eat more calories than you use and underweight if you eat less. There are a number of variables involved, including how well you digest and absorb foods, the influence of appetite hormones, leptin resistance, insulin resistance and probably many other metabolic influences we have yet to understand.

Scientists have observed in mice and humans that people who gain weight more easily have more of a certain kind of bacteria in their gut than people who don't: a group of bacteria called Firmicutes. They also have fewer of a quite different group called Bacteroidetes. A human study just a few years ago showed that adults with 20% more Firmicutes and 20% fewer Bacteroidetes extracted an average 150 extra calories from their diet.[121]

A type of bacteria called Akkermansia muciniphilia has also been identified to be more prevalent in lean people than in overweight people. A Belgian scientist called Cani explored this further and found this microbe seems to aid the gut wall to protect itself by helping to maintain a healthy layer of mucus. This mucus seems to help prevent a substance called LPS from getting into the bloodstream. LPS is a coating on certain types of bacteria that is toxic once it's in the bloodstream, and Cani found that obese people had higher levels of LPS in their blood.

It's what happens next that's really interesting. The LPS drives the body to store more energy as fat – not just by increasing fat cells, but by cramming existing fat cells with even more fat. What's more, these cells contained high levels of inflammation-triggering immune cells.

Mice supplemented with Akkermansia lost weight. Their LPS levels lowered, their fat tissue became healthier and their leptin sensitivity improved so they naturally wanted to eat less.

Interestingly, high fat diets lowered Akkermansia levels in mice, while fibre-boosted diets raised levels. So you still don't want to be eating huge quantities of fat, especially with a sedentary lifestyle, but eating more vegetables may help you to burn the fat you eat more efficiently rather than send it to your waistline.[122]

Your microbiome and the rest of the iceberg

This all really is just the tip of a very deep and broad iceberg, and research is ongoing into the microbiome's relationships with Alzheimer's disease, Parkinson's disease, autism, diabetes,[123] cancer, cardiovascular disease, bipolar disorder,[124] liver disease[125] and so much more. The list and the research will be endless, because your microbiome is a deeply entrenched part of you, who you are and how each aspect of you behaves. So let's skip to the practical: how to keep your internal microbial ecosystem in balance.

Action plan

- *Actively try one new recipe this week that uses vegetables that you don't often eat. Aim to do this at least once a month.*

- *Get an organic vegetable box, so you take delivery of seasonal vegetables each week that you may not have thought to buy. Note that most veg box companies give you the option to tell them if you don't like or want any particular vegetables, and some let you add things you definitely want that week. So getting a veg box doesn't have to mean giving up control of your shopping!*

Reflection time

- *How much diversity is there in your current diet? Do you tend to eat the same things over and over again, or is there variation throughout the week/month/year?*

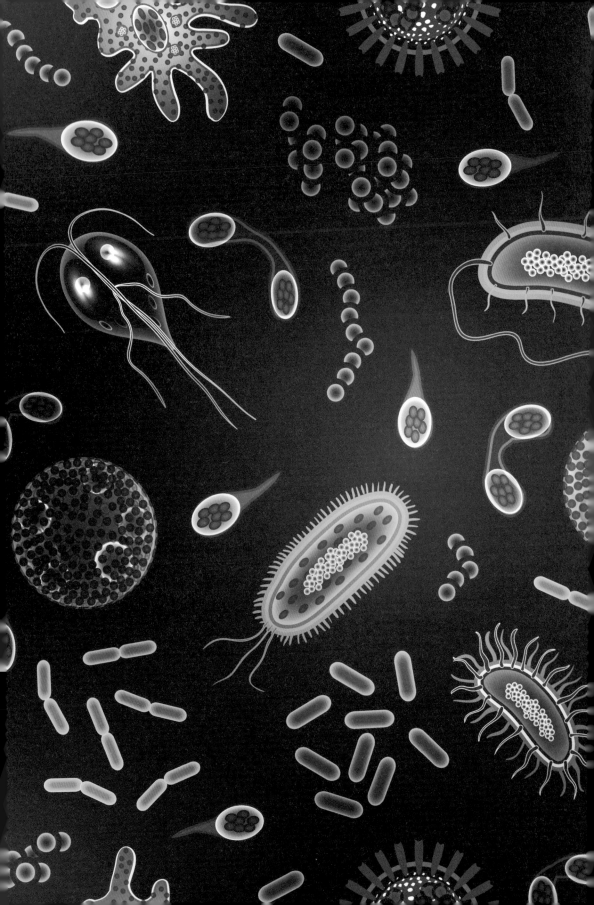

Chapter 12

Nourishing your microbiome

The easy answer: eat foods and take supplements that enrich your gut with beneficial microbes ("probiotic"). Is this the correct answer, though?

Indeed, good quality probiotic foods and supplements can be helpful in all sorts of situations, but before I go on to talk more about those, I just want to point out there is often more to it than just popping a pill. And there may be pitfalls to taking high levels of probiotic supplements or fermented foods too quickly.

Your microbiome is an ecosystem, and just like the earth and ponds and oceans, its bacterial balance depends on and affects the environment. Those bacteria considered to be beneficial tend to thrive in a slightly acidic environment, and will help to create that for themselves. While we often talk about the body needing to be alkaline, your skin and mucous membranes strive for varying degrees of acidity. Beneficial bacteria help with this by excreting acids as part of their normal metabolic processes. Most harmful (pathogenic) bacteria can't survive in such an acidic environment.

So when you add beneficial bacteria to your gut – whether via probiotic supplements or fermented foods (see below) – you also help to create an environment where more beneficial bacteria can thrive, and pathogenic microbes die. At the same time, a sudden influx of beneficial bacteria will crowd out at least some of the pathogenic microbes, starving them of food and resources, and in some cases spraying them with deadly bacteriocins.

When a pathogenic microbe dies, it releases inflammatory toxins that your body needs to be able to deal with. This seems to be the case whether it's been killed by antibiotics, probiotics or changes to your diet that quickly alter your internal environment.

If you introduce too many (antibiotics/probiotics/changes) too quickly, then you essentially create a messy morgue in your gut, which at the very least will be uncomfortable, with gas, bloating, cramps, fatigue. This is often known as "die off."

"Too many" and "too quickly" are relative to each individual, and while some people seem to be able to fare well with a high intake of beneficial bacteria, for others even the tiniest amount can cause extreme die off. In people with very weak and vulnerable guts and immune systems, this can make the problem a whole lot worse. I have seen people with chronic gut and immune problems who, in desperation (or often on recommendation from a health professional), take high dose antibiotics or probiotics, or large amounts of fermented foods, which then plunge them into a much deeper health mess than before.

A serious effect was first noted by two dermatologists called Jarisch and Herxheimer, when treating syphilis with mercury, and later with antibiotics. They noted a non-fatal and yet severe reaction that included fever, chills, low blood pressure, palpitations, hyperventilation, headaches, muscle pain, anxiety and skin lesions. Syphilis is caused by a spiral-shaped bacterium in the same family as the borrelia bacteria that cause Lyme disease, and in fact this "Herxheimer reaction" is also reported among people treating their Lyme disease with high strength antibiotics and/or probiotics.

Similar symptoms have been reported to a greater or lesser degree in the treatment of candidiasis (candida albicans overgrowth) and general dysbiosis, and the following symptoms (and more) have been added to the list:

- Flu-like symptoms
- Acne
- Skin rashes
- Vaginal itching
- Depression
- Lethargy
- Insomnia

It is often difficult to assess whether someone's symptoms are due to toxic overload as a result of microbes being killed off, or whether other options need to be considered. It's very easy to blame the slightest thing on die-off when actually there may be a quite different culprit. At the same time, people are often encouraged to push through their die-off, perhaps without realizing the full implications of what this means. For some it may mean success at the expense of temporary unwellness and discomfort. For others, pushing through may put a strain on their body that is difficult to fully recover from.

There is unfortunately little solid research around this that I can find. However, from my own experience in the field, and the wisdom of some of the amazing teachers I have had from around the world, I am inclined to subscribe to an approach of gentle, patient and sensitive progress. A more gung ho approach will work for some people, but I am less of a risk taker when it comes to health. There are some really amazing high dose supplements available with support for varying aspects of your microbiome, but most people need to work up to these gently – and some, very gradually indeed.

So bearing this in mind, here are a few considerations on an approach to keep your microbiome in balance.

Microbiome nourishing diet

The key aims with diet are to:
- make changes gradually, continually listening to your body to register how it feels
- be hydrating
- help provide an environment that is pH friendly
- be low in irritating, inflammatory components, and rich in anti-inflammatory foods
- provide small amounts of fermented foods to contribute further sources of beneficial bacteria
- provide food for these bacteria
- provide appropriate levels and forms of carbohydrates.

Hydrating the digestive tract

Your body needs water for pretty much everything, from structural integrity to enabling chemical processes. Specifically in your digestive tract, you need adequate levels of water to make digestive fluids and for your digestive enzymes to work. If this isn't in place, you will most likely have a sluggish digestive system and poorly digested food particles that may well be contributing to inflammation.

Human beings lose on average four litres of water a day – largely through breathing (and in my case, talking!), and also through weeing, sweating and other secretions. You don't need to drink four litres of water a day, however, and in fact doing so may put a strain on your kidneys. However, you probably need to ensure that you drink around a couple of litres of fluid, and that your diet is hydrating enough to provide the rest. The exact amounts will vary according to each individual, what they've done that day, the climate and more.

In terms of *what* to drink, there is ongoing debate about whether a cup of tea or coffee will hydrate you as much as a glass of water. The thing to remember here is that tea and coffee are diuretics, which means they make you wee more. Most (if not all) herbal teas are also diuretics.

Fruit juice may seem like a good option, but remember that you may want to avoid too much concentrated fructose for reasons explained in the chapters about sugar and energy. A little fruit juice (not from concentrate) diluted with water may be a good option for those who don't like drinking plain water. Another great option is to add a slice of cucumber to your water. Drinking warm water is often easier than drinking cold water, especially in winter.

Perhaps most helpful in getting people to drink more plain water, however, is getting a decent water filter. The change perhaps as much in quality as in taste seems to make it much easier to go down. What do I mean by "decent"? Well, it really depends on your budget, and I, for one, am grateful for whatever water I can get hold of in any situation. However, remember the gold standard is pure mountain spring water that has been eddying around rocks and stones in a pollution-free environment – so the closer to that you can get, the better!

In terms of hydrating foods, consider how a bowl of porridge or even soup might be a more hydrating start to the day than a slice of toast or many of the dried, extruded breakfast cereals available (even if you add milk). The extrusion process used to make those hardened flakes and dry puffs of cereal exposes the grains to super high heat and pressure that may damage their proteins as well as making them just really dry.

A pH friendly environment

When it comes to pH and the human body, this is where people tend to get confused. Aspects of the nutrition world are so fixed on "alkalising", and yet the digestive tract needs to be acidic. And can we really alkalise through diet anyway?

I prefer to speak of pH balancing, rather than alkalising, for this very reason. The levels of pH in different parts of your body are really crucial to your health, and to staying alive. Just as it is necessary to be hydrated for the fundamental biochemistry in your body to happen, you also need the various pH readings to be just so. It's so important that your body has a number of mechanisms to control this. But first, what is pH?

The pH of a substance refers to the amount of hydrogen ions (H^+) it contains. On the pH chart, anything with a number less than 7 is acidic, and anything higher is alkaline. Substances with a pH of 7 are considered to be neutral. If something has a pH of 6, this means it has 10 times more hydrogen ions than a substance with a pH of 7; something with a pH of 5 has 10 times more H^+ than something with a pH of 6 etc. And going the other way, a substance with a pH of 8 has 10 times fewer H^+ than a neutral substance.

Here are the pH ranges of various parts of your body:
- Cells: 7.2-7.4 (slightly alkaline)
- Blood: 7.34-7.43 (slightly alkaline)
- Saliva: 6.5-7.5 (between slightly alkaline and slightly acidic)
- Stomach: 1.5-6.5 (between slightly and very acidic)
- Small intestine: 7-8.5 (between neutral and alkaline)
- Large intestine: 4-7 (between neutral and acidic)
- Skin: 4-4.5 (acidic)
- Urine: 4.6-8 (between acidic and slightly alkaline)

You'll notice that sometimes the range is very narrow – for example your blood and cells, both of which absolutely need to be slightly alkaline all the time. At other times the range is wider – for example the stomach will reach its greatest levels of acidity when it has proteins to digest.

As these ranges are so crucial to wellbeing, and being alive, your body has several mechanisms for regulating it all. Your blood uses acid buffering systems to mop up the acid, preventing it from affecting pH.

Natural pH balancing systems

One of these involves attaching (acidic) hydrogen ions to (alkaline) carbonate ions to form carbonic acid, and then converting that to carbon dioxide and water to be breathed out. Equally, carbonic acid can be converted back to hydrogen ions (for example, when the stomach needs acid to digest proteins) and carbonate ions (for the pancreas to then make alkalising fluids).

The blood can also use protein to help buffer (reduce) a little of its acidity, and cellular fluid can use phosphates as an acid buffer.

Finally, a number of minerals, such as potassium, magnesium, calcium and zinc, are alkaline and can be used to buffer acidity. Plus there are other substances in your diet that can have an alkalising effect. Citrates, for example, are converted to alkalising bicarbonate in the liver.

Diet, urine pH and health

You can assess your saliva or urine pH with testing strips, but this may not fully represent what is going on with the pH of the rest of your body. Your urinary pH may, however, indicate what you are excreting through your urine, give clues to your kidney health, and warn of ketoacidosis in diabetics. It may also signify a degree of insulin resistance and therefore metabolic syndrome, i.e. increased risk of heart disease and diabetes.[126]

There is certainly a correlation between diet and urine pH, as demonstrated by a large-scale study of over 20,000 men and women in Norfolk in the 90s.[127] The study showed that eating foods that contain more carbonate salts, magnesium and potassium (i.e. vegetables and fruit) led to more alkaline urine than diets higher in hydrogen ions (protein-rich meat and cereals). The study also demonstrated that men seem to be able to maintain a more alkaline urine reading with slightly higher levels of meat than women, and that a younger cohort with lower BMIs generally had more alkaline urine. This confirms that while diet will have an impact on urine pH, it's not as straightforward as at first glance.

Are men more efficient at excreting hydrogen ions? Are there aspects of male biochemistry that require more acidity? I would pose the same questions for younger adults with lower BMIs. And does more alkaline urine even equate to better health?

Indeed there are studies that demonstrate a relationship between bone density and diet that point to pH being a factor. Pre and post menopausal women with a more acidic diet have poorer bone strength.[128, 129] This is interesting in view of the fact that many of your acid buffering substances are the same minerals you need to make bone tissue. If you are deficient in any of them, then you use your skeleton as a mineral pool to draw from. We tend to think of bones and teeth as solid, fixed structures, but actually you continually break them down and build them up again. In the process, you can divert some of the minerals to processes deemed more important, like pH balance. This is why osteoporosis is often a pH issue.

Acidity in the digestive tract

So how does all this help the acidity of your digestive tract? Well, the aim is not to have exclusively alkalising ions in your body, but instead to be able to keep alkaline and acid ions in an appropriate balance. The carbonic acid system is able to produce both at the same time, so that it can use carbonate ions for your blood, pancreatic fluids and elsewhere, and hydrogen ions for your stomach, saliva, skin and so on. Your body will be able to do all of this more efficiently if it has sufficient access to alkalising ions, and seems to struggle on a number of levels if it doesn't. So if you feel you have low stomach acid, that doesn't mean you need to avoid alkalising foods.

Equally, there is no need – and in fact it may be dangerous – to focus just on alkalising foods. The macrobiotic diet brought over from Japan with its awareness of balancing acid and alkaline emphasised avoiding extremes. So a purely meat-based diet would usually put too much strain on pH balancing and protein-metabolising systems, while a long term diet of just lettuce and celery might be just as damaging for their lack of proteins. This may seem obvious, but I have witnessed people doing both: the first in fear of carbohydrates, and the latter in fear of acid-forming proteins. Another example of how fear-based diets will get you nowhere.

So the simplest approach here would be to ensure you have contained amounts of protein and carbohydrates in your diet, together with plenty of alkali-rich vegetables. If you are male, you may do well on slightly higher levels of protein, and slightly lower levels of carbohydrate. Helpful ratios will vary from person to person, but most people seem to have a surprisingly low vegetable intake.

Many people I interview consider eating meals that are one third vegetables (not counting potatoes) to be a veg-rich diet, where for me I'd sometimes even double that – gradually of course!

Fruit – acidic or alkalising?

Fruit is generally considered to be alkalising. My view (naturally!) is that it depends on a number of factors.

Oranges and lemons may be rich in alkalising minerals and citrates, but their juice is highly acidic. There is an argument that their ash is alkaline, and so that's the effect they will have on your body once digested, but that argument makes little sense to me – we don't just eat the ash, and burning foods does not precisely simulate what happens when we digest them. I would also suggest that the overall effect of eating an orange in the middle of a north European winter will be quite different to doing the same in a hot desert. Unfortunately the immense Norfolk study mentioned above didn't separate fruit and vegetables out when analysing everyone's diet – in fact most research lumps them in together, so it's difficult to get a clear picture of their differences.

One study looking at risk factors for kidney stone formation found that orange juice was helpful in reducing risk, probably due to its potassium citrate content (providing both an alkalising mineral, and a citrate ion that can be converted in the liver to alkalising bicarbonate).[130] The authors also noted mixed results with citrate-rich lemon and cranberry juices in other studies, possibly due to the citrates being accompanied by a proton, which would negate the amount of bicarbonate produced. So it seems that the varying alkalising and acidic components of fruit may work individually to both benefit and scupper pH balance. Someone with irritable bowel syndrome, however, might find that orange juice produces too much inflammation in the gut to be helpful.[131]

As is often the case, when your fruit was picked and how it has been stored may also be important. Blackberries, for example, get a little more acidic as they start to ripen, and then a little less acidic as they continue to ripen.[132] The South American cherimoya fruit, when studied, became more acidic the longer it was stored, unless it was kept at 1° C.[133]

Additional influences to pH

Your body's buffering systems rely upon more than the acid/alkaline content of your diet. Again, hydration will be an important factor, alongside communication systems that trigger certain activities in your body. Alkalising minerals will be depleted by stress, overuse of diuretics and stimulants, and other factors. The competence of your kidneys and lungs play their part in all this, as well as other factors that determine mineral placement, such as your thyroid activity. So some or all of this may need attention too. The previous chapter on adrenal support and the information through this book on anti-inflammatory nutrition may offer a helpful degree of support.

Finally, remember that your gut bacteria take a certain amount of responsibility for maintaining their own environmental pH. The more beneficial bacteria you have, the more likely your gut will be adequately acidic; the more pathogenic microbes, the more alkaline it will be. So introducing small amounts of fermented foods to help gently influence this balance not only seems sensible, but is also a feature of traditional diets all over the world.

The sugar wheel

One of the stimulants that may be depleting your alkalising minerals is sugar. So there's another argument for focusing more on vegetables than fruit in a quest to maintain pH balance.

In addition, if you're having regular sugar cravings, be it for fruit or biscuits, this could be a clue that your microbiome needs support. Could it be that your microbiome is out of balance, and the pathogens are screaming out for more food? And then the more you feed them, the more their colonies grow, and the more they will be demanding you feed them? If this is the case, then the only real way to address those sugar cravings is to rebalance your gut bacteria.

The classic anti-candida diet takes out all sugars: refined sugars in sweets, pastries, chocolate, biscuits and cakes; honey, molasses, rice syrup and other less refined sugars; fruit; refined grains in white bread, white rice etc. This is on the basis that candida uses sugar to survive and grow.[134]

It can be helpful to at least reduce sugars to small amounts of raw honey or molasses, but for real long-lasting change, you need to work on the environment, including hydration and pH balance. If you're doing this, then such an extreme approach to "starving the candida" may not be necessary.

Fermented foods

Fermented or cultured foods and drinks have undergone a natural process that fosters a colony of varying species of bacteria and other microbes that are generally beneficial to your gut and overall health. You may have come across, or even regularly enjoy, some if not many of these:

- yoghurt (cultured milk)
- buttermilk (cultured milk)
- cheese (cultured milk)
- kefir (cultured milk or water)
- sourdough bread (cultured grains)
- beer (cultured grains)
- sauerkraut (cultured vegetables)
- kim chi (cultured vegetables)
- apple cider vinegar – with the "mother", i.e. unfiltered (cultured fruit)
- balsamic vinegar – unfiltered (cultured fruit)
- wine (yeast cultured fruit)
- soya sauce and tamari, the wheat-free option (cultured soya)
- tempeh (cultured soya)
- fermented tofu (cultured soya – note that most tofu is not fermented)
- miso (cultured soya, sometimes with grains)
- kombucha (cultured green tea)

This list is by no means exhaustive, but offers a great variety of options for enriching your diet. Many of these are as easy to make as they are to buy. They are all acidic in nature, as the microbes need an acidic medium to grow on. The "mother" referred to in apple cider vinegar is the culture – other refined vinegars will have had this component filtered out.

Note that some of these, for example wine, beer, kombucha and kefir, will contain added sugar to feed the community of microbes – how much sugar is left when you drink it will depend on how much of it has been eaten by the bugs. And there will be a resultant alcohol content that may range from negligible (less than 0.1% in kefir for example) to high (about 12.5% in wine).

When to avoid fermented foods

It is often suggested that people with candida overgrowths should avoid fermented foods and yeasts in case it contributes to the yeast overgrowth. More recent approaches encourage the introduction of small amounts of beneficial yeasts and bacteria via fermented foods and drinks to help outweigh pathogenic microbes.

Some people may find they are intolerant to fermented foods as a result of an inability to break down histamines. Histamine is one of the substances released by your immune system in response to allergens – which is why people with hay fever and other allergies may choose to take anti-histamines to counter this response. Histamines trigger inflammation, and can make your eyes and nose run, your skin itch and welt, and your lungs struggle to breathe.

Certain foods also contain histamines, including fermented food and drinks. If you lack the enzymes to break them down, then you may experience unpleasant symptoms including headaches, diarrhea, asthma, low blood pressure, palpitations, itchy skin or anus, flushing, runny nose, streaming eyes and more.[135]

Other foods on the high histamine list are processed meats, chocolate, vanilla, spices, eggs, spinach, aubergines and tomatoes.

You can help your production of one of your anti-histamine enzymes, DAO, through topping up vitamins C and B6 to your diet,[136, 137] as well as ensuring adequate soluble fibre.[138] On the other hand, the long chain fatty acids found in most fats and oils help more histamine to be released during digestion,[139] and so should probably be reduced – note that coconut oil, as a predominantly medium chain fatty acid, may be useful here.

Supplements: probiotics

The most ubiquitous supplements for rebalancing your microbiome are probiotics. Probiotics are described as beneficial gut bacteria that are able to survive the extreme conditions of your stomach and find their way to the bulk of your microbiota in your intestines. Their quality has improved vastly in recent years, with options for freeze-dried powders with a long shelf life, and controlled liquid cultures. In the past, supplements have focused largely on the well known L. acidophilus, while now you can find probiotics containing a broader range of 4-6 or sometimes over a dozen different species.

I prefer to use lower doses of multiple species, but I have also seen people benefit from high doses of just two or three species. A supplement that feels nourishing and helpful in some instances may feel inadequate or too strong at other times. Your microbiome is a very intimate and personal thing, and so your choice of probiotics needs to reflect that.

My best advice is:
- choose supplements with no unnecessary additives
- start with low doses and build up gradually
- be prepared to try a few before you find one that suits you right now.

Supplements: prebiotics

Prebiotics contain a form of soluble fibre that is said to feed your beneficial bacteria. The most common is inulin, which is naturally found in chicory and Jerusalem artichokes – otherwise known as "fartichokes". When your gut microbes ferment inulin, they produce gases relatively quickly. Some people are particularly sensitive to this, and may need to avoid inulin-rich foods and supplements.

Inulin contains fructooligosaccharides (FOS), which have been shown to increase levels of Bifidobacterium and Lactobacillus in the gut,[140] in one study up to ten times the colon's previous amount.[141] Some companies prefer to use galacto-oligosaccharides (GOS), which are similar to a substance found in breast milk. More research is currently needed to confirm that such substances feed only the beneficial bacteria, but it's certainly an aspect of gut health worth exploring.

Supplements: Saccharomyces boulardii

S. boulardii is a yeast rather than a bacteria, and you'll see it in some supplements either on its own or together with other probiotics – and also in kombucha tea. It was discovered in the 1920s in a fermented tea in Indo-China, where those drinking it seemed to be protected from cholera.

A review of 27 trials involving over 5000 people found S. boulardii to be strongly effective for the prevention and treatment of several different kinds of diarrhea, including antibiotic induced and travellers' diarrhea. In addition it showed promise for treating IBS, Crohn's disease, giardiasis, HIV-related diarrhea, acute adult diarrhea and for preventing the recurrence of C. difficile disease.

What's most impressive is how it does this. The author identified multiple ways in which S. boulardii protects the gut, including behaving as an antidote to E. coli endotoxins, C. difficile toxins A and B and cholera, as well as having general antimicrobial action. In addition it helps to preserve the tight junctions of the intestinal wall (and so helps prevent leaky gut syndrome), increases short chain fatty acids, increases enzyme activity to complete the breakdown of sugars and carbohydrates, and reduces inflammation.[142]

Supplements: serrapeptase and lactoferrin

Certain enzymes that break down proteins (proteases) may also be useful. Serrapeptase, for example, is the enzyme that silkworms produce in order to break down their cocoon – it only dissolves non-living tissue, so it is able to destroy the raw silk cocoon without harming the newly emerging moth. Serrapeptase can now be produced artificially, without killing silkworms, and has been found to be incredibly anti-inflammatory, as well as useful in dissolving blood clots and even arterial plaque due to its ability to break down a protein called fibrin.[143]

Nattokinase is a similar enzyme produced by fermenting soya beans. Its particular superpower is also breaking down fibrin, the protein involved in blood clotting, and so it too has been suggested for use in cardiovascular disease.[144]

In more recent years, interest has turned to their potential role, alongside that of other proteases, in dissolving the biofilm that many microbes live in.[145] Biofilm is a fibrin-rich matrix produced by the microbes themselves, that makes for a much stronger colony of microbes that can stick to the mucous layer on the intestinal wall – as well as in the mouth and in other areas of microbial activity. Certain proteases have been found to break down this matrix, while serrapeptase seems to be effective in preventing food-borne Listeria bacteria from even forming biofilms in the first place.[146]

Another substance called lactoferrin has also been shown to block biofilm development, even at low levels. The study in question looked at lactoferrin's effect on biofilm production by a specific pathogen called Pseudomonas aeruginosa, which is associated with hospital acquired infections and hot tub rash. Lactoferrin is found in most bodily secretions, including saliva, snot, sweat and tears. It is most abundant in breast milk, especially colostrum (the first milk expressed), and you can buy supplements made from cow's milk. Its main activity is to bind iron in the gut, which prevents bacteria from using it and instead makes it easier for you to absorb it. As it binds to iron, it stimulates twitching, which causes bacteria to move across surfaces rather than cluster together and form biofilms on them.[147]

Lactoferrin has other hidden talents too. It seems to be able to stimulate the intestinal wall to grow healthy new tissue, so that it can absorb more nutrients, while inhibiting the growth of cancerous tissue.[148] It also forms part of white blood cells called neutrophils that are involved in your normal anti-inflammatory response – so a high lactoferrin level in a stool test may indicate inflammation in the intestines. Lactoferrin levels in faeces are therefore often used to help diagnose colitis and Crohn's disease.

Although proteases and lactoferrin have been found to be effective at reducing pathogenic biofilms, there are still questions around how to use them without destroying colonies of beneficial microbes that also form biofilm in your digestive tract.

More on your biofilm

Biofilm is everywhere, inside and outside of us: in water and soil, on plants and solid objects, in insects, animals and humans. There is now growing research about biofilm in the mouth and throughout the digestive tract, and indeed the body, and their association with ulcerative colitis, pneumonia, vaginosis, urinary tract infections, Lyme disease and more.

Microbes that produce biofilm are a little bit like Spiderman. Except that the web they shoot out connects them to other "spidermen" to form a goo of supermicrobes. When this happens on a grand scale, a formidable colony of microbes is formed that can adhere to the mucous barrier throughout your digestive tract. This biofilm matrix not only connects them, but also *switches their state*, so that they are even stronger than when swimming around on their own.

Not all microbes form biofilms, but many do, even the beneficial ones, and they are an incredibly clever and resilient way to form a close-knit, self-protective community that can communicate with each other more readily.

Biofilms usually house multiple species of microbes, but single-species colonies have been found on medical implants, tubes and stents, leading to stubborn infections. Biofilms, by their design, are highly resistant to both antibiotics and your body's usual antimicrobial defense systems, including macrophages, your toxin-munching cells.

Biofilm in your digestive tract

There's nothing wrong with having biofilm growing in your digestive tract – as long as it contains an appropriate and diverse balance of microbes.

Dental plaque is one such biofilm. In a healthy mouth, plaque provides a home for a balance of microbes that help to maintain that flourishing state. However, oral biofilms containing an overgrowth of pathogenic microbes are extensively involved in tooth decay, gum disease and oral cancer.

A sugary diet may help to increase pathogenic plaque, but perhaps more due to the excessive acidity sugar creates than to the sugar actually feeding the microbes.[149] This degree of acidity is favoured by bacteria such as mutans streptococci, which not only causes tooth decay, but also secretes further acids to maintain the pH it loves. The acids then attack the tooth enamel, and may be as much of a problem as the bacteria itself. This is why dentists often recommend using mints or gum sweetened with xylitol after a meal, which, together with the saliva flow this stimulates, brings the pH back to a more mildly acidic range, which is healthier for your mouth and teeth.

Generally your oesaphagus, stomach and small intestine have very low amounts of microbes, so any biofilm there is associated mainly with disease. For example, ulcers are caused by H. pylori biofilm[150] in the stomach, and leaky gut syndrome and malabsorption may be caused by pathogenic biofilm in the small intestine. This is where biofilm prevention such as serrapeptase supplementation may be of most use.

The mucus in your large intestine is much thicker, and allows for greater biofilm colonisation by the huge amounts of both beneficial and pathogenic microbes found there. Pathogen-dominant biofilm has been found to completely coat the mucous lining of the large intestine in ulcerative colitis.

One group of scientists found it useful to encourage biofilm production in the large intestine so that beneficial bacteria can take hold there and not be flushed so easily away. Here, hydrogen sulphide (e.g. from garlic) was used to promote biofilm production in the colon, so that certain colitis symptoms might be improved.[151] Conversely, hydrogen sulphide has also been shown to be a possible causative factor for colitis,[152] and is notably produced by pathogenic bacteria such as Pseudomonas, E.coli and salmonella.

Confused? Essentially, it seems that biofilm is a fantastic thing when it is strengthening colonies of beneficial bacteria, but a problem when pathogenic microbes dominate using the same skill and intelligence. So how can you influence which of your gut bugs get to use their spiderman powers?

Essentially, I keep coming back to the principle that to try and manipulate the delicate and intricate balance of over 10,000 different types of living microbes is a difficult task. It is far easier to work on the environment these microbes inhabit, help to re-seed with beneficial bacteria where you can, and then trust your internal ecosystem to find its own balance.

The lining of your digestive tract is described as a mucous membrane, and is formed of a layer of protective epithelial cells covering a sheet of connective tissue. In the next chapter, we'll look at how to nourish your epithelial and connective tissue, not just for gut health, but also to benefit your joints, bones and indeed whole body.

Recipes

- **Sauerkraut (and variations)** – p.271
  So simple and tasty, a spoonful of raw sauerkraut daily will help replenish the friendly bugs in your gut.

- **Apple cider vinaigrette** – p.273
  Apple cider vinegar "with mother" is the unfiltered version: the "mother" is the ferment of magical microbes

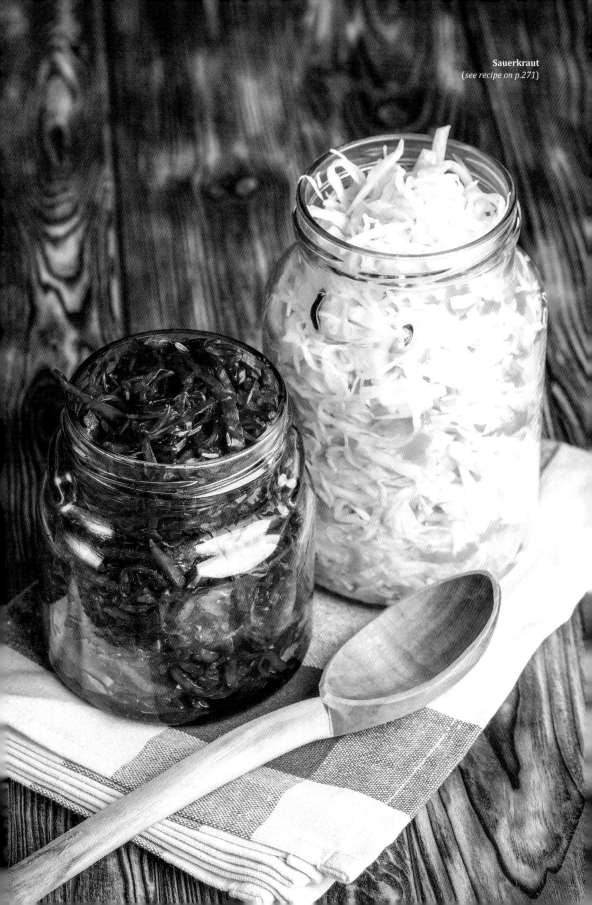

Sauerkraut
(*see recipe on p.271*)

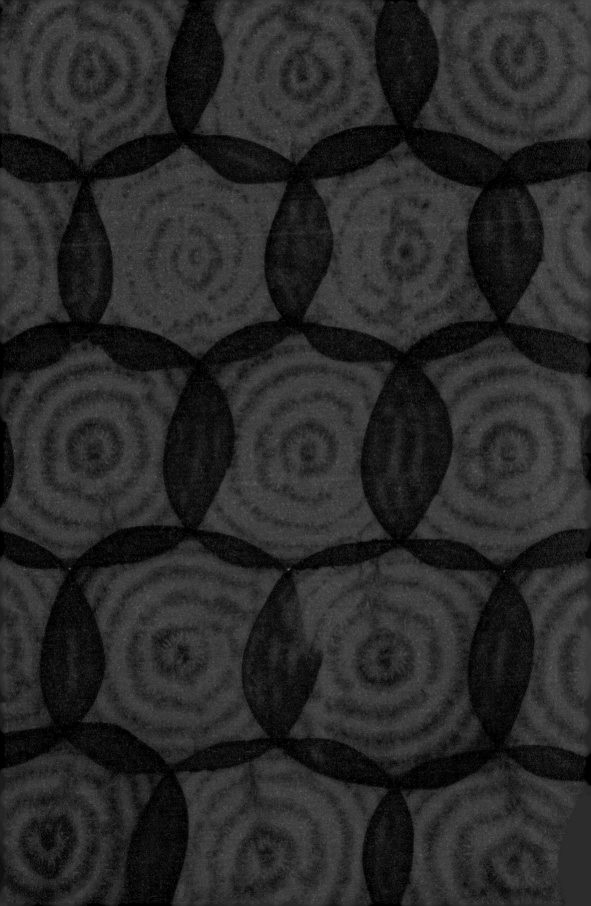

Chapter 13

Tissue protection and repair
for your gut, joints, skin, bones and everywhere

People often talk about "healing your gut", and one of the aspects of keeping your digestive tract in good health involves nurturing the tissue that it is made up of.

Your body is predominantly made up of different kinds of tissue: muscle tissue, nerve tissue, epithelial tissue and connective tissue. This chapter contains a particular focus on the health of your epithelial and connective tissue – but I'll also include some key support for nerve and muscle tissue.

All tissue is made of cells that are ultimately formed of proteins, fats and sugars – and predominantly water. Those cells house your DNA (the set of patterns your body is made from), your mitochondria (energy factories) and many other structures involved in responding to hormones, transporting and using nutrients, waste and other substances, and more.

Muscle tissue is what makes up the muscles you use to move when walking, dancing, blinking, breathing or poking your tongue out. Your heart is a large muscle that pumps blood around your body, while your blood vessels have a thin muscular layer which controls how narrow or dilated they are, and so affect blood pressure and circulation. The walls of your digestive tract also contain muscles that help to squeeze and stretch, easing foodstuff gradually downwards.

Most bodybuilders need post-workout protein to help build up their muscle mass. That's not the only nutrient your muscles need to be effective, however. To contract and relax effectively, your muscle cells need ongoing access to magnesium, potassium and calcium, among other nutrients. To communicate effectively with your brain and nerves, and recover well after exercise, your muscles need to have additional nutrients, such as B12 (found in animal products), phosphatidyl choline and phosphatidyl serine (in egg yolks, liver and some pulses).

Nerve tissue makes up your brain and nerve cells. They need a similar range of nutrients to muscle cells, plus extra essential fatty acids. Many nerve cells (neurons) are coated in an omega 3 fatty acid rich sheath (called the myelin sheath). Your brain cells also have an increased demand for EPA and DHA, the omega 3 fatty acids found in fish oil. For electrical signals to flow through your nervous system, your neurons need access to appropriate quantities of sodium, potassium and calcium.

Epithelial tissue is what makes up the outer coating of the skin and digestive tract, as well as lining other organs. It allows for specific modifications, such as goblet cells that secrete mucous, sweat glands on your skin and the finger-like microvilli in your small intestine that absorb nutrients.

In your intestinal wall, epithelial cells are held together by tight junctions to form a strict border control – except in the case of leaky gut syndrome, where these junctions lose their integrity.

A layer of epithelial tissue lining a thicker sheet of connective tissue is sometimes referred to as mucous membrane. There are mucous membranes lining and protecting your digestive tract, your sinuses and wherever you have inlets, crevices and tunnels.

Connective tissue makes up everything else: the flesh between and surrounding areas of epithelial and muscle tissue, your bone tissue, the cartilage, tendons and fluids that surround your joints, and even blood. It was named such as it was originally thought just to connect things to each other, but much more has been learnt about this fascinating tissue in recent years.

You may also have heard of fascia, which is essentially a network of connective tissue running through your whole body, surrounding and infusing your muscles and organs. It links your ankle to your hip to your armpit, your feet to your groin to your neck. It is just as involved in your structural alignment and stability, and your body's freedom of movement, as your muscles and nerves. In fact, in some cases of muscle tightness, it may be the fascia that is tense rather than the muscle itself.[153]

Fascia contains a high number of nerve receptors that respond in different ways to different kinds of pressure, for example as pain, as relief from pain, by thickening and stiffening or by relaxing and loosening.[154] Some bodywork therapists have trained to work with myofascial techniques that seek to release the fascia surrounding and infusing muscles.

Connective tissue plays additional roles in hydration, nutrient delivery and removal of unwanted substances. It is essentially a nurturing, elastic, supportive, shock absorbing web. It is useful on so many levels to make sure it's in great shape, so there's a section below on how to do that.

Keeping your epithelial tissue healthy

For your gut to be healthy and absorb the nutrients you need, the epithelial tissue there needs to be in top condition. You also have epithelial tissue lining your lungs, sinuses, vagina (if you have one!), bladder, kidneys, liver, brain, heart, blood vessels and more.

We have already looked at how your microbial balance affects the health and activity of your mucous membrane, and vice versa, so support there is crucial, as described in the previous chapter. Fermented foods and/or probiotic supplements may be useful in appropriate amounts.

In addition, there are specific nutrients that your epithelial tissue needs to regenerate itself, in addition to the base ingredients of proteins, fats, carbohydrates and water:

Vitamin A helps epithelial cells to differentiate, which basically means to develop in a specific way to do a specific job. Where vitamin A is deficient, epithelial tissue might, for example, become mucus-secreting where it needs to be protein secreting, or vice versa. In some cases, cells might go even further astray and become carcinogenic.[155]

Food sources of vitamin A (retinol) include liver and fish. Beta-carotene can be converted into vitamin A, and so is described as pro-vitamin A, and is found in carrots, sweet potatoes, spinach and kale.

Vitamin B12 is required alongside folic acid to keep the DNA of epithelial, and all tissue, stable.[156] In fact, one study of the epithelial tissue in the mouth suggested that vitamin B12 deficiency may alter the cells in a pre-cancerous way, and noted a case where B12 supplementation returned a woman's oral tissue to a healthy state.[157]

Meat, fish, eggs and dairy are the main viable sources of vitamin B12, and even then, absorption may be difficult. Vegan diets are particularly low in B12,[158] and it is difficult to make up the shortfall with diet alone.[159]

Vitamin D protects your epithelial tissue against infection and inflammation, and helps to protect the mucus barrier in your digestive tract.[160] Vitamin D deficiency therefore has attracted interest in the study of conditions such as asthma[161] and colitis (inflammation and ulceration in the large intestine), and supplementation has been shown to reduce colitis symptoms and the risk of colon cancer.[162]

The absolute best source of vitamin D is sunshine. A cholesterol-based substance in your skin converts the UVB rays to vitamin D. Note that if the sun is less than 50 degrees above the horizon, the UVB rays won't reach you – which is for about seven months of the year in Northern Europe. However, from spring, we start to have a short window around noon, and as we move into summer, a longer window of several hours, where vitamin D production is possible.

Standard advice these days is to spend around 20 minutes in the sunshine during this time, with as much bare skin as possible, and no sun cream – and to cover up as soon as you start to go pink. Note that cloud cover, rain, pollution, clothing, glass and, of course, sun tan lotions and sun blocks, all interfere with the necessary UVB rays getting to your skin. People with darker skin will usually need longer than 20 minutes, as skin pigments also slow down vitamin D production and absorption. The other option is to supplement, and/or to eat substantial quantities of oily fish. Other sources of vitamin D (mushrooms, eggs etc.) are too low to really be useful.

Vitamin E and selenium are both antioxidants, and have been shown to protect epithelial tissue in the intestinal wall from heat stress, preventing signs of leaky gut.[163] They are also needed to create both pro-inflammatory and anti-inflammatory cytokines, and as such, deficiency will also affect wound healing and your gut's ability to calm inflammation.

Avocados are a great source of vitamin E, as are sunflower seeds, almonds and green leafy vegetables.

Selenium is a vital to the health of your mucous membranes, the epithelial tissue lining your gut, airways, lungs and more. Selenium-deficient lung epithelial tissue grown in a laboratory was more mucus producing than the same kind of lung tissue grown with selenium, and also was less able to fend off the flu virus.[164]

Research into selenium and cancer suggests that your epithelial tissue is very sensitive to this mineral, with many studies showing selenium to be beneficial, while others show the opposite. We also know that excessive levels of selenium supplementation (i.e. higher than 400mcg daily in adults) may lead to adverse epithelial tissue symptoms, such as rashes and skin lesions and diarrhea, in addition to hair and nail brittleness and loss and nervous system abnormalities. High levels of selenium toxicity can lead to more acute gastrointestinal and respiratory conditions, among other severe symptoms.[165]

So I would suggest keeping your selenium-rich food intake adequate, with regular portions of fish, or even just a brazil nut or two a day, rather than dosing up on high strength supplements.

Zinc is known for its anti-inflammatory and antioxidant activity, and zinc deficiency can be a key factor in leaky gut syndrome – while zinc supplementation has been shown to heal your gut wall tissue[166] and tighten junctions between the epithelial cells.[167] In fact, zinc is one of the first minerals I think of when addressing gut, lung, skin and even hair health – i.e. issues connected with the epithelial and connective tissues.

Pumpkin seeds are my favourite source of zinc, and if you soak them overnight in water, the zinc becomes more available. Nuts, seeds, lentils, chickpeas, beef and lamb all contain good levels of zinc.

Iodine is found in the tissue lining your digestive tract, and so is considered to have a role in maintaining the health of mucous membranes. Indeed, healthy gastric mucosa seems to have higher concentrations of iodine than that of people with chronic gastritis.[168]

Indirectly, it governs the health of your tissue and body generally by providing (together with the amino acid tyrosine and co-factors such as selenium) raw ingredients for your thyroid hormones. Your thyroid governs metabolism, which is essentially all the chemical reactions that happen in your body. It influences temperature, pH and heartbeat, and even how quickly or slowly food passes through your digestive tract. A sluggish bowel may improve with thyroid support.

The best source of iodine is kelp, or kombu, a form of seaweed. You can buy this in supplement form, or buy dried sheets of kombu. A classic way to use dried kombu is to add a strip to a soup or casserole at the start of cooking, and then remove it before you serve it up – many of its nutrients will now be enriching the sauce, so you don't need to actually eat the seaweed.

Vitamin C is necessary for the production of the collagen in connective tissue, and also has a protective effect on all your bodily tissues, including your epithelial cells. This is partly due to its antioxidant activity, protecting cells from damage, and additionally because it helps you to make more glutathione. Glutathione has crucial roles in transporting and using amino acids, DNA synthesis and repair, cell death (apoptosis), detoxification and tissue protection.

Fresh, raw fruit, vegetables and herbs are good sources of vitamin C.

Flax seed lignans have been found to reduce the colitis symptoms of erosion, ulceration, crypt abscesses and oedema, as well as to restore gut permeability where the gut barrier has been damaged.[169] Other studies have found that flax seeds irritate acute colitis, however.[170] In my experience, lignan-rich flaxseed tea (or linseed tea) is usually helpful for most kinds of digestive upset and irritability, including colitis. (You can find out how to make Linseed tea on page 293, in the Recipes section.)

Berberine is a strong yellow pigment found in the stems, bark and root of herbs such as goldenseal, as well as barberries, a jewel-like berry used in Iranian cooking. It has been well studied for its ability to heal damage to the intestinal mucosa barrier,[171] and has long been used as a herbal remedy for a number of gastrointestinal complaints, including diarrhoea.

Glutamine is an amino acid (more on these in the next chapter) with a specific role in gut mucosa health, and so you may have come across glutamine supplements for gut healing. It does indeed help keep your intestinal barrier functioning during injury and infection, so that you can continue to absorb the nutrients you need. Glutamine has also been shown to stimulate the growth and development of the intestinal mucosa and help the epithelial cells in your intestinal wall stay healthy.[172]

Glutamine is found in all animal protein sources (meat, fish, eggs and dairy) as well as pulses, nuts, seeds, grains and some vegetables – in particular cabbage. Bone broths are a great source of glutamine, and so are recommended to help gut healing in protocols such as the GAPS diet (Gut And Psychology Syndrome).[173]

The role magnesium and other anti-inflammatories play will be discussed more in chapter 17. For now I'd just like to highlight that calming and soothing inflammation in the gut is crucial to the health of the epithelial tissue there

Keeping your connective tissue in shape

Your connective tissue is made up of a matrix in which various types of cells may reside (e.g. cartilage cells, bone cells, red blood cells, white blood cells etc.). This matrix is gel-like: a more liquid gel in your blood, and a much firmer gel in your bones. It has as its base material something called ground substance, which is made up largely of water and hyaluronic acid, as well as the protein fibres collagen (to hold everything together) and elastin (to make it more flexible).

Vitamin C is necessary for the production of the collagen in connective tissue. This is why vitamin C has been such a strong area of focus for Ehlers-Danlos Syndrome (EDS),[174] a connective tissue disorder where the skin and tissue may be so stretchy that the joints may become hypermobile. With EDS skin is easily bruised and it can take a long time for wounds to heal. Vitamin C is also recommended to promote wound healing[175] in general, after accidents and surgery, for example.

Minerals are also vital ingredients in making collagen, including zinc, magnesium, boron, copper and iron, and then silicon to strengthen the crosslinks in its structure. Zinc deficiency has been shown to have a detrimental effect on collagen production. Adding magnesium to collagen gels has been shown to soften connective tissue, and help prevent calcification[176] where tissue has been hardened or made more brittle due to calcium deposits. In addition, *boron* deficiency has been noted in the synovial fluid and the heads of some bones of arthritis sufferers, and boron supplementation found to reduce pain.[177]

Certain proteins are fundamental to collagen production, in particular the amino acids glycine, proline, hydroxyproline and arginine. These specific amino acids are released from bone tissue when making bone broths, alongside the minerals connective tissue are rich in, which is another of the reasons why these broths have become so popular in recent years. They give you easy access to the fundamental ingredients you need to make your own collagen, for healthy bone, joint and connective tissue throughout your body. You can also buy gelatin powder or collagen powder for making sweet and savoury jellies as well as adding to hot and cold drinks and broths.

One study of athletes given a gelatin and vitamin C rich drink suggested that their collagen producing ability improved compared to those given a placebo. The optimum time for taking the drink seemed to be an hour before exercise, and then it took only six minutes of rope skipping to stimulate new collagen production. Those who had the most amount (15g) of gelatin had twice as many collagen-producing proteins in their blood. When samples of this blood were added to engineered ligaments in the laboratory, the ligaments became stronger and more flexible.[178]

If you find your joints are giving you trouble when you exercise, try having a smoothie modeled on this experiment an hour before you train. You could blend berries with banana, plant-based milk and a good quality gelatin powder. Or for a savoury, low-sugar option, I love avocado with plant-based milk, fresh parsley (for the vitamin C) and gelatin powder.

Glucosamine sulphate is frequently recommended for joint and connective tissue health, and here's why. It has to do with something called ground substance. Ground substance is an interesting component of connective tissue, in that it is understood to hold a remarkable amount of water – often quoted as up to 1000 times its own weight. It attracts water to itself like a magnet, and so is responsible for keeping your connective tissue well hydrated, and so able to nourish and cleanse itself. Being so hydrated also enables it to respond to pressure and nerve signals and behave as a protective shock absorber. It is made up of substances called GAGs (glycosaminoglycans), and it is for this reason that glucosamine is so popular for joint health.

N-acetyl glucosamine is a precursor to GAGs (i.e. a vital ingredient), but it has been suggested that it's the sulphate aspect of glucosamine sulphate that is most useful in joint health, as it makes GAGs more hydrophilic – that is, more of a water magnet. Sulphates are also needed by the liver for detoxification processes, and anything that helps keep your toxin levels low will help with tissue health. You can also increase your sulphate intake with Epsom salt baths. Epsom salts are magnesium sulphate, so you would benefit from the muscle relaxing qualities of magnesium together with the fascia hydrating qualities of the sulphate.

Chondroitin sulphate is another GAG, but is poorly absorbed in the gut.[179]

Joint health

So for general joint health, you would want to ensure you have a great supply of all of these connective tissue nutrients, including water. At the same time, you would need to ensure your epithelial tissue is in great condition, so that you can absorb everything you need.

A key focus for both gut and joint health is inflammation, and so I'll revisit this in a later chapter. As we have already seen, a balanced microbiome (gut bacteria etc.) and calm adrenals and HPA axis (your stress response system) are involved with resolving inflammation, and there is also further support you can put in.

If your adrenals have been overworking or depleted for a while, your thyroid might start to feel the strain. There has been some interesting research linking thyroid activity with the structure of your connective tissue,[180] which ties in with the well-documented association between the thyroid and frozen shoulder. There is also a known link between low thyroid and rheumatoid arthritis, so it may be wise to ensure an adequate intake at least of iodine and selenium. Most seaweed contains all the nutrients you need to nourish your thyroid, and I encourage its use on a daily basis (unless you are on thyroid medication).

Joints and the Wood Element

Finally, joints and tendons are governed by the Wood Element in Five Elements Theory. We've already looked at Fire, Earth, Metal and Water, and if they're all flowing beautifully, then your Wood Element will be in a great place too. Or you could see the Wood Element as the point in the cycle where things begin, as the inspiration and drive of springtime. This is when seeds have sprouted and are shooting upwards with determination. After the stillness and reflectiveness of winter (Water Element), this is when things really start happening again, momentum builds, plans are afoot and there's a tangible shift in energy.

A well-watered and well-fed tree will be able to harness this energy to grow straight and tall, and with flexible branches. It will be able to sway in the wind without breaking, and eventually bloom and grow fruit. A poorly nourished tree will grow perhaps gnarled and brittle, snapping in the wind and less fertile. This is a useful metaphor for how your bodily structure develops, the strength and flexibility of your joints – and also for how you face the world and deal with situations in life. Do you tend to be stubborn and inflexible, or break easily under stress, or are you adaptable and able to bounce back easily?

Part of looking after your joints will involve taking care of your Wood Element organs and their functions: your liver and your gallbladder. You can find out more about this in chapter 18. Your cartilage certainly needs to be well hydrated in order for your joints to stay healthy and recover from injury. Of all your soft connective tissues, cartilage is among the firmest and is the least connected to your blood supply. Any stagnation will further affect its ability to nourish and cleanse your joints, and as your liver is at the hub of your stagnation-shifting processes, it makes sense to give your liver some love. As you will see later on, Five Elements theory relates the colour green to the Wood Element, so you could start by ensuring you include green leafy vegetables with as many meals as possible.

Bone health

Your bones and teeth are made of an even firmer connective tissue matrix than your cartilage, and it's easy to think of them as a solid, lifeless mass. In actual fact, they are a living, dynamic reservoir of minerals that come and go all the time, so that your bone matrix is continuously freeing up nutrients and then rebuilding itself. The bone cells that live in this matrix are largely cells that are involved in this task of demolition and reconstruction.

The primary minerals in your bone matrix are calcium and phosphorous, but there is also magnesium, sodium, zinc, boron and other minerals. How strong your bones are at any given moment in time relies on a number of factors.

The first question often asked is: is there enough calcium in your diet? The answer is usually (but not always) yes. We think of dairy as being our main source of calcium (thanks at least in part to the success of the Milk Marketing Board's campaigns), but actually we can obtain fantastic levels of calcium from green leafy vegetables, nuts, seeds and other foods. So vegans and those avoiding dairy, you don't need to worry on that front if you have a varied diet.

The next question to ask is: how well are you absorbing calcium? Which goes back to everything we have looked at in terms of improving digestion and absorption of nutrients.

Perhaps the most important question might be: what is your body doing with that calcium? It will put it into your bones and teeth to make them nice and strong where possible, but that's not its top priority.

Calcium is also one of your body's key acidity buffers. This means that if any of your cells are in danger of becoming too acidic to carry out their important tasks (i.e. keep you alive), then calcium will be quickly sent there to help keep them within a safe pH range. If necessary, calcium will be taken out of your bones to do this. This is why osteoporosis (weak bone density) should be considered a pH issue as much as a calcium deficiency issue.[181]

The usual treatment for osteoporosis is high doses of calcium carbonate (the cheapest, although not the best absorbed form of calcium supplement), together with vitamin D, which helps you absorb more calcium.

However, that may carry with it the risk that your tissue becomes over calcified.[182] Hypercalcification of the soft tissue in your body has been reported in breast tissue, lung tissue, heart structures, blood vessel walls, the stomach, kidneys and more. Calcified tissue is a feature of tuberculosis, cancer and general inflammation. Vitamin D3 alongside the following nutrients may be more useful, perhaps together with a little calcium citrate if required.

Vitamin K2 is greatly involved in triggering bone tissue formation and helping to keep it stable, and as such, has been noted to also help prevent hypercalcification of tissue.[183] In fact, in a 2-year study where people with osteoporosis were given either 150mg calcium a day, or 150mg calcium plus 45mg vitamin K2, the K2 group had less than half the amount of fractures and more sustained bone strength.[184] For this reason, I would suggest that all vitamin D and/or calcium supplementation should be accompanied with vitamin K2.

Food sources of K2 are difficult to access, the main one being a fermented Japanese dish called natto. Egg yolks and pasture-fed butter contain limited amounts.

Magnesium is also hugely influential in calcium placement and bone formation. We know that magnesium deficiency is a key factor in osteoporosis, and it saddens me that GPs aren't trained to assess this. Magnesium is essential for the crystalline structures in bones to grow in a way that they can bear loads. In addition, magnesium is associated with low levels of PTH, the parathyroid hormone that triggers bone formation (see below). Osteopaenia (low bone density) can additionally be caused by low-grade inflammation, which is a notable feature of magnesium deficiency.[185]

Unsurprisingly, magnesium supplementation has been found to reverse low bone density in women with osteoporosis, and to help strengthen bones of pre-pubescent girls with typical Western diets low in magnesium. In fact, magnesium supplementation has been found in some instances to even aid in the normalisation of vitamin D levels, which would then assist calcium absorption.[186]

Magnesium can be found in many sources, including green leafy vegetables, nuts and seeds, but like many minerals, soil content is low and so levels in the food chain are not optimal. Added to that, magnesium is depleted with stress, fizzy drinks and high intakes of sugar and other stimulants.

So I usually recommend supplements, perhaps magnesium citrate or bisglycinate or a magnesium chloride spray for the skin.

Zinc, silicon and **boron** are also crucial to bone formation and strength. Zinc, as I have mentioned, is to be found in nuts, seeds, lamb and beef. Silicon is rich in green beans, various other vegetables and grains (especially beer!) – and also banana, although we don't seem to absorb the silicon in bananas so well.[187] Boron can be found in beans, artichokes, sweet potatoes, avocados, berries, cherries and other fruit.

The actual process of bone formation and loss is controlled via your thyroid (a butterfly shaped hormone-secreting gland in your throat) and your parathyroids (two smaller glands nestling on the butterfly wings). If your body wants to put more calcium into your bones, your thyroid secretes the hormone calcitonin to trigger this. If your body wants to pull calcium out of your bones for use elsewhere, your parathyroids will secrete parathyroid hormone (PTH) to trigger this. It therefore makes sense to give your thyroid some attention, perhaps with some regular sea vegetables in your diet, not just for the iodine, but also for the co-factors that help your thyroid to produce its iodine-rich hormones.

Seaweed is also one of the main foods that relate to the Water Element, which governs bones and teeth. You can remind yourself of the basics of how to support the Water Element by revisiting chapter 7. You can add a strip of Icelandic kombu when making bone broths, or try making kombu and ginger tea, which you will find in the Recipes section on page 293.

Nerve tissue health

You have nerve tissue in your brain, along your spine and branching out to all your organs, limbs and wherever you have senses (touch, taste, sight, smell, hearing). There are different types of nerve cells in this nervous system network, but those driving the communication are called neurons. Neurons are uniquely shaped for speedy communication of sensations and commands. These messages take the form of electrical signals that pulse from one end of a neuron to the other, and then jump across to the next neuron.

These electrical signals ride on a kind of Mexican wave of sodium and potassium ions ebbing and flowing across the nerve cell wall. And they jump across to the next nerve cell with the help of calcium ions. So although we think of nerve signals as electrical in nature, they very much rely on the right kind of chemicals being around. We know that magnesium plays a major role in calcium placement, and also that magnesium acts to block certain receptors of abnormal pain signals.[188] So at least four of your electrolytes, sodium, potassium, calcium and magnesium, are directly involved in pain and sensation, as well as all the other signals telling your heart to beat, your lungs to breathe and your hand to pull away from the fire. A balanced diet with plenty of vegetables should help you to provide these, but I usually find that most people seem to be lacking in magnesium, even with a well balanced diet.

Your neurons are mostly covered by a fatty white coating called the myelin sheath. This protects and insulates your neurons, much like the rubber coating on electrical wire. Your myelin sheath is made largely from oils (70%) and proteins (30%), both of which I'll talk about more in the next couple of chapters. Brain levels of oils called essential fatty acids influence the process of myelination, i.e. coating the neurons with myelin.

There are two types of nervous cells that are responsible for myelination: oligodendrocytes in your brain and Schwann cells in the rest of your body. These are types of glial cells, or glia, and there are more, including:

- microglia, which are involved in immune response and repair
- astrocytes, which nourish and protect via the blood brain barrier
- ependymal cells, which create, secrete and circulate cerebro-spinal fluid.

We sometimes forget this family of glia when talking about the nervous system, and yet you have three times as many glia in your brain than neurons. For a long time their role was underplayed to that of just supportive and protective, but now we know that at least some of them also get involved in communication.

Food: more than energy

This is a neat reminder that eating isn't just about calories and energy. For all the different kinds of tissue in your body to keep growing and renewing, stay healthy and perform well, you need all the vitamins and minerals mentioned above, plus many more of these and other co-factors, antioxidants and anti-inflammatories on a day to day basis. Equally, your structure needs more than just building blocks. However, we do need to look at the "bricks" that make up your cells too, so the next two chapters are devoted to proteins and oils. I have already written a considerable amount about sugars, the end product of carbohydrates, and they will also sneak their way in again, as they can also form structures such as glycoproteins (sugar and protein) and glycolipids (sugar and fat). Glycoproteins and glycolipids are part of the fabric of every cell in your body, alongside proteins and lipids in other forms.

Before we delve into the fascinating "legoland" of cell structure, here's an opportunity (if you would like it) to reflect on and review this chapter, and what you might do to strengthen, protect and support your muscles, nerves, joints, gut lining and other areas of connective and/or epithelial tissue.

Reflection time

- *Do your joints regularly feel stiff or achy?*

- *Are you concerned about your bone strength or density?*

- *Do you experience signs of inflammation or discomfort in your gut, your lungs, your skin or other mucous membranes?*

- *Now consider how your body is continually making new tissue cells, and you have daily opportunities to influence the health of the fabric that makes up your body.*

Action plan

- *Consider regular weight bearing exercise, such as walking, hiking, dancing, skipping, tennis, badminton, weight training etc.*
    - *This kind of exercise helps to increase bone strength, joint strength and fitness*

- *Consider regular stretching and toning exercise, such as yoga or pilates.*

- *Pay attention to how much water you are drinking daily*
    - *Aim for around 1.5-2 litres of the best quality water available to you.*

Recipes

- ***Bone strengthening carrot and sea spaghetti salad** – p.266*
  Rich in calcium and many of the other minerals you need for bone strength, and completely dairy free.

- ***Kombu and ginger tea** – p.293*
  Great for the bones, teeth, kidneys, bladder, adrenals, thyroid and more.

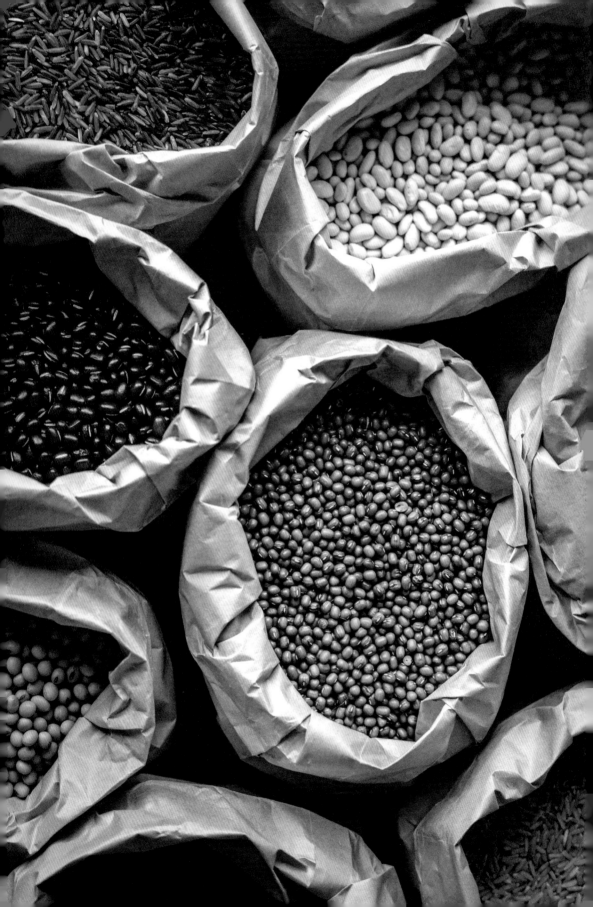

Chapter 14

Protein power

Proteins – part of the fabric of your cells

We tend to think of protein as being primarily for muscle tissue, and that is one of the reasons that protein shakes have become synonymous with trips to the gym. Dairy protein in particular has been shown to help build muscles when taken soon after exercise, and so many protein shakes therefore contain whey powder. It should also be noted that many of them also contain an excessive amount of sugar and other additives, so it's always wise to check the labels. You can easily make very delicious protein shakes by blending pure whey powder – or hemp or pea protein powder, for example – with a glass of almond milk, ¼ avocado and either a few berries or some green leaves (e.g. spinach, mint, parsley or rocket.)

It's not just muscle cells that need protein, though. Every cell in your body does. The cells that make up your eyes, your knees, your bones, your skin and your heart.

Proteins form structures within your cell membranes (the outer walls) that help to transport substances in and out, as well as provide antennae and docking stations for hormones such as insulin and cortisol. Proteins also help to form structures within your cells, and deeper still, your very DNA (which contains the architectural plans for all of this) is made of protein.

In addition, many of your hormones are made from protein, including insulin and leptin, which are involved in energy regulation and how hungry you feel. The antibodies in your immune system are also protein-based, so your fundamental wellness depends on what's in your diet.

As mentioned in the last chapter, sometimes proteins bind to sugars to create glycoproteins. There are many other substances in your body that are made from proteins, including the enzymes, methyl donors and many of the hormones that trigger essential processes involved in the day-to-day running of the human body. So without enough protein, for example, you can't make the digestive enzymes you need to digest protein!

Because the same is true of animals, and plants, every time you eat you are probably consuming at least a little protein.

Proteins and plant-based diets

As we shall see, it's perfectly possible to get plenty of protein from a vegetarian or vegan diet. That doesn't mean everyone does, though. I frequently meet veggies and vegans whose diets are rich in carbohydrates, fruit and vegetables, but their protein intake isn't enough to fully support good health.

Sometimes there is a problem with the digestibility of plant-based proteins. Beans, lentils and peas are famous for creating bloating and wind, which in itself is perfectly normal. However, some people experience excessive, painful bloating, cramps and wind. This is not only unpleasant, but puts a stress on your digestive system and may contribute to long-term inflammation. To reduce this effect, try soaking pulses overnight – or even a day or two, changing the water frequently – rinsing well, then cooking them thoroughly with a strip of kombu seaweed or some bay leaves. If this doesn't help, you can buy enzymes supplements that help you break down substances such as cellulose – or reconsider your choice of main protein.

Fermented pulses can be easier to digest, such as tempeh, which is made from fermented soya beans. Nuts and seeds are another vegetable protein to consider including (see below), but best in moderation. Some may also find it helpful to add protein powders, such as pea or hemp protein powder, to smoothies, pancake mixtures, energy ball snacks, soups and other recipes.

Conversely, I see a lot of meat and fish eaters whose protein portions are way larger than they need to be, or is indeed healthy. So I wanted to take some time to look at which proteins you need and roughly how much of them. To do so, we first need to take a look at how different protein sources offer different kinds of proteins, and how that might affect your choices.

Essential amino acids

Proteins are made up of their own little building blocks, called amino acids. There are dozens of different kinds of amino acid, nine of which are said to be essential – which in the nutrition world means you cannot make them, so you have to have them in your diet. The nine essential amino acids have mythical sounding names:

Histidine	Lysine	Threonine
Isoleucine	Methionine	Tryptophan
Leucine	Phenylanaline	Valine

In addition, the amino acids cysteine, tyrosine and arginine are needed in the diets of infants and growing children.

Leucine is the dominant essential amino acid rich in whey powder and other dairy products that helps muscles to grow after exercise. Methionine helps to create cartilage, new blood vessels and much more. Lysine is needed to make, among other things, collagen, bones and muscle tissue. You need tryptophan to make your happy chemical, serotonin. The gifts of the essential amino acids are endless.

A food or combination of foods that contains all nine essential amino acids in a useful amount and ratio is called a complete protein. All animal proteins fall into this category, but there seems to be a great deal of debate as to which vegetarian proteins are considered to be complete. This is partly due to how they are measured, for example just by content, or by how well we absorb them. There is also a great deal of difference between the quantity of amino acids in meat and those in grains and vegetables. To give you an example, in the following chart, approximate amounts of each amino acid (in mg per 100g of food) is compared:[189]

	Broccoli	Brown Rice	Oats	Quinoa	Sunflower Seeds	Chickpeas	Fish	Chicken
Histidine	78	197	292	288	345	531	665	521
Isoleucine	186	300	526	432	635	891	900	1069
Leucine	236	648	1012	720	954	1505	1445	1462
Lysine	218	299	517	672	536	1376	1713	1590
Methionine	61	183	234	240	283	209	539	502
Phenylalanine	177	406	698	492	662	1151	737	800
Threonine	161	307	462	420	547	756	861	794
Tryptophan	46	101	230	170	202	190	580	205
Valine	210	433	711	540	754	913	1150	1018

So while all of these foods contain all of the essential amino acids, animal proteins generally contain much greater amounts and in ratios that are more in line with your body's needs.

Rice, for example, is considered to be too low in lysine to be considered complete. The fact that its lysine content is in such short supply means that it may limit your body's ability to work with other amino acids. Lysine is therefore said to be a "limiting amino acid" in rice. Chickpeas are sometimes described as a complete protein, but their methionine and tryptophan levels are considered to be too low, or more accurately, as "limiting."[190] However the lysine content of chickpeas can help make up for the lack of lysine in rice.[191]

By eating a varied diet that includes plenty of pulses alongside some grains, nuts and seeds, vegetarians and vegans can obtain an ample supply of essential amino acids without relying on animal proteins. In addition soya (and therefore tofu and tempeh) as well as quinoa and amaranth are complete proteins.

Protein portion sizes

The chart on the previous page also helps us to understand one of the reasons why animal protein consumers don't need to eat huge portions of it: meat, fish and dairy are much denser in amino acid content, while the proteins in vegan sources are often diluted with higher levels of carbohydrates and other nutrients.

Current government advice for daily protein is 45g for female adults and 55g daily for male adults. Of course some women will need more and some men will need less, depending on body size and type, but an approximate amount for most adults eating 3 meals a day would be between 15-18g of protein per meal.

In practical terms, this roughly equates per meal to (all raw weights except baked beans):

- 50-60g chicken or beef (NB a chicken breast is usually about 150g)
- 60-70g cheddar cheese
- 60-75g salmon
- 70-85g sunflower seeds
- 80-95g chickpeas
- 110-130g quinoa
- 2 large eggs
- 135-165g oats
- 190-225g lentils
- 300-360g baked beans
- 350-420g kale (5-6 cups)
- 535-645g broccoli (6-7 cups)

So you can see that while chickpeas and sunflower seeds, for example, have a similar protein density to fish, other protein sources show much greater differences. Quinoa is often described as protein-rich, but you need to eat twice as much of it as you would chicken to get the same amount of protein. It contains a ratio of amino acids that means it can be described as a complete protein, but additionally contains relatively high levels of carbohydrate.

And while kale has been touted as a super protein source for vegans, you would have to eat an awful lot of it to get the same amount of amino acids. That amount of kale smoothie would provide more fibre than may be healthy for most people – and in fact when vegetable smoothies became more popular, I had a spate of new clients complaining about constipation and bloating as a result of having several kale-based smoothies a day.

Interestingly, many people seem to find that animal proteins have a denser *quality* about them, too, which can make you sometimes feel heavier after you eat them. This can at times be useful, for example, when you want to feel more grounded; for the most part, this heavy quality may be another reason to keep animal protein intake low. Sometimes, however, animal proteins feel lighter and easier to digest. Always listen to your body and follow its cues when deciding on the quality and quantity of protein to eat.

There are, of course, moral, ethical and environmental arguments around protein sources, and that is something you need to make your own decisions about.

Heating proteins – and brassicas to the rescue!

You don't lose proteins during cooking in the same way that you can lose vitamins and minerals (e.g. through leaching into water/steam). However, you can denature, or damage proteins when cooking at high heats. It has long been known that meat cooked at high temperatures for a long time forms a group of toxic substances called HAAs (heterocyclic aromatic amines). Foods particularly high in HAAs include well done and very well done steaks, pan fried burgers and pan fried sausages, as well as grilled and barbecued chicken,[192] and microwaved fish and chicken.[193] HAAs are being increasingly linked to cancer, and are in the same group of chemicals as the cancer-causing aromatic amines formed when tobacco is burned in cigarettes, pipes and cigars.[194]

Using spices and black pepper, for example in marinades and rubs, seems to help reduce the amount of HAAs formed.[195] Scientists have also noted that the incidence of cancers associated with HAAs is lower when people regularly eat brassica vegetables (broccoli, cauliflower, cabbage, kale, Brussels sprouts, kohl rabi, mustard greens, etc.). Brassicas, also known as cruciferous vegetables, contain anti-cancer compounds called ITCs (isothiocyanates), and one study showed that cooking meat with cabbage reduced HAA formation by 17-20%.[196]

ITCs are formed (from compounds called glucosinolates) when you chew or chop brassicas, which is another reason to chew your food well, shred cabbage into casseroles and sauerkraut, and smash cauliflower into root vegetable mash. There are different types of ITCs, including sulforaphane in broccoli and allyl ITC in kale, and they trigger your liver's detoxification processes, and so may also help to deactivate HAAs and clear them from your body. Indeed several studies have shown that adding brassicas to mealtimes can up to double the amount of deactivated HAAs in the urine, and also reduce damage to white blood cells.[197] They are responsible for the pungent taste in these vegetables, and so tie in beautifully with the Chinese Wood and Metal Element, where green foods nourish the liver and gallbladder, and white and/or pungent foods support your processes of elimination.

Rice cakes – as innocent as they seem?

Rice cakes seem to be everyone's go to for dieting, general health, and snacks for children and babies. The labels make them seem fairly virtuous, and they're just rice, right? I hate bursting bubbles, but rice cakes have always seemed so artificial and highly processed to me, that I had to do some research into how they are made.

Extrusion is a process used in food manufacturing to create a wide range of processed foods, from dog biscuits through to puffed rice through to vegetarian meat substitutes.

In its simplest form, extrusion works in a similar way to a masticating juicer, where vegetables or fruit are cold-pressed by being driven through a tube by a rotating screw-shaped shaft and then forced through a mesh. In juicing we are interested in the liquid that is released from the food. In extrusion, it is the dried product, and in most cases, the pressure and heat are much higher. The degrees of pressure and heat, in fact, directly impact the nutritional value of the output.

When rice is extruded to make rice pasta, for example, the pressure and temperature are relatively low, but still high enough to denature the proteins. Here, this actually makes the proteins more digestible. At the same time, enzyme inhibitors are deactivated, which makes other nutrients more available too.

The kind of high pressure and heat required to make rice cakes, however, reduces the availability of amino acids and other nutrients. At the same time, rice starch is converted to dextrins with a high glycaemic load, which means rice cakes (and similarly extruded cornflakes and other breakfast cereals) are much more likely to mess with your blood sugar than oatcakes (and good old-fashioned porridge), for example.[198] This stronger effect on your blood sugar (higher glycaemic load) may affect not just your energy, but also levels of inflammation throughout your body[199] – including those epithelial and other tissues you are trying to keep healthy.

Extruded breakfast cereals

Unfortunately this goes for many breakfast cereals, too. Puffed rice cereals, crunchy flakes, funky shapes... they've all been extruded, and most of them in a similar way to rice cakes.

Remember that, to keep blood sugar and energy levels stable throughout the day, most people fare best with a protein-rich breakfast. With extruded cereals, however, the small amount of proteins these often contain are harder to digest, and have to compete with the effects of high GL dextrins.

So if you would like your breakfasts and snacks to sustain you, rather than create spikes, crashes and inflammation, think twice about the puffed, dried and heavily processed cereals you may have been brought up with. These relatively recent trends have been marketed as healthy options for babies, toddlers, children and adults, and yet their very substance is of questionable nutritional value – that's before you take into account sugary coatings and other additives. More sustaining and nutritious options might include soft poached eggs with wilted spinach on sourdough rye bread, oat porridge with tahini or almond butter, or an avocado and fresh herb smoothie with almond milk and a little pea or hemp protein powder.

Protein-powered: animal or vegetable

To make sure the quantity, quality and variety of proteins in your diet works for you, you may need to experiment a little and introduce some new ingredients or recipes into your week. The ultimate test of all of this is how you feel: your energy levels; your ability to recover well from exercise, injuries and illness; your hormonal health and your overall health.

Vegetarian sources of proteins, such as pulses and grains, often benefit from some form of gentle processing to help you digest them – this includes soaking, rinsing and cooking well, as well as fermentation. Tempeh and yoghurt are both great examples of how fermenting a food can make it much more digestible. But too much processing can have the opposite effect, as happens with rice cakes and many breakfast cereals.

Animal proteins, such as meat, fish and eggs, can be harmful when overcooked, but these effects can be softened with marinades and side orders of cabbage, broccoli and other brassicas. It is usually the case – but not always – that meat eaters could benefit from eating a lot less meat and other animal proteins. Eating smaller quantities may then enable them to source their food from organic and high welfare sources, and farms that have a lower impact on the environment. It is sometimes the case that someone who doesn't usually eat animal protein finds substantial health benefits in eating a little from time to time – and then may or may not choose to do this, depending on how well that sits with them.

Your ethical considerations around this are your own, and it's not my intention to influence them here. My personal approach is to try to make decisions that include consideration of my own health, animal welfare and the environment. Some of my decisions have shifted over the years and may well shift again as I continue to reassess my values alongside evolving research and information. Nothing is ever as straightforward as it seems, so I aim to respect whatever approach individuals choose. Sometimes one's ethics can appear to be at odds with one's health requirements – and all of these seem to be challenging on the wallet – but there are usually ways to navigate this, and I try to help people do this in a way that fits with their own values and choices.

Reflection time

- *Take a little time to consider your current protein intake:*
    - *Is it enough / too much?*
    - *Are you getting a variety of amino acids?*
    - *If you eat animal produce, does it ever make you feel too heavy, dense or lethargic? Or light and energised? Or satisfied and reassuringly grounded?*
    - *If you eat pulses (e.g. beans and lentils), do you feel lighter and more energised? Satisfied, or wanting more? How do they affect your digestion?*
    - *Do you notice any changes in your health and wellbeing if you eat more nuts? Fewer nuts?*
    - *How does it feel when you change the protein content of your breakfast?*

Recipe

- **Coriander houmous** – *p.278*
  Houmous contains both pulses (chickpeas) and seeds (sesame seed paste a.k.a. tahini), and this is a fresh take on this reliable dip.

- **Superseed crackers with rosemary** – *p.280*
  The perfect protein-rich cracker to dip into your houmous.

- **Broccoli and almond soup** – *p.247*
  Vegetable soups are often very low in protein, so adding ground nuts is a tasty way to make them more sustaining. Add a side of coriander houmous and your proteins are complete!

- **Cauliflower and hazelnut soup** – *p.247*

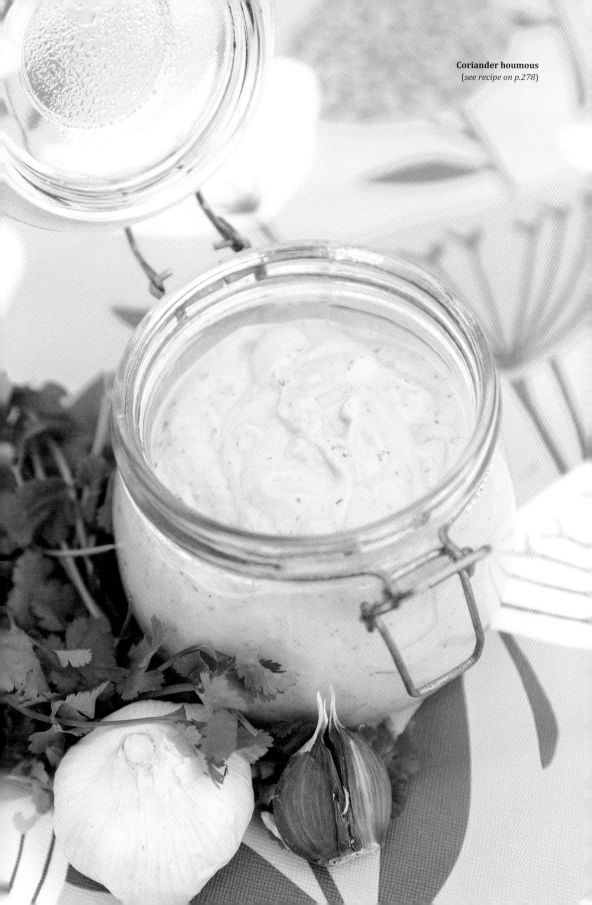

Coriander houmous
(*see recipe on p.278*)

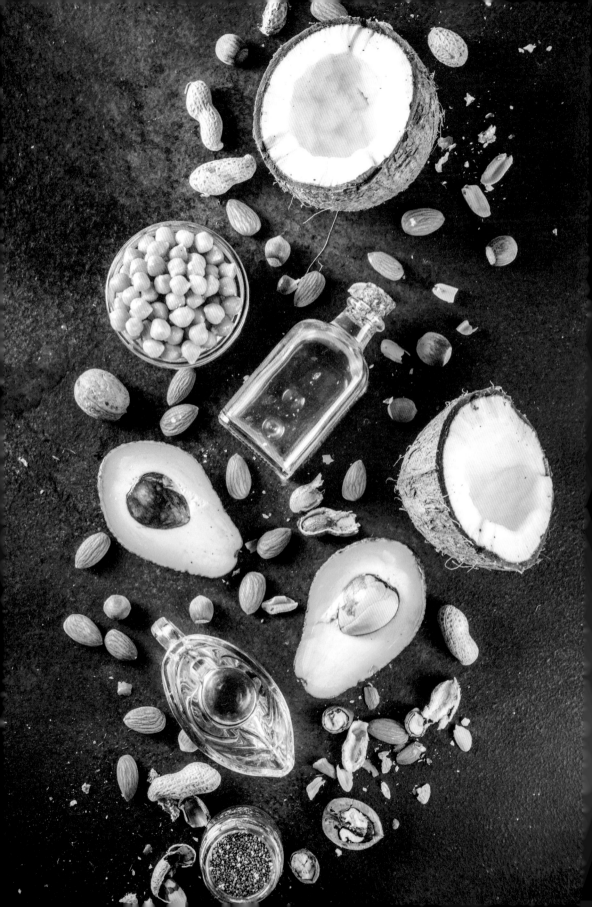

Chapter 15

Oils
~ structure and light ~

Magical lipids (fats and oils)

A great deal of attention is paid to the part proteins play in providing the raw material for your physical structures, but fats and oils are often overlooked.

Your cell membranes are largely composed of fats and oils (lipids), so while proteins are usually credited as being the building blocks of our bodies, lipids are much more than the mortar between them. In fact, lipids are the main component both in the external wall of each of your cells, and in the more internal wall that surrounds the nucleus of each cell, where your DNA lives. In addition, we've already seen how your neurons are protected by an additional lipid-rich myelin sheath.

The lipids in your cell membranes play more than a structural role. They strongly influence the transport of substances and messages (e.g. hormonal signals) in and out of each cell, for example, and so help to regulate pretty much everything that happens in there.

These lipids are in special structures called phospholipids. A phospholipid is essentially a phosphate group with two lipids, or fatty acids, attached. There are many different kinds of fatty acids, as we shall soon see, and a phospholipid might contain any of these. The type(s) of fatty acid it contains will influence how straight and firm, or how wiggly, the phospholipid and by extension that part of the cell wall will be. A mixture of different types is necessary to make sure the cell has a stable structure, but can still allow things to move in and out when necessary.

Lipids are not just part of your cell membrane make-up. They also form part of other structures in your body, for example the myelin sheath that is wrapped around nerve cells, and also the lipoproteins that carry your cholesterol to where it needs to go. Additionally, some specific lipids are crucial to the processes of triggering and reducing inflammation, right at the site where it happens.

There is also some fascinating and ongoing research into oils and light that I'd like to explore with you. This is where the realms of biochemistry, physics and magic overlap.

Controversy, confusion and jigsaw puzzles

The topic of fats and oils has perhaps caused more controversy and confusion in nutritional science than any other. Saturated fats are "bad", then maybe not so "bad", then perhaps "bad" again. We're told to cook with sunflower oil, olive oil, rapeseed oil or coconut oil, depending on who you listen to and sometimes changing by the week. Margarine is better than butter, then evil, then cholesterol lowering. Low-fat diets are the only way to lose fat/are dangerous/ are fattening. Who knows what to believe anymore?

It's not just magazines and newspapers that create confusion, the scientific research seems all over the place too. So we can't just blame sensational reporting and fad diet mongers. I think there are a number of reasons we've got in such a tizz.

Firstly, we all like things to be black and white, good or bad. If we can put things into simple boxes, then we know where we are, and we can be "good" or "bad" depending on what we're eating. However, what is becoming increasingly clear with fats and oils is that there is no "good" and "bad". Instead there is a rich diversity of options that we've only been exploring for a few decades, and there's still so much more to understand.

So let's remember to banish "good" and "bad", and instead understand that there are many different kinds of fats and oils, each with their qualities, functions and benefits. Like any foods, there are times, amounts and ways in which you would and wouldn't want to eat them.

Secondly, science is a bit like doing a jigsaw puzzle. At the beginning, a group of scientists might find a couple of blue jigsaw pieces, and make an assumption that they belong to some sky at the top of the puzzle. Perhaps as they get further into the puzzle, a few trees and birds add weight to that assumption, and they become pretty fixed on the idea. They make an announcement, the press and other organisations get involved, and this whole story about blue skies lights up our collective imaginations.

Then another scientist comes along, slots a few more pieces into place, and declares that it's a sunrise scene and the sky here is orange. However, there is a person in the picture, and the pieces of blue most likely belong to their coat. For a while there is an argument, with some scientists still insisting the blue pieces are sky, and the new scientist insisting they're part of a coat. Equally, some journalists and other organisations stick doggedly to the party line that the sky is blue, while others stick their necks out and declare the sky to be orange and the person's coat blue. Some change their mind each week, some weeks giving tips on how jigsaw puzzles are always easy to do once you've located the blue bits (which are sky), and other weeks talking about blue coats and how to look for bits of orange for the sky. Others lose confidence in jigsaw puzzles altogether, and denounce all puzzle solvers as charlatans.

Actually the coat will turn out to be green, and the blue pieces part of a parrot, or perhaps some sky after all, but in a picture hanging from one of the trees... but my point is that we can only really work with what we've got, and should always keep an open mind to the possibility that we may have missed a detail or two along the way. In a similar way, we have discovered saturated fats, declared them to be responsible for heart disease and other health problems, discovered more information that contradicts this, and are now yo-yoing between bits of research that seem to declare either that it's good or it's bad. In the meantime, people have staked their reputation, cemented national and global health policies, and built up companies and industries – all of which makes it even more difficult to admit the sky might not be blue.

So let's look at the jigsaw pieces that we have, and instead of trying to finish the picture (we probably don't have enough pieces of information yet), enjoy what's there and do with it what we can. We can start with some basic definitions.

Fats, oils and lipids

Fats are solid at room temperature, while oils are liquid. Simple as that. Except in the summer or a hot country, where fats might melt. So to be more precise, fats are solid at temperatures at or below "average room temperature", which is around 20°C to 25°C (68°F to 77°F).

Lipid is the technical term for both fats and oils. Fats are predominantly made up of saturated fatty acids, while oils are mostly comprised of unsaturated fatty acids. Let's have a look at what that actually means.

Fatty acids

Fats and oils (lipids) are both made up of different chain lengths and types of fatty acids. For example, olive oil is made up of 13 different types of fatty acid.

A fatty acid is a chain of mostly carbon atoms, all or most of which are "holding hands" with hydrogen ions. Short chain fatty acids (SCFAs) can have as little as four carbon atoms in the chain, while long chain fatty acids can have as many as 28. At the end of the chain is a structure called a carboxyl group (COOH, i.e. comprising of one carbon, one hydrogen and two oxygen atoms), which is the bit of it that makes it an acid.

Saturated fatty acids

Saturated fats are so called because *all* of their carbon atoms are "holding hands" with hydrogen ions. I use the term "holding hands" because I often get students to stand in a line pretending to be a carbon chain to illustrate this point. They imagine being connected to each other like a convoy of elephants, trunk to tail, and then they usually each have a hand free on either side to mimic the opportunity to bond with ("hold hands with") something else. In the case of a saturated fatty acid, each and every hand is holding, i.e. bonded to, a hydrogen ion. There are no free hands. This makes saturated fatty acids incredibly stable, as they don't have the capacity to interact with anything. You can expose them to oxygen and they won't go rancid. You can heat them and they won't easily damage.

The saturated fatty acids that sit in your cell membranes provide a dependable integrity. Their structure forms a straight line, and they won't bend or change. This is a positive thing – you need an aspect of that in your cell wall.

Many fats and oils are made up of a mixture of saturated and unsaturated fatty acids, but the ones that contain predominantly saturated fatty acids are known as saturated fats. These include animal fats – such as *goose fat, duck fat, lard, dripping, bacon fat, butter, ghee* – plus *coconut oil* and *palm oil*. To reiterate: none of these are "bad fats." It may not be wise to eat lots of them all of the time, but their link with heart disease is an increasingly grey area.[200]

Short chain fatty acids (SCFAs)

We spoke about SCFAs in the chapter about your microbiome, as your gut bacteria produce these when they eat fibre. Examples are acetate, proprionate and butyrate, and they provide your colon wall with energy. There is also increasing evidence for the ability of these SCFAs to regulate glucose metabolism and potentially prevent obesity (and they are technically saturated fatty acids!). They seem to have a number of roles here, including how the liver stores glucose as glycogen, how well muscles take up sugar, and how much insulin is triggered in response to a meal.

Unsaturated fatty acids

With unsaturated fatty acids, one or more pairs of carbon atoms in the chain are connected by an additional "hand", as well as being connected trunk to tail. We call this a double carbon bond. You could perhaps think of this additional connection as a hand resting on each other's shoulder, like a gentle hug. Their other hand is still bonded with a hydrogen ion.

This changes the structure of the chain: there is now a kink at the double carbon bond, so the fatty acid now has a bend in it (and sometimes more than one). These wiggly fatty acids are not so easy to stack up in a straight line, and so when they form part of your cell wall, they help it to be more permeable and less rigid.

Examples of oils rich in unsaturated fatty acids: *flax oil, hemp oil, olive oil, sunflower oil, pumpkin seed oil, wheatgerm oil, corn oil, walnut oil, rapeseed oil and fish oil.*

Monounsaturated fatty acids (MUFAs)

MUFAs have only one kink. Oleic acid, which makes up much of the lipid profile of olive oil (and some other oils), is a monounsaturated fatty acid.

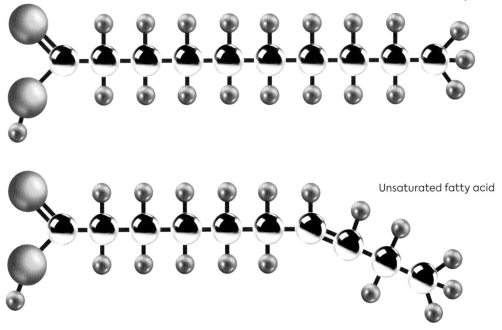

Saturated fatty acid

Unsaturated fatty acid

Polyunsaturated fatty acids (PUFAs)

These are unsaturated fatty acids that have more than one kink (double carbon bond), so are extra wiggly. Flax oil, fish oil, sunflower oil and corn oil all have high levels of these, as do many oils. Butter contains a small amount of PUFAs, but is largely made up of saturated fatty acids and also some MUFAs.

Essential fatty acids (EFAs)

Two PUFAs, alpha-linolenic acid (ALA) and linoleic acid (LA), are known as "essential" because your body can't manufacture them at will, it can only get them from your diet. ALA is one of the omega 3 fatty acids, because its first kink is at the 3rd carbon from the omega end of the fatty acid structure. LA belongs to the family of omega 6 fatty acids, as its first kink is at its 6th carbon.

You can obtain them from nuts and seeds, which usually contain more LA than ALA, with the exception of flax and chia seeds, which contain more ALA. You can convert these essential fatty acids to longer omega 3 and 6 PUFAs, but this requires a lot of work, and you may not be very efficient at this, particularly with converting ALA to EPA and DHA.

EPA and DHA (found ready-formed in fish oil) are anti-inflammatory as well as having other very special roles. In fact, there are some great tricks the unsaturated fatty acids in general have up their sleeves we'll explore a little later. However, with that potential comes a certain degree of instability – which makes them a little more exciting than saturated fatty acids, but not without risk.

When "good" fats go "bad"

Yes, I know I banished those words, but I couldn't resist a cool subtitle.

So these double carbon bonds in our unsaturated fatty acids are vulnerable in a key way. Double carbon bonds can be interfered with by oxygen in the air or free radicals in your body. When this happens, the lipid is damaged and will usually smell and taste off: it has gone rancid.

This can happen to cooking oils, salad dressing oils, nuts, seeds, grains, flour, butter – anything with an unsaturated fatty acid content. The more heat and/or light present, the faster the oil will go rancid. Which is why *unsaturated fatty acid rich oils are ideally cold-pressed, kept in cool, dark cupboards, and used raw rather than for cooking.* And yet the oils with the highest unsaturated fatty acid content are the nut, seed and vegetable oils that we have been encouraged to cook with for several decades now, including olive oil, sunflower oil, rapeseed oil and corn oil.

So what harm can rancid fats do? The truth is, we don't really know the full extent. A recent review has highlighted how we haven't even fully identified all of the substances produced when oil goes rancid, let alone how toxic they are. Added to this is the issue that most research uses oils that have been used in frying, and so it's difficult to tell which effects are from oxidation (rancidity) and which are from heat damage. Some of this research does suggest, however, that rancid oils are more difficult to digest, and these undigested lipids may have a negative impact on the epithelial tissue in your gut wall and on your balance of gut bacteria and other microbes. So we can perhaps add these to the list of pro-inflammatory foods that it may be wise to limit or avoid.[201]

And in fact research has measured worryingly high levels of cancer-forming toxins called aldehydes in heated unsaturated fatty acid rich oils. These aldehydes are formed through oxidation when the oils are heated – and the more unsaturated fatty acids in their lipid profile, the more aldehydes they form.

Professor Grootveld and his team compared sunflower oil, corn oil, extra virgin olive oil, butter and coconut oil – of these coconut oil has the fewest unsaturated fatty acids in its make up, butter the next fewest and so on, with sunflower oil containing the most. Even after 10 minutes of heating, the sunflower oil, corn oil and extra virgin olive oil showed levels of aldehydes several times greater than the butter and coconut oil. After 20 minutes, only the coconut oil had levels less than 1 millimole per litre of oil. After 30 minutes, the levels of carcinogens in coconut oil and butter were still at a similar level to 20 minutes (comparatively low), while levels in the other oils had shot up. This piece of research seems to back up what some scientists have been suggesting for years now: only cook with fats/oils that have low levels of unsaturated fats.

Professor Grootveld comes to a similar conclusion: "People have been telling us how healthy polyunsaturates are in corn oil and sunflower oil. But when you start messing around with them, subjecting them to high amounts of energy in the frying pan or the oven, they undergo a complex series of chemical reactions which results in the accumulation of large amounts of toxic compounds."[202]

Heated oils and heart disease

Further research carried out by scientists such as Professor Hermann Esterbauer[203] in Austria and Professor Grootveld in the UK link the toxic aldehydes in unsaturated fats to heart disease. According to Grootveld, this may explain the low prevalence of cardiovascular disease in areas like Sri Lanka and Southern France who primarily use saturated fat, and the dramatic rise in cardiovascular disease in countries like the US as they have switched from using saturated fats to unsaturated fats in cooking. His team also points out previous research that shows how the toxic aldehydes in heated PUFA-rich oils negatively impact the growth of cultured human and bacterial cells, prevent proteins being formed, deactivate enzymes, destroy white blood cells and more.[204] The public health messages to cook with sunflower, olive and corn oils seem to have been misguided.

Scientists have been questioning the standard health messages around fats, oils and even cholesterol for many years, however. The above research was similar to a project published over 20 years ago, with Grootveld on the team.[205] And in fact Dr. Johanna Budwig[206] was questioning the quality of highly processed unsaturated fats and the low-fat, margarine-touting diet industry back in the 1950s. Then Dr. Uffe Ravnskov[207] and Dr. Malcolm Kendrick[208] both took time to revisit and review the research over a decade ago, producing books that throw into doubt everything we've been brought up to fear around saturated fats and cholesterol. Finally it feels like at least part of this message is drip-feeding through, but progress seems patchy and slow.

In fact a 2015 article in the British Medical Journal accused the committee behind the US Dietary Guidelines for Americans (which influences dietary guidelines worldwide) of ignoring recent research when it continued to promote the restriction of saturated fats. Nina Teicholz, who wrote the BMJ article, points to a number of significant trials and reviews that had been ignored or misreported by the committee, including:

- a meta-analysis and two major reviews that showed no association between saturated fats and cardiovascular disease
- the Women's Health Initiative, a controlled clinical trial of nearly 49000 women who reduced their saturated fat intake, and yet failed to show

reductions in incidence of coronary heart disease events (both fatal and non-fatal) or cardiovascular disease
- a meta-analysis that was actually looking at polyunsaturated vegetable oils, not saturated fats
- three meta-analyses that shared the conclusion that saturated fats do not increase cardiovascular fatalities
- two meta-analyses that showed saturated fats to be more artery clogging than PUFAs, but less so than MUFAs and carbohydrates.

Teicholz laments that, "Despite this conflicting evidence, however, the committee's report concludes that the evidence linking consumption of saturated fats to cardiovascular disease is 'strong.'"[209]

While saturated fats continue to be denounced as "bad", there is a great deal of persuasive research out there that appropriate levels of saturated fats within the context of a balanced diet are healthy. What constitutes appropriate is likely to vary, like most nutrients, according to body type, lifestyle and other factors, so this isn't carte blanche to start devouring mountains of lard, dripping and other saturated fats. However, it is a great reason to strip saturated fats of their negative reputation and look at them with a fresh pair of eyes. After all, you do at least need a little of them for the structure of every cell in your body.

The truth about trans fats

A trans fatty acid is similar to a saturated fatty acid, but with a key difference: it has a double carbon bond without a wiggle. They do occur in very small amounts naturally, but most trans fats have been artificially produced through hydrogenation, and so are also called hydrogenated fats, or more accurately, partially hydrogenated fats. It's a process that takes an unsaturated fatty acid and straightens out its kink. The result is an unsaturated fatty acid that is now more solid at room temperature.

This is very convenient if you'd like to make a spreadable margarine out of a largely unsaturated fat, such as sunflower oil or olive oil. However, a trans fatty acid is neither truly saturated nor truly unsaturated, and so has its own behaviours and attributes. Many of which seem to be detrimental to your health.

A 2015 review published in the British Medical Journal compared a swathe of studies on saturated fats and trans fats that involved many hundreds of thousands of people. They looked for associations with a number of chronic health conditions, including cardiovascular disease (CVD), chronic heart disease (CHD), stroke and type 2 diabetes. The scientists noticed that naturally occurring trans fats (from ruminant animals) did not carry the same health risks as artificially produced trans fats, and in fact the higher the levels of ruminant trans fats, the lower the risk of type 2 diabetes. Their overall conclusion was:

"Saturated fats are not associated with all cause mortality, CVD, CHD, ischemic stroke, or type 2 diabetes, but the evidence is heterogeneous with methodological limitations. *Trans fats are associated with all cause mortality, total CHD, and CHD mortality,* probably because of higher levels of intake of industrial trans fats than ruminant trans fats."[210]

Partially hydrogenated fats are not just found in margarines, they appear in many different kinds of ready meals, convenience foods and processed foods. In addition, partially hydrogenated fats are often used for deep fat frying in the fast food and food processing industries. In recent years, with trans fats gaining a bad reputation, many companies have switched to palm oil instead, which is a predominantly saturated fat. Although this might be welcome in terms of health benefits, there are major issues with deforestation and loss of orangutan habitat.

So what fats/oils are best to cook with?

Olive oil and other unsaturated oils are best cold-pressed for a reason – they damage when heated. So why spend extra money on cold pressed oils and then heat them?

Some chefs seem to think the answer to this is to cook with cheaper olive and sunflower oils that haven't been cold pressed – but they are missing the point. These cheaper oils haven't been protected during processing, so I would avoid these as much as possible.

On the other hand, there is some interesting enquiry into whether cooking with garlic and/or herbs protects the oil to some extent, and allows a greater range of cooking possibilities. The antioxidants in herbs, spices and garlic may help to protect the oil somewhat. Until there is more clarity on this, my answer (and I am not alone in this) is to cook only using saturated fats – or just water – and then use cold-pressed oils as dressings. Professor Grootveld advocates cooking with butter or lard. I prefer coconut oil for the most part, as it feels lighter and my diet is generally low in animal produce.

I do have some exceptions to this. If I'm cooking pizza, for example, then I'll occasionally drizzle on some olive oil – but then it's in the oven for ten minutes or less. Generally, though, I save it for salads, dips and pesto, and enjoy the intense flavour of high quality, cold-pressed extra virgin olive oil made by traditional methods.

Olive oil – the MUFA of all salad dressings

Olive oil is one of the most studied and lauded of the vegetable oils. Its benefits were highlighted by Ancel Keys when he promoted the Mediterranean diet in the 1950s and 60s as a result of his Seven Countries Study. Keys used the study's findings to promote a Mediterranean style diet that was supposedly low in saturated fat and used olive oil instead in an attempt to halt the growing rate of cardiovascular disease in the US. It's one of the main reasons so many people cook with olive oil today. The study has been criticized for poor methodology, including Keys's selection of only countries that suited the outcome he wanted, and using a study cohort during Lent, when their cheese intake would have substantially dropped. A wealth of further studies has cast a shadow over his belief that saturated fats are a major cause of cardiovascular disease. And yet, I do believe he was onto something with promoting olive oil, even if I don't want to cook with it.

Olive oil is made up of the following fatty acids[211] – note that a range is given, as many different factors can affect the overall balance:

Fatty acid	Structure*	Percentage
Oleic acid	18:1n9 omega 9 MUFA	55–83%
Palmitic acid	16:0 saturated	7.5–20%
Linoleic acid	18:2n6 omega 6 PUFA	3.5–21%
Stearic acid	18:0 saturated	0.5–5%
Palmitoleic acid	16:1n7 omega 7 MUFA	0.3–3.5%
α–linolenic acid	18:3n3 omega 3 PUFA	0–0.9%
Arachidic acid	20:0 saturated	0–0.6%
Eicosenoic acid	20:1n9 omega 9 MUFA	0–0.4%
Margaric acid	17:0 saturated	0–0.3%
Heptadecenoic acid	17:1 MUFA	0–0.3%
Behenic acid	22:0 saturated	0–0.2%
Lignoceric acid	24:0 saturated	0–0.2%
Myristic acid	14:0 saturated	0–0.05%

* For those of you interested in chemical structure: the numerical symbol in the Structure column refers to the number of carbon atoms, followed (after the colon) by the number of double carbon bonds (kinks) and then the position of the first one. So oleic acid has 18 carbon atoms in its chain, with just 1 double carbon bond (making it a MUFA) at the 9th carbon atom (making it an omega 9 fatty acid).

So olive oil is largely a monounsaturated fatty acid, with a substantial saturated fatty acid portion (palmitic acid), and an often equally substantial portion of an omega 6 polyunsaturated fatty acid (linoleic acid) – which is why it is a little more stable to heat than sunflower oil, for example, but still unwise to heat for very long.

Oleic acid, which makes up at least half, and sometimes most, of olive oil, has been credited with a great many benefits, including preventing ulcerative colitis,[212] breast cancer[213] and cardiovascular disease. A 2014 meta-analysis collated the results of 42 studies, which included a total of 841,211 people whose dietary intake of a variety of MUFAs, including oleic acid, was measured, alongside various indicators of health status. Those with the highest intake of oleic acid from olive oil had 11% reduction in death from any cause, a 12% reduction in death from a cardiovascular event, 17% fewer strokes and 9% fewer cardiovascular events than those with the lowest. People with a high intake of MUFAs other than oleic acid didn't seem to enjoy this protection.[214]

Olive oil polyphenols

In addition to the lipids in olive oil, there are a great many other exciting and exotic compounds with impressive health benefits. The most abundant of these are polyphenols, a vast group of interactive plant chemicals that provide protection and colour. They are anti-inflammatory, anti-bacterial, anti-oxidant and often directly anti-cancer, and you find them in fruit, vegetables and throughout the plant kingdom. They are the pigments that absorb some colours from the light spectrum and reflect others, and so provide your food with its rainbow hues. Olive oil, especially when unfiltered, has over 100 different types of phenols.

One of these, secoiridoid, is unique to the oleaceae family, and is noticeable by its bitter taste. The more bitter the olive or olive oil, the more secoiridoid, and so the more health giving properties, it contains.[215] Secoiridoids such as oleocanthal and oleuropein have been studied for their anti-cancer activity. They have been shown to inhibit cancer development at both initiation and progression phases, as well as being able to prevent proliferation and trigger cell death in cancer cells. Some studies have also suggested a protective role for DNA.[216]

So drizzling a little strong-tasting, cold-pressed, unfiltered olive oil on your lunch or dinner might be a habit you want to adopt.

Or you may want to go a step further and get hold of one of the by-products of olive oil pressing: olive mill wastewater. Not the most glamorous sounding of products, but OMWW has been found to contain over 20 times more polyphenols than olive oil itself, and actually looks a little like wine. Recent studies have shown it to be effective against colon cancer cells[217] and to have a strong anti-angiogenic effects in endothelial cells – which means it can prevent tumours creating their own blood supply and even destroy any connection it has already made to the blood supply.

The most abundant polyphenol in OMWW is hydroxytyrosol (HT), but there seems to be something special about the combination of HT with the other phenols, as OMWW has been shown to be more powerfully anti-angiogenic than HT on its own.[218] Sorry – lots of long, chemical words all in one place. In plainer English, there's a substance in the wastewater from olive mills that stops cancer in its tracks, and it works even better when the whole liquid is drunk than when the substance is extracted.

This happens a lot in nature – so that it can sometimes be useful to concentrate a nutrient, but actually the true magic happens when nutrients work together as a family, in a whole food.

There is also a substantial amount of polyphenols in olive leaves, in particular the anti-inflammatory, anti-viral oleuropein, which has been shown to protect against high blood pressure, Alzheimer's disease and Parkinson's disease, as well as cancer, HIV and non-alcoholic fatty liver disease.[219] So you can get olive leaf extract in various powdered and liquid forms to supplement your diet.

Polyphenols aren't oils, but I couldn't resist mentioning them in this chapter as they are such very special nutrients. Their anti-inflammatory nature and special relationship with light reminds me of the next category of lipids I'd like to explore: essential fatty acids.

PUFAs, EFAs and sunlight

Remember that EFAs are the polyunsaturated fatty acids that are essential to your diet – i.e. you can't manufacture them, you have to get them from food. Your cells and liver have the ability to make oleic acid, for example, if they need to and have the right resources, but you can only get EFAs from your diet.

They take their place in every cell in your body as part of the phospholipid membrane (cell wall). They are also used to make a group of substances called eicosanoids, which are responsible for creating or calming inflammation; we'll look at this more closely in the next chapter. Some eicosanoids (called prostaglandins) are also involved in other activities, such as triggering labour in pregnancy.

EFAs are part of a collection of omega 3 and omega 6 polyunsaturated fatty acids (PUFAs):

Omega 3	Omega 6
α–linolenic acid (ALA) – 18:3n3	Linoleic acid (LA) – 18:2n6
Eicosapentanoic acid (EPA) – 20:5n3	Gamma-linolenic acid (GLA) – 18:3n6
Docosahexaenoic acid (DHA) – 22:6n3	Dihomo–gamma-linoleic acid (DGLA) – 20:3n6
	Arachidonic acid (AA) – 20:4n6

Remember that the first number indicates the length of the carbon chain, so these are all long chain fatty acids. The second number shows how many wiggles, or double carbon bonds, there are. And the final number shows the position of the first wiggle, which makes it either an omega 3 or an omega 6 fatty acid.

The second number shows not just how wiggly the structure is, but also how many double carbon bonds there are – and wherever there are double carbon bonds, there are magical subatomic particles called pi electrons. Pi electrons carry an electromagnetic charge that is essential to the bonding of the carbon atoms. They are also, like many plant polyphenols and other compounds, able to absorb light. This is interesting not just from the perspective of providing colour, but also in terms of harnessing energy directly from the sun.

Biologists have studied this in plants for many years, but there is a possibility that humans are also able to be energised directly by light.

The chlorophyll that makes plants green is best known for its role in photosynthesis, which is how plants get their energy from sunlight. Light can be measured either as a wave, or as a particle called a photon. The electrons in chlorophyll, on meeting photons from light with longer wavelengths, absorb the energy from those photons. These electrons are now in a high energy state, and the plant uses that energy to split water (H_2O) into hydrogen and oxygen. Interestingly, the polyphenol beta-carotene, which makes carrots orange and can be found in many plants, has nine double carbon bonds in its structure, and also seems to trap longer wavelengths of light.

Even more fascinatingly, scientists have studied the ability of the double carbon bonds in polyunsaturated fatty acids to do the very same thing, with different PUFAs able to trap different frequencies of light. UV light, for example, can be trapped by the omega 6 linolenic acid.[220] If you consider that each cell in your body has a membrane that is PUFA-rich, what better way to bring energy to the very place you need it – for chemical reactions and communication at cellular level.

This is truly groundbreaking research. It means we may be nourished by light as much as we are by food, air and water. It means light provides so much more than vitamin D and something to see by – plus it knocks counting food calories forever out of the ballpark.

Feel the lipid love

So the take home message here is: don't be scared of fats. They are your friends. All of them. Well, maybe keep an eye on the artificial trans fats, but the rest of them are all super important in your life. As usual, it's getting the balance right that's important: small amounts of saturated fats alongside moderate amounts of raw, cold-pressed oils, making sure you have good levels of omega 3 fatty acids – especially EPA and DHA. This may mean you consider eating more oily fish or taking a good quality fish oil, or you may choose to supplement with a vegan DHA and EPA supplement.

You might want to take a moment to revisit chapters 3 and 4 to remind yourself why fat free diets are not the best approach to losing weight, and how too many refined carbohydrates and sugars is more likely to get you piling on the pounds.

Your liver and lymph can, however, get overloaded by too many fats, so if you are noticeably sluggish, nauseous, itchy or lumpy, this could be something to consider. Sometimes it might be helpful to substantially reduce fats for a short time, to give your system a break, but I've never seen this be helpful to do for long periods of time. Your fatty acid friends are just too important for your physical and cognitive health. Liver support is never a waste of time and can be really helpful here, and there is more on how to do this in chapter 18. If you suspect you're not digesting and absorbing fats well (perhaps your stools float and are greasy), then sprinkling lecithin granules on meals may help with this, as they will emulsify the fats and help you break them down.

So make friends with fats and treat them with respect.

Reflection time

- *What oils do you use for cooking? Dressings?*
- *How often do you fry foods? Are their times when you could grill, steam or bake instead?*

Action plan

- *Find out where you can get good quality, cold pressed oils to use in dressings.*
- *Experiment with coconut oil and ghee (unless you are vegan), and see which you prefer.*

Recipes

- ***Salad dressings** – p.273*
  Salad dressings are the easiest thing in the world to make, and are so much nicer (and better quality!) homemade than out of a bottle. Here are a few ideas to get you going.

- ***Pesto** – p.275*
  The most versatile of pastes. Stir into (gluten-free) pasta and risotto dishes, swirl into soups, or mix with yoghurt for a superquick dip.

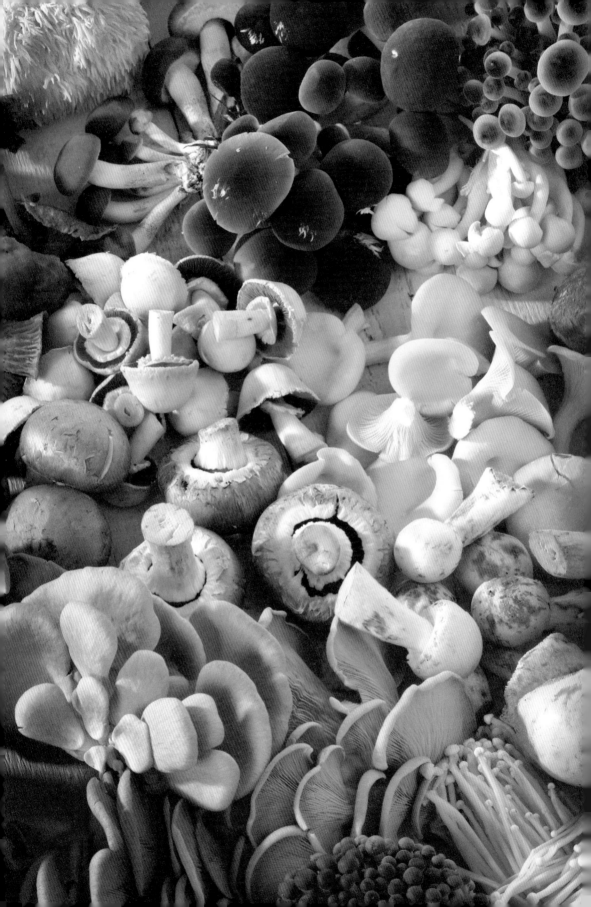

Chapter 16

Inflammation, chronic disease and your immune system

We constantly hear and talk about boosting the immune system – but what does this actually mean? And what is your immune system, anyway?

Your immune system is quite a vast network that involves various sorts of cells called leukocytes, or *white blood cells*, each with their own abilities and roles. Plus a whole series of processes and substances that trigger and counter inflammation.

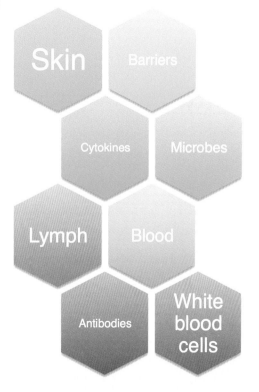

However, before you even get to that layer of immune support, you have various *membranes* and barriers to help prevent pathogens from entering specific areas. So you have your *skin*, which allows tiny particles through, like magnesium, but not larger particles, like water (which can only get into the outer layer). Your skin also produces *antimicrobial peptides* (AMPs) that help keep pathogenic bacteria and fungal infections at bay, and help with wound healing and the processes of inflammation. Some toxic chemicals are too large to enter, but others are small enough, unfortunately.

Then there is your *gut wall*, with its epithelial layer of tissue and mucous secretions that help your gut to be similarly selective. Food that has been fully broken down to amino acids, simple sugars and fatty acids can enter; undigested food particles and pathogens cannot.

Oh, and let's not forget your *microbiome*, the bacteria and other microbes at the front line of your immune response, guarding, protecting and relaying information to your leukocytes. They populate all your mucous membranes and your skin, providing an additional physical and functional barrier.

Going deeper, you have membranes and walls protecting internal organs, and for one of your most crucial organs, you have the *blood brain barrier*. This is formed by endothelial cells with tight junctions (i.e. closely packed together, like those in the small intestine), which will let some substances through, but protect the brain from as much as it can. This activity is assisted by some of your brain cells, including *neurons and microglia*. If there is any damage to the blood brain barrier, a mass of microglia will rush to the site and can quickly repair it.

In pregnancy, there is also the *placental barrier*, which adds an additional line of protection for the developing baby.

Then in your *blood stream* and *connective tissue* you will find some of the leukocytes mentioned above, also known as white blood cells (WBCs). Some of these are continually circulating, looking out for things that aren't supposed to be there, while others are triggered when they're needed. They have various jobs, including clearing up dead cells, neutralising and eating up infections and even parasites, helping to calm down inflammation and triggering other immune activity.

Shadowing your system of blood vessels are similar channels of *lymph vessels*. The fluid in your lymph vessels has been drained from your tissue and bloodstream, and contains toxins and waste. It is eventually dripped back into your bloodstream, and then carried to your liver and kidneys to be processed and filtered. Every now and then, your lymph passes through clusters of *lymph nodes*, perhaps under your arm, around your groin or in your neck or chest. These lymph nodes are jam-packed with certain types of white blood cell called lymphocytes, whose job is to clean up as much as it can before the lymph enters the blood. Your *spleen*, an organ tucked away in the left hand side of your ribcage, performs a similar role as lymph passes through it, like a giant lymph node.

All of these systems, and more, comprise your immune system. They work together in complex ways, many of which are still being explored. Despite their complexity, there are some simple and specific ways that you can use nutrition to support their work.

We've already looked at how to maintain healthy epithelial membranes and their tight junctions and keep other types of tissue healthy too, so all of this information will be useful for keeping the barriers and membranes involved in good shape. We've also looked at how to keep your microbiota in a balance that contributes to your health and immunity. In this and the next chapter I'd like to focus on two more key areas:

- How to regulate white blood cell (leukocyte) activity
- How to help your body regulate inflammation

Leukocytes – the Luke Skywalkers of the immune system?

Perhaps not a completely accurate analogy, but your leukocytes, like the Jedi of Star Wars mythology, are there for your protection. They are also known as white blood cells (which may be confusing in this analogy, being of course the colour of the Stormtroopers, but let's not take this too literally!).[221]

You have five different types of white blood cell: neutrophils, eosinophils, basophils, monocytes and lymphocytes. They all have different and overlapping jobs, and interact in various ways.

Some of them continually roam your inner galaxy like a frontline guard, acting against anything that seems to be problematic. These form what is called your *innate immune system*, together with your epithelial barriers (skin, gut, blood brain barrier etc.), and certain types of proteins like the AMPs described above. Others are more like special task forces that are activated in response to specific threats that your body has learnt to recognize. They probably overwhelmed your innate immune system at some point, and your body has created a memory of this. These white blood cells include most of your lymphocytes, and are described as *your adaptive immune system*, as they adapt to new knowledge and experience.

There are several different types of lymphocyte, most of them T cells, and some B cells. While B cells and T cells are both produced in your Bone marrow, T cells mature in the Thymus in your chest. They are both stored in your spleen (alongside your monocytes).

There are additional lymphocytes called Natural Killer cells, best known for destroying cancer cells and viruses. These differ in that they belong to the innate immune system, and so are continually on the prowl. While we're back on the innate immune system, monocytes deserve a special mention. When a monocyte enters the tissue where it is needed, it turns into a macrophage, the Pac Man of the immune system, eating up dead cells and pathogens, and helping to regulate inflammatory processes. There are hundreds of billions of macrophages munching away on debris in your body right now. Monocytes can also turn into dendritic cells, which are involved in instructing the adaptive immune system (e.g. T cells) what to attack.

White blood cell counts – what do they mean?

Doctors will sometimes look at levels of white blood cells in blood tests. Both a low and a high reading can indicate that your immune system is or has been working harder than usual. A high WBC count is called leukocytosis. This may indicate that your body is fighting infection, or that there is inflammation or an allergic reaction present, or a stress or trauma. It is also one of the symptoms of leukaemia, characterized by (sometimes extremely) excessive levels of abnormal leucocytes. Some medications can elevate your WBC count, including corticosteroids, lithium and beta-agonists such as Ventolin inhalers. Sometimes WBCs are higher in the late stages of pregnancy as well.

A low count is called leukopaenia. This can also be caused by infections, plus there is a long list of additional associations. These include vitamin B12 or folic acid deficiency, liver disease, an enlarged spleen, cancer, bone marrow disease, HIV and more. Leukopaenia can also be caused by chemotherapy, radiotherapy, anti-epilepsy drugs, the anti-psychotic clozapine, immunosuppressive medication given mostly to people who have received transplants, as well as other medications.

In either case, you want to be making sure that your body is able to produce plenty of healthy leucocytes, both the innate ones that are always on duty, and the adaptive ones, as and when you need them – and then reduce them as appropriate too.

What to eat for healthy leucocyte production

There really are too many nutrients involved to mention them all, but here are some particularly crucial ones: vitamins A, C and D, selenium and zinc.

Vitamin A

Retinoic acid, the active form of vitamin A, is essential for the healthy development of white blood cells. It helps T cells, for example, to evolve into the specialised form required right now to counter the threat your body has just identified, and attach to the tissue where they are most needed.

Numerous studies have shown that vitamin A deficient children are more likely to get infectious diseases such as measles and diarrhoea, as well as weakened, degenerating lymphoid tissue, such as the spleen, thymus and lymph nodes.[222]

Incidentally, retinoic acid provides a great deal of protection for the blood brain barrier where its integrity is affected by inflammation.[223]

The best food sources of vitamin A are liver and eggs, but you can also get a precursor to vitamin A, beta-carotene, from carrots, squash, sweet potatoes and green leafy vegetables.

Vitamin C

Ascorbic acid, or vitamin C, has been shown to support the activity of your innate immune function.[224] White blood cells contain a high concentration of ascorbic acid, which is believed to help them in their job of tearing apart and devouring pathogens.[225] This is why fruit, salad, raw herbs and raw green leafy vegetables (including salad leaves) are essential to your diet.

Vitamin D

White blood cells have vitamin D receptors, so we know vitamin D is important to their activity. It has long been noted that vitamin D deficiency goes hand in hand with poor health, and a 2013 review of the science gathered so far found:

"Adequate vitamin D status seems to be protective against musculoskeletal disorders (muscle weakness, falls, fractures), infectious diseases, autoimmune diseases, cardiovascular disease, type 1 and type 2 diabetes mellitus, several types of cancer, neurocognitive dysfunction and mental illness, and other diseases, as well as infertility and adverse pregnancy and birth outcomes. Vitamin D deficiency/insufficiency is associated with all-cause mortality."[226]

Monocytes, for example, produce AMPs (antimicrobial peptides) as part of your immune response to bacteria. One of these is called cathelicidin antimicrobial peptide (or CAMP). Its production is triggered by vitamin D,[227] and in one study, supplementing 4000IU of vitamin D daily led to a dramatic increase in CAMP production where it was most needed after just three weeks. The study involved people with atopic eczema, and CAMP levels in their skin multiplied by around eight in affected areas, and by just a little where there was no eczema.[228]

We also know that vitamin D can directly influence the activation of T cells and dendritic cells,[229] and are learning more every day.

It's very difficult to get enough vitamin D from diet, and our main source of this vitamin has always been sunshine. You absorb UVB rays into your skin, and a cholesterol-based substance converts them into vitamin D. These UVB rays are only available to you when the sun is over 50 degrees above the horizon: i.e. never in a Northern European winter. The sun only starts to reach the right height in late spring and then dwindles again in the autumn. Early morning sunshine in the summer probably won't suffice either. You need as much skin exposure as possible in sunshine when it's high enough in the sky (when your shadow is shorter than you) for around 20 minutes depending on a number of factors – but stop before you start going pink. People with darker skin may need longer, and be aware that various things interfere with UVB absorption, including sunscreen, clothing, glass, pollution, clouds and rain.

UVB – isn't that dangerous? It seems that the more vitamin D you make from sunshine, the more mechanisms you trigger which protect your DNA from sun damage.[230] So don't burn, but don't be scared of a little sunshine either.

Selenium

Selenium plays an integral role in your immune function, from helping T cells to multiply and develop, to regulating your macrophage activity. If you are deficient in selenium and contract a mild flu or even the Coxsackie virus (associated with hand, foot and mouth disease and viral meningitis), the virus is able to mutate to a highly pathogenic strain.[231] So you really don't want to be low in selenium. This is easy to avoid, with just three or four brazil nuts daily.

Zinc

Zinc is also crucial to the number, function and balance of practically all your leukocytes, and so deficiency will have severe effects on how well your immune system works.[232] In one trial, supplementation of 45mg of zinc gluconate daily very effectively reduced the number of infections in a group of 50 men and women between 55-87 years of age.[233] In another, 10mg of zinc daily almost halved the incidence of lower respiratory infection in a group of 298 toddlers aged 6-35 months (compared to 311 in the control group) after just four months.[234]

Pumpkin seeds are particularly zinc-rich, but you can find it in all nuts and seeds, and the zinc is more bioavailable from them if they are soaked overnight. Chickpeas, lamb and chicken are also good. So make sure you have at least one of these in your daily diet.

The inflammatory cascade – an impressive firework display

When I hear the word cascade, I think of bursts of silver, pink, purple, gold and green in the night sky, one after the other, until the heavens seem filled with showering blooms of fireworks. When we talk about cascades in biochemistry, we are describing an effect where an event triggers a response, which triggers other responses, which may then trigger further responses. It's an escalation of events, which means that your body can respond in many exciting and resourceful ways from perhaps a single trigger.

In the inflammatory cascade, your white blood cells are activated in response to a situation as described above. They release a host of protein structures called cytokines. Pro-inflammatory cytokines call for and activate more white blood cells. Which produce more cytokines etc.

So if you cut yourself on something covered with pathogenic bacteria, your body does what it can to deal with the situation swiftly, and from a number of angles. Firstly remember inflammation in itself is not a bad thing – in fact it can be life-saving; it's a critical part of your immune system response to injury, trauma, infection and stagnation. Wherever your body perceives a threat to health, it calls the emergency services, and it's inflammation that fast tracks them with their lights flashing and sirens wailing. White blood cells, cytokines and other substances released cascade, crowd round the area and sort it out. You might feel this, at least to begin with, as an internal pyrotechnic display, with fiery activity and pain. But when their jobs are done, the fireworks calm down and all becomes quiet again.

Sometimes, however, the cascade seems heavy handed compared to the actual situation. If your immune system is already in a state of alert, then it doesn't take much to trigger it to a full, overblown response.

This is why just a few grains of pollen might end up with your eyes and nose streaming, or having a cat sit on your lap might give you an asthma attack.

Such a response may be an indication that your inflammatory cascade hasn't quite calmed down from the last time – or the time before that. So it might be over sensitive to new triggers. Sometimes its very activity, if prolonged, might even cause damage to the tissue around it, which then keeps you stuck in your cascade of reactions. This may be the case in autoimmune diseases such as rheumatoid arthritis, SLE (lupus), MS and psoriasis (see below).

Inflammation therefore becomes an issue when it fails to calm down – when it becomes chronic. A chronic condition is simply one that has been around for a while (technically, three months or more). It may be a slow burner, it may have flare-ups every now and again, but it's there, simmering away for months if not years. All the while using up energy and resources that you might want for digestion, fertility, bone strength, memory, concentration and more.

So it's important that you support your body's ability to regulate its inflammatory activity as much as possible. In the next chapter there's a collection of foods and nutrients that actively help with this. So read on for some practical ways you can support your immune system.

Reflection time

- *How many times have you cut, bruised, sprained, broken something or been ill, and then healed?*

Action plan

- *Practise gratitude for your miraculous body! Thank it often for doing such an amazing job of keeping you alive.*

Recipe

- *These dishes contain specific nutrients to help you make leukocytes, the white blood cells so important to your immune system.*
    - ***Roasted squash with pumpkin seeds and rosemary*** *– p.259*
      Serve it with salad and a little quinoa, or fish/meat and steamed greens.
    - ***Mighty egg salad*** *– p.268*

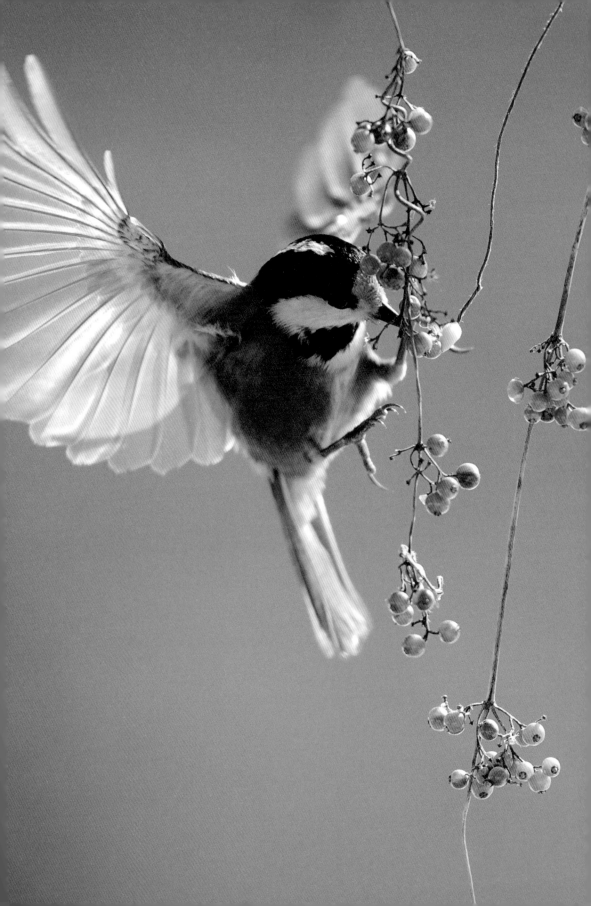

Chapter 17

Strengthening your immune system

Helping your body get back to its routines

So that's a lot of chemicals and complex cascades of activity. If you feel like you are drowning in all of this, then the first thing you need to do is step back and take a look at the bigger picture. Do you have any kind of chronic inflammation or long-term illness? Do you feel your body is using up a lot of energy managing a situation rather than resolving it?

Boosting your immune system might include helping your body to make enough good quality white blood cells. In cases of chronic disease and conditions, it also means a great deal of anti-inflammatory support; both avoiding things that trigger inflammation, and including anti-inflammatory nutrients. We'll look at foods for all of this in this chapter.

By working holistically – ensuring that you are putting both general and specific support in where you personally need it – you can often help your body get back to good health, and its usual routines. In the process, you may need to address at least one if not all of the following:

- Resolve, remove or reduce the reason inflammation is there to begin with (stressors, irritants etc. – see below)
- Calm and support your adrenals (see chapter 10)
- Keep blood sugar stable (see chapter 5)
- Ensure you have enough of the right kind of essential fatty acids for anti-inflammatory eicosanoids (see below)
- Increase your intake of natural anti-inflammatories and immune system modulators (see below)
- Ensure you are generally hydrated and nourished enough for everything to be working properly
- Resolve stagnation and get everything flowing again (see chapters 6, 7, 18, 20)

First let's have a look at the some of the ways you might be able to resolve or reduce any irritants or stressors that may be continually provoking an immune response.

How to stop poking the wound

You wouldn't expect a cut or a sore ankle to heal if you kept prodding and poking it. The same is true for all inflammatory and immune responses. You have to minimise anything that might be aggravating the situation.

Work/life/relationship stress – sometimes it may help (or even be essential) to just walk away from it all. But first ask yourself:

- will this just throw up a whole load of new stresses?
- is the current stress a repeated pattern that you might just take with you?
- are there any patterns, behaviours or responses you can start to address in yourself to make the situation more enjoyable and better functioning for all concerned?
- are there any emotions from old events that you have either suppressed or clung to, that you can now work to release?
- is there anything you can do or say to help restore the situation to one that is more balanced and nourishing?

Chemical stress – this may include pollution from:

- your environment, be that cars, aeroplanes, factories or crop-spraying;
- your food, where pesticides and fungicides have been used, and from other toxins in the soil;
- your household products, including cleaning products, air fresheners, paints, varnishes and glues;
- your personal hygiene and cosmetic products, such as shampoo, hair products, shower gel and soap, moisturiser, deodorant/anti-perspirant, make-up and perfume.

None of us live in an oxygen bubble, but you may be able to reduce this chemical load considerably with your shopping habits. Buy organic products where you can, not just to reduce your own immediate exposure to toxins, but also to help reduce the amount of harmful chemicals going into the water, air and soil. Choose more natural household and personal hygiene products, again that are friendlier to both you and the environment.

If that's too expensive an option, there are many fabulous and effective options you can make yourself from cheap ingredients that you may even already have in your cupboard. Lemon juice, bicarbonate of soda and spirit vinegar, for example, have a multitude of uses around the home. You can make great toothpaste from coconut oil and bicarbonate of soda, and there are whole books and websites devoted to making your own hair, face and body products.

Food stress – there will be some foods or nutrients that your digestive system sometimes or always struggles with. That list will be fairly unique to you, and you may be able to reduce that list by working on your digestive processes. Common food stressors and irritants include:

- Nightshade family – potatoes, tomatoes, bell peppers, aubergines – due to the inflammatory alkaloids they contain
- Gluten in wheat and wheat products, and in smaller amounts in rye and barley
- Casein (a protein) and lactose (a sugar) in dairy products
- Caffeine and xanthines in tea, coffee, chocolate, cola etc.
- Alcohol
- Sugar
- Citrus fruit
- Grains
- Pulses – e.g. peas, beans, lentils
- Fructose and fructans – e.g. in fruit, onions, garlic, chicory, artichokes and beetroot
- Polyols – including the sweeteners sorbitol and xylitol
- Onions and garlic
- Cruciferous vegetables – e.g. broccoli, cauliflower, cabbage, kale, Brussels sprouts
- Allergy triggers e.g. peanuts, shellfish, eggs
- Processed meats
- Artificial additives

This doesn't mean you should avoid every food on the list! There may be some that you are aware are problematic, or you may not have noticed an issue with any of them. However, it may still be worth investigating if any of these are creating digestive issues and inflammation. This sometimes isn't as easy as it sounds.

Elimination diets were brought about to help. Essentially, you eliminate all suspected foods until you feel nothing is irritating you. (This stage can be tough!) Then you bring back each food or food group one by one, assessing each time what your body's response is.

Sometimes this is a really useful process to go through. However, it has its limits. You don't always have an immediate response to the food you eat. It can take hours, or sometimes days, for you to feel an effect. Bloating after breakfast might be due to something in your breakfast, something you ate the night before or something from two days before. Or it may be more to do with how you ate, what time you ate or even something unrelated to food. So sometimes it can take a few months of meticulous food/mood/symptom diaries to figure out some of what may be causing irritation.

Or there may be a low key effect that your nervous system isn't really alerting you to. So you don't have any obvious symptoms at all. However, after years, this low level of irritation can insidiously build up and contribute to ill health.

This difficulty in pinpointing offending foods has led to the rise of food intolerance tests. These, however, vary widely in their approach and reliability, and none are bullet proof.

For most people, I suggest slow, leisurely elimination diets, as a playful and curious exploration of what your body feels best eating. I additionally recommend mindful eating, as this helps you become more aware of what your body wants and doesn't want, likes and doesn't like, right now in this moment. Practise being intuitive, and this will help guide you calmly through what can otherwise become a stressful minefield.

As and when you identify foods that are problematic, adopt a "now/not now" approach, rather than a "my life is over, I'll never be able to enjoy X again" approach. For example, one of my known stressors is sugar. If I eat too much sugar, or consistently eat sugar – or if other things in my life are creating stress and I have sugar on top of that – then I often get skin reactions. These might show up as dry, flaky areas, or sometimes red itchy patches, usually on various parts of my face or hands. I could decide to give up sugar completely, but that approach feels too stern and punishing for me. It feels that it might disrupt my Earth Element just as much as having too much sugar. I'd also just think about sugar all the time!

So instead, if I am in a situation where I want or am offered something sugary, I check in to how my body feels and make an assessment:

- Will I actually fully enjoy this, or is it just the thought of it that seems appealing?
- Is my body in a good position to handle this right now?
- Does it feel nourishing on *every* level?

If the answer is yes to all 3, then I say a resounding yes, and savour each morsel, guilt-free and relaxed. If I get a possible or definite no to any of these questions, I generally (but not always!) politely decline.

Having this approach has definitely helped me reduce my sugar intake enormously. I can go for days, weeks and sometimes months without any refined sugars at all, and sometimes with extremely low or zero unrefined sugars too. No willpower required!

Emotions around this can sometimes be tricky, as we have already explored. You may be familiar with those voices complaining:

- "But I deserve a treat!"
- "Why can't I eat normally like everyone else?"
- "It's not fair!"

Or conversely:

- "I don't deserve that, I haven't been good enough,"
- "I'm too fat already."
- "People will think I'm a greedy pig if I eat that."

I have found it's good to acknowledge such thoughts, thank them for their point of view, and then remind myself they're not the only voices to listen to. There are also the ones from my body saying things like:

- "I'm not sure I want to deal with a sugar hit/crash right now,"
- "I'm going to feel a lot more energised and nourished by X"
- "I'm in a really good place right now, I don't actually need anything to feel good or give me more energy."

Why are so many people now gluten-free or dairy free?

Gluten is a family of protein structures found in larger quantities in wheat, spelt, kamut and other wheat varieties, and in smaller quantities in rye and barley. Oats contain a form that is not usually a problem, but oat production means that oats are also often contaminated with a little gluten from wheat products.

When partially digested gluten reaches your small intestine, it has the potential to cause damage and inflammation there.

Gluten has not always been part of the human diet, and we seem to be in various stages of adapting to it. For some people, eating gluten can be extremely serious, causing such damage to the villi lining the small intestine that it severely affects absorption of other nutrients, as well as triggering an immune response that can often be debilitating. This is known as Coeliac disease. With others, gluten may trigger an inflammatory response that can feel mild, moderate or severe but doesn't damage the gut lining or have the same long-term impact as Coeliac disease. This is known as gluten intolerance. Symptoms can include pains, spasms, bloating, constipation, diarrhoea, fatigue and headaches, and may be immediate or hours later. So sometimes it's difficult to make the connection.

With dairy products, there is a similar protein called casein. The casein in some types of dairy is easier to digest than others, which is why some people find sheep and goat dairy more digestible. The casein in Jersey and Guernsey cows is also gentler, and you may have heard this referred to as A2 milk.

Another potential issue in all dairy products is lactose, a milk sugar. You most likely produced good amounts of lact*ase* in the first couple of years of your life, as this is the enzyme that helps to break down lactose in breast milk. After that, your lactase production may have reduced – or you may be one of those born not making sufficient lactase in the first place. Without being able to break down lactose, all dairy products can cause gut problems, and this is known as lactose intolerance. Fermented dairy products, such as yoghurt, contain lower levels of lactose, so if you find you can tolerate yoghurt better than milk, lactose may be the issue.

Unless you have serious symptoms, or indeed Coeliac disease, it may not be necessary to completely avoid gluten and dairy. However, there is a possibility that these foods may be contributing in part to some of the inflammation in your body, and this can be difficult to measure or pinpoint. So it might be wise to at least experiment with keeping your intake moderate to low.

As long as you have a balanced and varied diet, being gluten or dairy free will not lead to nutrient deficiency – if anything, it may help you absorb nutrients more efficiently. Be wary of gluten-free products however – always read the label before you buy any! Some of them are great, but I find many of them astounding in terms of how many extra sugars and additives there are trying to make up for the gluten. You're usually better off making something yourself. My favourite go-to is gluten-free pancakes, and there is a recipe for these on page 282, in the Recipes section.

Natural anti-inflammatories

Actually the list of anti-inflammatory foods is much longer than the list of potential pro-inflammatories, and a lot of them are pretty delicious too. Below is a list of some of my favourites, together with the primary anti-inflammatory compounds that have been identified in them.

It's worth noting that usually there are a number of anti-inflammatory compounds in each food that work together. This means that it may not be helpful to rely just on, for example, a resveratrol supplement – it may be wiser to find your resveratrol in food, or in food but with a supplement to top up. Topping up with a supplement is worth considering where growing conditions and other factors may limit the amount of that compound in the food. For example, most foods are low in zinc and magnesium these days due to soil depletion – even in organic farming. Also, supermarket varieties of blueberries may be much lower in antioxidants than homegrown or wild varieties.

Anti-inflammatory food	Example anti-inflammatory compound
Turmeric NB turmeric's anti-inflammatory compounds are difficult to absorb, but are made more bioavailable by adding black pepper and a little oil	Curcuminoids (e.g. curcumin)
Nuts and seeds (especially pumpkin seeds), chickpeas, chicken, lamb	Zinc
Green leafy vegetables, green superfood powders, nuts, seeds	Magnesium[235, 236]
Blueberries, cranberries, bilberries, blackcurrants, grapes, red cabbage, red onions, cocoa, cinnamon	Proanthocyanidins
Blueberries, cranberries, bilberries, blackcurrants, grapes, red cabbage, cocoa	Resveratrol
Onions, green leafy vegetables, cruciferous vegetables, dark berries and cherries	Quercetin
Ginger	Gingerol, zingerone
Brown seaweed, e.g. kombu, wakame, bladderwrack	Fucoidan
Green tea, cinnamon, cocoa, acai berries, broad beans	Catechin
Oily fish (or fish oil supplements, or vegan EPA/DHA supplements)	EPA, DHA

So I'm thinking a chickpea, wakame, and spinach stir-fry with ginger, turmeric and black pepper. Or gently grilled salmon with a pumpkin seed crust served with broccoli and a broad bean mash. Or perhaps mixed berry and cinnamon pancakes made with brown rice flour and coconut milk.

Remember that these foods, too, have their appropriate and inappropriate times. For example, a bowl of wild foraged blackberries might be refreshing in the late summer and will provide a burst of anti-inflammatory nutrients – but frozen blackberries (even when defrosted) in the middle of winter might challenge a weak digestion and cause more inflammation that they actually help to reduce.

Omega 3 and 6 oils have garnered a lot of flattering publicity in recent decades, and I'm not about to buck that trend. But there are a few caveats that it's important to be aware of:

1. **You need to have the right ratio, which is probably about 1:1, i.e. roughly equal amounts.**[237]

   Omega 3 fatty acids and some of the omega 6s can be used to make anti-inflammatory eicosanoids. These are the substances triggered by many other anti-inflammatories, so without them, it's hard to cool inflammation down. Some of the omega 6 fatty acids, however, are used to make pro-inflammatory eicosanoids.

   So in theory, if your diet contains a lot of omega 6s and not many omega 3s, then it may be harder to switch off inflammatory processes, and therefore be a factor in chronic disease.[238]

   Note that a diet rich in margarines, vegetables oils, nuts and seeds (except flax and chia seeds), is likely to contain much higher levels of omega 6 than omega 3. A number of studies also show that livestock fed on natural pastures is likely to produce meat, dairy and eggs that contain healthier ratios than their largely grain-fed counterparts. In fact, Western diets have been estimated to contain up to 25 times more omega 6 than omega 3 fatty acids.[239]

2. **You need to have the right types of omega 3.**

   Remember that the omega 3 fatty acids in flax seeds, chia seeds and all other plant sources are in a "parent" form called alpha-linolenic acid that you can't necessarily use to make anti-inflammatory eicosanoids. You first have to convert it to another form of omega 3 called EPA. This is possible with the help of enzymes such as delta-6-desaturase (D-6-D), so you can absolutely produce EPA on a standard vegan diet. However, humans are really quite inefficient at doing so, and therefore can't usually rely on this to produce optimum EPA levels.

   This is why fish and fish oil can be so important. The EPA – and similarly anti-inflammatory DHA – are ready formed and in good quantities.

   Sadly, fish consumption isn't without problems of its own. The levels of heavy metal and other toxicity in both wild and farmed fish is really unacceptable, both for the fish and for our consumption of it, and in addition, it's becoming harder to maintain sustainable stocks. Plus, of course, eating fish is just not an option for vegans and vegetarians. (If you think of yourself as a "vegetarian who eats fish", then technically you are a pescetarian.)

   Fortunately you can now get vegan EPA/DHA supplements that are concentrated extracts of algae, which are plant-like microbes that live in water. This is one of the supplements, together with vitamin B12, that I frequently recommend for people on a vegan diet.

3. **If your liver and lymph are overloaded, you may not be able to process a larger intake of oils.**

   Many fats and oils are transported from the digestive tract to the liver via the lymph first, and then the blood, rather than directly through the blood like the other macronutrients. So the health and flow of your lymphatic system as well as that of your liver may impact on how well your body works with oils.

   If increasing your fat or oil intake leads, for example, to nausea, vomiting, headaches, itchy or lumpy skin, sluggishness or greasy feeling eyes, then you may need to address this. See the next chapter for more on liver health and general flow.

Regulating your leukocyte response

There are many more anti-inflammatory compounds in foods, and continuing studies on their effects. There has also been some research into the effects of foods on your white blood cells, directly regulating their activity.

Chocolate

The rich combination of antioxidants and anti-inflammatories in cocoa has been shown to directly impact white blood cell activity. Cocoa influences the amount of inflammatory substances that are released from macrophages and T helper cells, largely down-regulating their activity.

There have been a number of studies feeding cocoa to growing rats and seeing their lymphocyte balance substantially affected both in the gut and throughout the body, but as far as I am aware, this hasn't been studied in humans yet.

Plus, of course, there is a world of difference between pure cocoa and sugar-laden chocolate bars, drinks and treats, so this is not an excuse to go out and gorge. Raw cacao might have these benefits (at least for rats) – personally I find raw chocolate far too stimulating to have regularly in my diet. However, you may be interested in my Avochocolate mousse recipe (page 288), which uses standard (roasted) cocoa, and so still has some antioxidants but less of a hit.

Ginger

Ginger has long been used as an anti-inflammatory, both in cooking and as a ginger tea. Studies have shown it to be beneficial for rheumatoid arthritis and other chronic conditions.

Scientists have additionally been able to observe how it reduces inflammation in tumour cells.[240]

Rosemary

The same scientists also looked at rosemary's activity, and saw how it reduces specific substances produced by white blood cells.

These substances are called tumour necrosis factor (TNF) and IL-1, and both belong to a large family called cytokines that have jobs ranging from causing inflammation to muscle loss to fever. TNF can both kill cancer cells and cause them to proliferate, depending on the conditions. IL-1 is involved in fever, pain, dilating blood vessels and other inflammatory processes.

Onions and garlic

Onions and garlic are well known for helping to keep colds and flu at bay – but do they really work? Well, it appears they probably do.

Various substances in garlic and onions have been shown to modulate both white blood cells and cytokines, stimulating macrophages, lymphocytes, natural killer (NK) cells, dendritic cells, and eosinophils.[241] In addition, they are "antimicrobial, antiviral, antifungal, anti-protozoal, hepatoprotective, cardioprotective, anti-inflammatory, neuroprotective, anti-amnesic, anticarcinogenic, antimutagenic, antiasthmatic, immunomodulatory, hypolipidemic, anti-hypertensive, anti-diabetic and antioxidant."[242] That's a lot of activity for a simple bulb!

The substances in garlic and onions that make them so beneficial to your immune system are a group of sulphur-containing compounds, including thiosulfinates and allicin. There are similar sulphur compounds in cruciferous vegetables, such as cauliflower, broccoli, Brussels sprouts and cabbage. If you get a lot of smelly wind after eating these, then you can probably blame the sulphur. In fact, some people are severely intolerant to sulphur, and may also experience pain and bloating – quite the opposite effect to the anti-inflammatory, immune-boosting effect we're after here!

A recent study of IBS sufferers noted that they tended to have higher levels of bacteria in their gut that converted certain sulphur compounds (sulphates) to hydrogen sulphide – the rotten egg smell you may sometimes notice in farts. Higher hydrogen sulphide levels could potentially mean more colon pain, constipation, plus more bloating and gas.[243] Working to improve the balance of gut microbes might help those IBS patients that struggle with sulphur.

Incidentally, onions and garlic belong to the most lyrical group of vegetables: the beautifully named liliaceous family. Which includes leeks, chives, aloe and, of course, lilies (although please don't eat these, as they are often toxic to humans and animals).

Medicinal mushrooms

These include oriental mushrooms such as shiitake, reishi and maitake, as well as chaga, cordyceps, coriolus and many more. Their medicinal properties are largely, but not exclusively, due to substances they contain called beta-glucans – so make sure any powdered form you are buying contains these.

Beta-glucans are known to modulate the effect of both the innate and adaptive immune systems – so both the more generalised protection they afford and their ability to target specific diseases and threats. They have also been studied for their anti-tumour abilities, which may be directly related to their effect on the immune system.

For a while it was thought by some that mushrooms were to be avoided by anyone with a candida or other fungal issue, and by anyone with cancer – but it seems, in fact, that the opposite is true. Mushrooms, whether categorized as medicinal or not, can have great benefits for fungal issues and the immune system.

Shiitake are perhaps the best known of medicinal mushrooms, and have been readily obtainable in the UK for many years now. Fresh shiitake mushrooms are making a regular appearance in some supermarkets, and dried, whole shiitake have been reconstituted in oriental soup and stir-fry recipes for several decades.

You can also buy shiitake powder, and other mushroom powders, either on their own or combined with other medicinal mushrooms, sometimes in capsule form to be taken like a supplement. However, I prefer to use all of these in cooking. I stir-fry whole mushrooms into stir-fries and mix the powders into soups, sauces, smoothies and even hot drinks, such as dandelion coffee (check out my Spiced latte recipe on page 292) and cocoa (try my Immune-boosting hot chocolate recipes, also on page 292).

It's not just the oriental mushrooms that have been getting attention. Mushrooms are now known to be the richest food source of a powerful pair of antioxidants: ergothioneine and glutathione.[244] Such compounds protect your skin, heart, blood vessels, nerves and DNA, and so are important in the prevention of conditions such as Alzheimer's, MS, heart attacks and strokes. Porcini mushrooms (or "ceps") have been found to be the best source. Ergothioneine and glutathione levels are maintained even when you cook them, so mushroom soup, grilled mushrooms and baked mushrooms are all excellent sources.

Ceps are also an excellent source of ergosterol, as are reishi, chaga and other medicinal mushrooms. Ergosterol has been studied for its anticancer effects in a number of different cancer cell types, including breast,[245] ovarian,[246] colon,[247, 248] laryngeal[249] and more.

And if that wasn't enough to get you reaching for some mushrooms, their polysaccharide content is excellent food for the microbes in your gut that form such an integral part of your immune system. Which brings us neatly to the next delicacy on our list...

Fermented and prebiotic foods

In taking care of your immune system, you need to be nurturing your microbiome. You may want to revisit chapters 11 and 12 to refresh your memory about what all this entails. With fermented foods (sauerkraut, kefir, kim chi, yoghurt, apple cider vinegar "with mother" etc.), prebiotic foods (fibre-rich) and both probiotic and prebiotic supplements, remember that less is often more. It can be tempting to pile in as much as possible, especially if you have digestive or chronic health issues. However, that is the time when you may need to be most gentle, so start small, and build up gradually and mindfully.

And this brings us to the next piece of the puzzle: how to give your liver the love and support it needs to keep everything processing and flowing through, from the nutrients you digest to the toxins you need to get rid of. Liver support also works best when done sensitively and considerately, so I have called this next chapter Liver Whispering.

Reflection time

- *Consider the levels of pro-inflammatory and anti-inflammatory foods in your current diet – without self-judgement!*
  - *Remember to adopt an attitude of curiosity, humour and self-love when assessing your habits and patterns*

Action plan

- *Choose one food that you suspect is contributing to your overall levels of inflammation, and try substituting it with a gentler alternative.*
  - *For example, if you notice you are eating a lot of bread and think it might be part of why you feel bloated, sluggish or constipated, try swapping sandwiches for soups or salads, and toast for oatcakes or gluten-free pancakes.*

Recipes

- **Superseed crackers with rosemary** – *p.280*
  The most delicious and superquick, gluten-free, nutrient-dense alternative to any other kind of cracker.

- **Gluten-free pancakes** – *p.282*
  I never need an excuse to make pancakes. These are incredibly versatile, a great alternative to bread and crackers. You can add extra egg or protein powder for a more sustaining dish, or spread with houmous or nut butter, or serve with berries and yoghurt, or mushrooms and avocado... my mouth is watering already!

- **Gram flour wraps with mushrooms and avocado** – *p.260*
  This is a really great lunchbox option as well as a quick and tasty dinner, and you can include traditional medicinal mushrooms, like shiitake, or any mushrooms for an anti-inflammatory and leucocyte-boosting effect.

- **Superberry chia pot** – *p.287*
  This is a really well balanced way to increase your berry intake in a snack that's super easy to make and carry around. It's also a great breakfast and dessert, so you can add nutrient-dense, anti-inflammatory foods at any time of day.

- **Immune boosting hot chocolate** – *p.292*
  This feels decadent and comforting while giving your immune system a boost.

- **Tahini sauce** – *p.274*
  This is an excellent alternative to cheese sauce in most recipes, and especially delicious on roasted vegetables.

- **Turmeric paste** – *p.275*
  I keep this in a jar in my cupboard and melt it into soups, sauces and porridge when I cook.

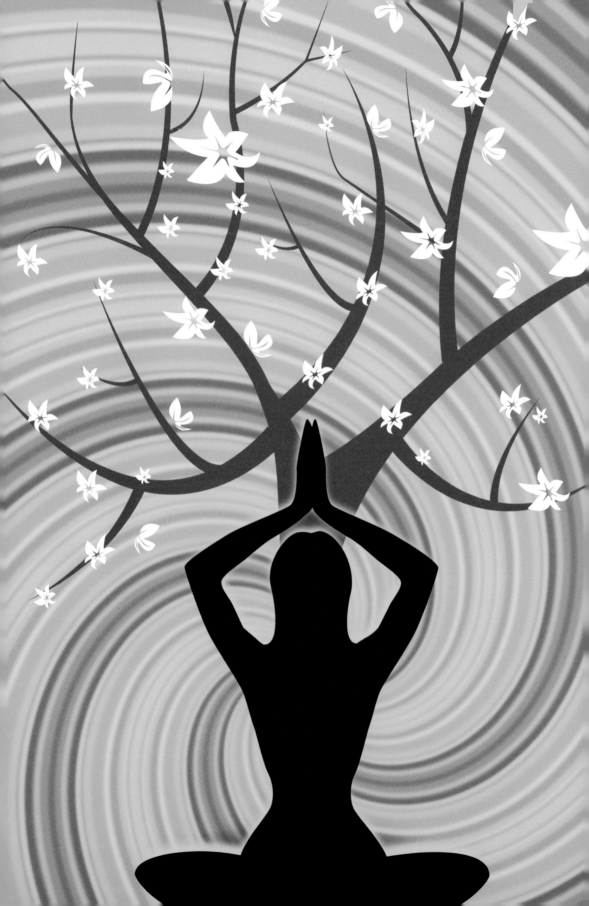

Chapter 18

Liver whispering

For this chapter, I am drawing on both Eastern and Western medicine to describe the functions and attributes of the liver and gallbladder, and they reflect each other beautifully.

The liver and gallbladder (which attaches to and assists the liver) both relate to the Chinese Wood Element. If they are vibrant and working effectively, this will contribute greatly to how well things are flowing through and around your body.

Remember that flow is important for:

- Nourishment: getting fluids and nutrients to where they need to go
- Detoxification: clearing toxins and waste materials
- Messaging systems: such as delivering hormones to their target cells
- Many other aspects of health

You need to be hydrated enough for things to be able to flow, so water is essential. However, stress and inflammation can create tension and blockages that then may prevent that water effectively flowing around the body – so drinking plenty of water is sometimes not enough. Your liver and gallbladder can be considered to be at the hub of all this, and have the ability to either facilitate or block this flow.

Planning and decision making

Your liver is described by Eastern medicine as your Planner. It certainly regulates what happens to the nutrients you absorb, your oestrogen levels, blood sugar levels and more.

It additionally processes fat soluble toxins, many of which come from environmental pollution, and converts them into water soluble substances that are safe to send into the intestines or kidneys to be emptied away. It likes to have a little space to do its many jobs, and can feel irritable when it's overloaded.

In fact, *you* might feel irritable when your liver's overloaded. You might also find life gets a little more chaotic around you – or you become a little obsessive about planning and ordering everything.

The liver's job description:

- Processes nutrients after they are digested and absorbed
- Balances levels of fats, amino acids and glucose in the blood
- Stores glucose as glycogen and releases it for energy as required
- Stores iron, plus vitamins A, B12, D, E, K
- Neutralises and clears toxins
- Makes up to a litre of bile a day
- Produces, breaks down and regulates a number of hormones including oestrogen
- Makes enzymes and proteins for tissue repair, immune processes and most of your bodily functions

Note that it's not just alcohol that can put a strain on your liver. I hear a lot of people say things like, "I don't drink much, so my liver should be fine." Your liver has daily exposure to traffic pollution, other sources of air pollution, water and soil pollution, pesticides, toxic chemicals in carpets, paints, household cleaning products, personal grooming products, cosmetics, plastics… the list goes on, and on. So just because your alcohol intake is low, that doesn't mean your liver isn't feeling under pressure.

Another thing I sometimes hear is, "I've had blood tests and my liver function is fine." That essentially means there is no identifiable liver damage. It doesn't mean your liver is coping with everything it's got to do.

Your gallbladder is described as your decision maker, and as the storage house for the bile your liver makes, it decides when to release that bile into your small intestine. It does this when you eat fats and oils, to help with their digestion. Bile has the additional benefit of carrying toxins and waste that your liver has processed to your intestines, so you can poo it out. It's like flushing your own inner toilet: your bile is the flush water that carries waste into the final part of your internal plumbing.

A struggling gallbladder can be mirrored by difficulty in carrying out decisions or activity. So while the emotion related to the liver is anger (or sometimes depression when anger is suppressed), that of the gallbladder is frustration.

If the work of your liver and gallbladder are disrupted, there may be a number of consequences, including a potential build-up of toxins. Your body's drive for survival will lead it to attempt to rid itself of toxins in other ways.

Plan A
This is when everything flows smoothly, nothing builds up excessively and excellent health is maintained. Your liver has the nutrients, energy and space it needs to do everything it needs to.

Plan B

If Plan A is your liver processing toxins and your bile helping to transport them out of your body, then Plan B is what happens when this route is overloaded. Plan B is your liver trying to find overflow pipes for the waste it can't handle. This might involve a rash, fever, spots or boils; temporary digestive issues; a cold or similar expelling of mucus from the lungs and airways; or perhaps a heavier period than usual.

Some might argue that the human body is opportunistic in this respect. It might make use of a passing infection, like a cold, flu or childhood disease, to have a bit of a clear out.

Of course, if a particular body doesn't have the strength or resources to properly manage that disease, there's sometimes the risk that the end result will be more damaging than helpful. Which may be why some people feel full of renewed vigour and clarity after a flu, where for others it might be the thing that triggers a long, chronic, debilitating illness, or even death. The stronger the immune system, and the more supported the liver, the less likely I believe this will happen. There is a lot to be said for preventative nourishment.

Plan B can also happen as part of a "healing crisis". This is essentially where some form of treatment, such as a massage, reflexology, or a herbal or nutritional programme, encourages or enables your body to start processing a few more toxins – but your liver and lymph can't handle the extra work so well. The strain may give you a headache, nausea, dizziness or sugar/carb cravings (as blood sugar drops), a rash or a sweat, for example.

Similarly, if you don't have the energy, nutrients and flow to process the healing crisis effectively, it may just contribute to the toxic load, and actually make things worse rather than better. I have studied with several teachers in a number of disciplines who repeatedly underlined the concept of "less is more". My favourite analogy of this is Japanese healer Akinobu Kishi's description of a person who recoils if you hit them with a hammer, but if you whisper, leans forward to hear.

Chronic illness

If Plan B has been overused, and/or there is a pronounced reduction in energy and flow in the body, then a condition is likely to become chronic. This essentially means long term toxic build up and overload, alongside systemic or localised inflammation as the immune system tries to keep up. It might show up as psoriasis, eczema, asthma, arthritis, colitis, fibroids, tumours, or other chronic conditions.

Most people have aspects of Plan B going on – who wouldn't with the levels of pollution and stress around these days? With many people, aspects of this are showing as chronic. So how do you get back to Plan A? What is it that we need to whisper?

Liver whispering

The liver likes space. It doesn't like to feel backed into a corner, or pushed for time. It has a lot to do, and it likes a measured, ordered approach.

I find my liver and my environment have a strong influence on each other. If I am overworking, living in chaos and rushing around, my liver struggles, and I feel a few of my usual Plan B symptoms on the horizon. It's good to get to know what your body's go-to Plan Bs are, so you can identify the early warning signs. If I keep a relatively clear and ordered diary, surroundings and headspace, then my liver seems to appreciate the space.

Similarly, if I actively work to support my liver, I find myself instantly tidying, cleaning, sorting, arranging and decluttering. Making the space I need. Even now as I write this, reminding myself of my liver's needs, I feel drawn to look up, stretch, breathe deeply, and create a pause in my day. So I just spent a few minutes at the door to my garden, breathing in the cool spring air and taking in the lively shades of green. Green is the colour of the Wood Element, and as such, nourishing to the liver, gallbladder, eyes and tendons. Green is also the colour of many of the foods that contain the nutrients the liver needs to thrive.

Liver detoxification phases I and II

Your liver detoxifies fat-soluble toxins, and converts them into water-soluble substances that can then be eliminated. This includes by-products from your body's own chemical processes, such as burning food for fuel, plus toxins from external sources like medication, drugs, food colourings, preservatives and flavourings, pollution from traffic, industry, agriculture and many substances in your own home (including carpets, furniture, cleaning products, non-stick pans, waterproof clothing, perfumes, hairsprays and much more).

This processing of toxins also happens elsewhere in the body, but your liver is the central hub for such activity. It carries out its detoxification duties using a two-part process: phase I and phase II.

A frequent criticism of nutritional "detox" programmes is that "you can't eat or drink something that detoxifies your body – and you don't need to, as your body can already detoxify what it needs to." I agree that most commercial "detox" programmes and potions are sadly lacking in the ability to help you clear toxicity. However, you absolutely need certain nutrients – such as B vitamins and vitamin C – to carry out your detoxification processes. In addition, there is now plenty of scientific research exploring the impact of a great many foods on how many and which detoxification enzymes you are able to produce, both for phase I and phase II detoxification.

Phase I detoxification

Phase I uses enzymes called cytochrome P450 (or CYP450), which are involved in processing 75-80% of medicines and drugs, including chemotherapy, as well as other substances. The amount of CYP450 you are able to produce may impact your interaction with medication, how well you break it down and what side effects you may experience.

You also make families of CYP1, CYP2, CYP3 and CYP4 enzymes to break down environmental toxins, some pharmaceutical drugs and products of normal metabolism (e.g. fatty acids), as well as hormones like oestrogen. Certain foods have been shown in various studies to influence how well you do this, and so are being investigated for their role in prevention of, for example, hormone receptive breast, ovarian and prostate cancers. Many substances in mostly plant-based foods are able to either promote or reduce the production of particular members of these families of enzymes.

These foods include leafy green vegetables (e.g. cabbage, spinach, watercress, kale), cruciferous vegetables (e.g. cauliflower, broccoli, cabbage, Brussels sprouts, kale), apiaceous vegetables (e.g. carrot, celery, fennel, parsley, parsnip), allium or liliaceous vegetables (e.g. garlic, leeks, onions), some herbs (including parsley, rosemary, peppermint, chamomile), berries, grapes, pomegranates, walnuts, peanuts, soy, green tea, coffee, chicory, turmeric, honey and coconut oil. Non-plant-based foods on the CYP enzyme regulating list are astaxanthin-rich foods (e.g. salmon, trout, algae) as well as fish oil supplementation.[250]

In some instances, a substance will have perhaps an enhancing effect in a smaller dose, and the opposite effect in a larger dose. This is another argument for keeping foods and supplements in balance and moderation, rather than just taking very high doses of one particular substance. However, most people who come to see me have a worryingly low intake of vegetables, and most would benefit from increasing the amount and variety of veg on their plate.[251]

Phase I tends to produce a lot of free radicals, and the liver will need protecting from those. High levels of antioxidants are needed for this, which are to be found in a high plant diet. Many of these antioxidants additionally regulate a substance called Nrf2 that in turn influences Phase II detoxification.

Phase II detoxification

Phase I sometimes makes the toxins more toxic than they were before, even carcinogenic – so phase II is essential in rendering these compounds safe. It does this through a process called conjugation, which adds a structure to the compound. This structure might be gluceronic acid (in a process called gluceronidation), a sulfuryl group (sulfonation or sulfurylation), glutathione, amino acids, an acetyl group (acetylation) or a methyl structure (methylation). Conjugation also makes them water soluble, and so able to be flushed out of the body, via either bile or urine.

Again, ingredients are required to make these and the enzymes involved. Specific foods have been shown to influence the activity of the enzymatic reactions involved. Foods that seem to regulate the enzymes that help add gluceronic acid to toxins (UGT enzymes) include cruciferous vegetables, berries, grapes, pomegranates, walnuts, olives, soy, whole grains, rosemary, curcumin (in turmeric), coffee and astaxanthin-rich foods. In addition, mung beans, adzuki bean sprouts and a great variety of fruits contain ready made UGTs.[252]

Enzymes that add sulfuryl groups to toxins are called Sulfotransferases (SULTs), and these have been shown to be enhanced by caffeine, vitamin A and provitamin A carotenoids. Barley, oats, lentils, peas, butterbeans, nuts (brazils, almonds, walnuts and peanuts), a range of vegetables (including cabbage, horseradish, Brussels sprouts, leeks, spinach and watercress), mustard, ginger, apricots and peaches all contain the sulphur needed to make SULTs.[253]

To add a glutathione group, you need a complex of GST enzymes (glutathione-S-transferase). Cruciferous and allium vegetables as well as resveratrol help you make these. The following may also be helpful: fish oil, purple sweet potato, curcumin, green tea, rooibos and honeybush tea, coffee, berries, pomegranates, grapes, walnuts and ghee; and for kidney GSTs: genistein, in soya products (e.g. miso, tempeh). Again, in higher doses, some substances may have the opposite effect, such as the genistein in soy, and quercetin.[254]

To make glutathione, you also need the following nutrients:[255]

Nutrient	Example food sources
Vitamin B6	Turkey, pork, chicken, beef, amaranth, lentils, pistachios, sunflower seeds, garlic, prunes
Magnesium	Nuts (especially brazils and almonds), seeds (especially pumpkin and sesame), green leafy vegetables, beans, whole grains
Selenium	Brazil nuts, pork, turkey, lamb, chicken, egg
Methionine	Turkey, pork, chicken, beef, egg, Brazil nuts, soy, sesame seeds, spirulina
Cystine	Pork, turkey, chicken, egg, soy, spirulina, sesame seeds, oats
Glycine	Turkey, pork, chicken, amaranth, soy, peanuts, pumpkin seeds and beef
Folate	Pulses, liver, sunflower seeds, quinoa, spinach, asparagus, avocados, mustard greens, artichokes
Alpha-lipoic acid	Spinach, broccoli, tomato, peas, Brussels sprouts, organ meats
Other	Turmeric, milk thistle, cruciferous vegetables, artichokes

Many of these are amino acids, and so found in protein-rich foods – hence the sudden inclusion of more animal-based ingredients. A range of amino acids is also used in other types of phase II conjugation, including glycine, taurine, glutamine, ornithine and arginine. So adequate protein in the diet is essential for a well-functioning liver.

Acetylation is used to process aromatic amines and hydrazines, found in a number of medications, pesticides, dyes, cosmetics, cigarette smoke and more. For acetylation you need types of enzymes that could potentially be enhanced by quercetin.

Methylation is a hot topic in the world of health, as it is fundamental for so many processes, including detoxification, regulating hormones – including oestrogens – healthy genetic expression and protection, your production of serotonin and dopamine, energy production and protection of your mitochondria energy factories, and general disease prevention.

For methylation, you need a number of nutrients (see the table below), and you also need to keep sugar levels in check.[256]

Nutrients to support methylation	Food sources
Methionine	Meat, poultry, fish, shellfish, eggs, Brazil nuts, sesame seeds, pumpkin seeds, spirulina, soy
B12	Meat, poultry, fish, shellfish, eggs
B6	Meat, pistachio nuts, sesame seeds, sunflower seeds, whole grains, chickpeas, lentils, garlic, prunes
Betaine (in supplement form, look for trimethylglycine or TMG)	Quinoa, beets, spinach, rye, kamut, bulgur wheat, amaranth, barley, oats, sweet potato, meat, poultry
Folate	Pulses, liver, sunflower seeds, quinoa, spinach, asparagus, avocados, mustard greens, artichokes
Magnesium	Nuts (especially Brazils and almonds), seeds (especially pumpkin and sesame), green leafy vegetables, beans, whole grains

Heavy metal detoxification

Finally, there is a substance called metallothionin that can bind to heavy metals such as lead, mercury, cadmium and arsenic, and help rid your body of them. Heavy metals are toxic to your body, able to cause organ damage and cancer. They can be found in traffic and cigarette smoke, pollution from industrial and agricultural processes, food sources (such as mercury in fish, arsenic in brown rice – which, incidentally, you can drastically reduce by soaking it and rinsing it well before cooking), amalgam fillings and more.[257]

Metallothionin is rich in cysteine, which can be found in soy, beef, lamb, sunflower seeds, chicken, turkey, oats and pork. Zinc supplementation also seems to increase metallothionin production, as do cruciferous vegetables, quercetin and the medicinal mushroom *Cordyceps sinensis.*[258]

Bile flow

So now you have successfully processed your toxins, they are able to be flushed out. Some will be directed to your kidneys and released when you wee. The majority, however, will probably travel in the bile your liver produces, which flows via your gallbladder into your intestines, and then out when you poo.

Your liver makes bile, and your tiny gallbladder stores it, releasing it into your intestines (via your common bile duct) when you have eaten something fatty. This, as you know, is because bile is made up of lecithin salts, which can emulsify those fats and help you digest them.

Certain bitter-flavoured foods also encourage bile secretion, including:

- Dandelion coffee
- Artichokes
- Dark green leafy vegetables
- Coffee
- Chocolate (but sugar-laden chocolate may stress the liver, so your average chocolate bar/cake/biscuit may not be that helpful!)

One of the potential benefits of coffee enemas is bile release – plus coffee seems to increase glutathione production and CYP4 enzymes. Coffee can often irritate the stomach, so enemas are a convenient way of avoiding that.

Gallstones

Your gallbladder can unfortunately get clogged up with gallstones, for a variety of reasons and with a number of possible outcomes. These outcomes range from you being blissfully unaware there's anything there, to extreme pain, sickness and potential for life-threatening infection. Because of the potential severity of the situation, people who have been diagnosed as having gallstones are frequently recommended surgery to take the whole gallbladder out.

In such a case, the liver then has to take on yet another role: that of deciding when to release bile into the intestines. Sometimes it is able to do that job well, while in some people it never seems to quite get the hang of it.

So what causes gallstones in the first place? Bile is mostly water, with various substances dissolved in it, including bile salts, bilirubin (a by-product of red blood cells being broken down), cholesterol, amino acids, fatty acids and other substances, as well as toxins the liver has processed.[259] Gallstones are made of the same substances, but out of solution, and can form tiny crystals or large stones. Some are more cholesterol based, others seem to contain a lot of calcium carbonate (chalk) or calcium bilirubinate.[260]

There has been a great deal of research into how gallstones are formed, and some common themes have appeared. In some cases, there are links with diabetes, obesity and/or aging, and there is also a higher risk in pregnancy and with oestrogen treatment. So there may be a link with chronic inflammation, insulin resistance and/or an increased need for antioxidants.

Observed dietary risk factors include a higher intake of sugar, cereals, meat and saturated fat, as well as low dietary fibre, fruit, fish, folate and magnesium, and in women in particular, a low intake of calcium and vitamin C.[261, 262] Gallbladder patients in one study were also more likely to skip meals, especially in the evening, and eat less generally, as well as sleep more and walk less.[263] More recent research has noted a key relationship between bile formation and the gut microbiome, and suggests that disruptions in the equilibrium between diet, the gut microbiome and the size and composition of your body's bile acid pool result in not just gallstones, but also liver disease and gastrointestinal cancers.[264]

With this information, it would make sense to aim towards:

- Eating regular meals
- Reducing sugar, cereals and meat
- Ensuring good levels of fish, vegetables and fruit
- Including fermented foods and general support for your balance of gut bacteria
- Following an anti-inflammatory diet (as described in previous chapters)
- Support for blood sugar and insulin pathways

So nutrition may be useful in helping to prevent gallstones – but what if you already have them? Firstly, it's important to note that gallstones can be a life-threatening condition, and so the consequences of refusing surgical or pharmaceutical treatment may be extremely serious. Having said that, not everyone needs to undergo gallbladder surgery, and if you are fortunate enough to have received an early diagnosis, then there may be some leeway to try a nutritional approach.

The pain associated with gallstones is usually felt when the gallbladder contracts to squeeze bile into the intestines. A low-fat diet will require less of this activity, and so is usually recommended to reduce the pain. However, this reduced bile flow may also contribute to a further build up of cholesterol and bile salts in the gallbladder, and so more or bigger gallstones. This ties in with research showing that people with obesity who follow low fat diets for weight loss are more likely to develop gallstones, while weight loss diets with higher fat levels reduce the risk of gallstones.[265]

As we have already seen, certain bitter foods may help improve bile flow, including coffee, dandelion coffee and artichokes. Milk thistle supplements may also be helpful in improving bile composition.[266] Lecithin supplements are often frequently advised to help dissolve gallstones, although studies on this are limited and give mixed results.

A plant-based supplement seems to have had greater success, however, at least with cholesterol-based stones. It contains 6 terpenes (a family of natural substances found in plants), largely consisting of menthol in a base of olive oil. The other 5 terpenes are menthone, pinene, borneol, camphene and cineol. In several studies where gallstone patients have used the supplement either on its own or together with a bile salt, gallstones have either partially or completely dissolved, usually with few or no side effects. In one of these studies, however, out of 31 patients, 8 had to receive emergency treatment for biliary colic, obstructive jaundice, pancreatitis, or cholangitis. All were treated successfully, and 7 of these 8 resumed the terpene therapy.[267]

I have known people to make general improvements to their diet and nutrition that include increasing vegetable intake, reducing refined and excessive carbohydrates and increasing hydration, and this seems to have had a general supportive effect that has kept their gallstones in check or even substantially reduced them. I do not have a magic formula for this, but would reiterate that everyone is different, and that the human body is a wonderfully intelligent and capable organism. Given the right conditions, ingredients and fuel, it is often able to resolve quite complex issues.

In addition, this kind of approach gives your body an opportunity to find its own safe pace to get bile flowing from the gallbladder again. Too direct or speedy an intervention may create more pain, aggravation or even harm, so handle your gallbladder with love and care!

Gallbladder flushes, also known as liver flushes, have become quite popular in recent years. There are a number of versions, but usually require drinking large amounts of olive oil together with either apple juice, lemon juice, apple cider vinegar or Epsom salts during a fast. Many people have reported passing multiple gallstones as a result, but I am not aware of any of these actually being analysed positively as gallstones. Some that have been analysed have turned out to be lumps of soap made from the olive oil.[268]

I never recommend these, but have met several people who have tried at least one. In some cases, people report feeling better afterwards – whether that is a result of the flush or the fast is unclear. In other cases, people have reported feeling terrible as a result, as if they have put too much strain on their liver, and have taken some time to recover. There is a concern that such flushes might increase the risk of stones dislodging in the common bile duct and causing pancreatitis; as far as I can tell, incidents of this are rare and anecdotal.

Nourishing your Wood Element

Prevention is, of course, better than cure, which means investing in your health when you feel good, not just when you are ill.

In holistic terms, that means keeping a sense of how well things are generally flowing – physically, emotionally, and energetically. For example, do you feel sluggish, constipated or physically toxic? Are you stuck in feelings of anger, resentment, grief or sadness that you can't let go of? Or frozen in fear? Do you feel generally stuck in life, unable to progress or evolve as a human being?

Chinese Five Element theory gives us tools to monitor this and work to create more flow again. Keeping your Wood Element happy is fundamental to this.

The Wood Element is expressed in springtime, when everything that has been lying dormant springs to life. New shoots push up through the soil, grass gets taller and greener, trees bud and blossom, while insects start buzzing around the flowers that appear.

This natural seasonal vitality affects each of us as well, and you may find your body responding to situations with renewed vigour. As much of what you digest and take into the body as well as much of what you detoxify and eliminate pass at some point through the liver, it is especially important at springtime that your liver is clear, vibrant and up to the job. If it is, then it will sing its way through spring into summer, and pave the way for a time of immense creativity.

Otherwise you may find your liver quickly overloaded, with a healing crisis type of response. To avoid this, the tips already provided for nourishing your liver are valid. Chinese Five Elements also recommends adding touches of sour-flavoured foods here and there to gently stimulate the functions of the liver and gallbladder – perhaps some

> **Some wood element foods:**
> Watercress, rocket, cabbage, kale, green lettuce, spinach, broccoli, spring greens, asparagus, fresh herbs, mung beans, green lentils, limes, lemons, sour plums, apple cider vinegar

lemon, lime, balsamic vinegar or apple cider vinegar (preferably "with mother" i.e. unfiltered, to obtain its probiotic benefits).

The colour green provides additional sustenance for the liver. This includes green coloured foods – such as limes, spring greens, fresh herbs, spinach, kale, watercress and broccoli – as well as wearing some green, having a little green in your environment and spending time in nature.

You don't have to wait for spring to do this, you can take care of your liver at any time of year. When you emerge from the stillness, cold and darkness of winter, however, it's a great time to check in a see what state your liver and gallbladder are in. Clues that they may need support might include: nausea, headaches, itchy skin, achy joints, itchy or sore eyes, bloating, constipation, menstrual problems, fatigue, irritability, resentment, depression, stubbornness, difficulty making decisions, or a general feeling of inflexibility, stuckness or sluggishness on any level.

Once more it's worth noting that emotions we consider to be negative, such as anger, often have their rightful place, and can be healthy catalysts for change and evolution. Equally, they can also be destructive, either to you or to others. The lesson of the Chinese Five Elements is in how to allow such emotions an appropriate and constructive voice, and then move healthily on.

It's also good to remember that painting and furnishing your entire house in green, wearing only green clothes and eating only green and sour foods is not an approach that fosters balance and harmony! In my garden right now there are green leaves and blades of grass, but also white, yellow, red and purple flowers, light and shade, hot spots and areas that allow through a cool, refreshing breeze.

Spring is considered to be the start of the seasonal year, so it was tempting to start this book with this chapter and move through the Elements one by one. But life and our passage through it doesn't need to be so linear and rigid, and this oriental approach to health also teaches how the Elements interact fluidly in many different patterns, not just in a seasonal circle. If I have piqued your interest, then you can explore more with other authors and teachers. In the meantime, liver support is hugely relevant for the next chapter on balancing hormones.

This focus on Spring and new beginnings leads lightly towards the final chapters, where you can put everything you have learnt and continue to learn into practice.

Reflection time

- *How much space and flow do you feel there is in your body, and in your life in general?*

- *Do you feel toxic/stuck on any level?*

- *Do you frequently feel irritable, frustrated, angry or depressed?*

- *What activities or environments or aspects of your life help you feel most free?*

Recipes

These liver-support recipes focus on nutrients for key enzymes used in your liver's detoxification processes, as well as some green for your Wood Element.

- **Methylating salad** – *p.263*
  A seedy beetroot salad rich in nutrients needed for methylation, glutathione production and more.

- **Cruciferous curry** – *p.257*
  Yes, it's back, my Friday night favourite, excellent for those pungent flavours that help you eliminate toxins (see chapter 7) – but also full of nutrients that help you process the toxins first.

- **Green up your grains** – *p.250*
  You can use this recipe whenever you serve rice or quinoa with anything, be it a salad, stir-fry or curry, or have it on its own. NB: quinoa isn't a true grain, but works well instead of rice here, and also contains some additional liver enzyme nutrients.

- **Wood Element soup** – *p.246*
  This is a true souper-green: cleansing, hydrating, warming and soothing all at the same time.

- **Lime zinger tart** – *p.288*
  I serve this up at dinner parties, especially when I've cooked something quite rich. It's sharp and light, but still feels luxurious – and provides some excellent liver support too.

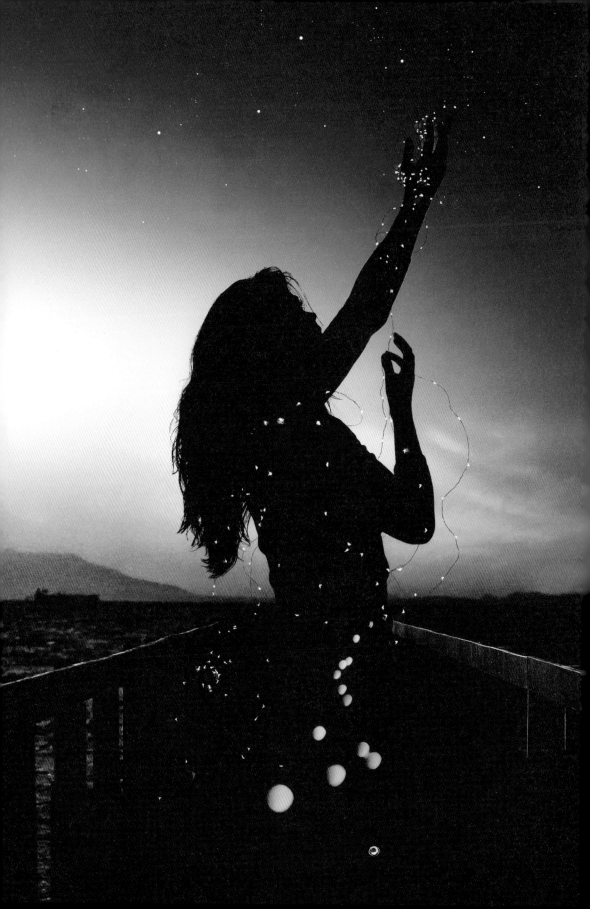

Chapter 19

Balancing hormones

We blame hormones for so much I couldn't finish this book without a focus on what they are and how to keep them as balanced as possible. Essentially, they help to keep you in balance by instructing processes to stop or start, speed up or slow down.

Hormones are the chemical substances that travel through your body delivering such messages. Like miniature postmen, with your blood vessels as their streets and road networks, and your cells the homes they are bringing the mail to. On each cell, there are lots of different letterboxes – or receptors – that can receive a particular type of message. We have already seen, for example, how insulin delivers the message "please let some glucose in" to take sugar out of the blood and into the cells for ATP (energy) production. We have also noted that if the insulin receptors are switched off (often due to glucose/insulin overload), it's like a nailed up letterbox, and messages can't get delivered.

Hormones are made either of amino acids (proteins) or cholesterol. You are continually making them, breaking them down and recycling them, so you need continual supplies of protein and cholesterol, as well as a lot of co-factors. So, as usual, vitamins and minerals are key.

Many parts of your body produce hormones, from your brain to your heart to your ovaries or testes. I'm going to focus on a specific set of organs called your endocrine glands, which secrete hormones directly into your blood network.

Adrenal glands – we've talked a lot about these already, they send out your stress hormones.

Ovaries/testes – these produce your reproductive hormones that regulate periods, sperm development, pregnancy and childbirth.

Pancreas – well, specifically the Islets of Langerhans, the 2-3% of your pancreas that releases blood sugar balancing hormones.

Thymus – this is near your heart in the centre of your chest. It makes hormones that stimulate your immune system's T-cells to develop. It's also where T-cells mature.

Thyroid gland – this butterfly-shaped gland is in your throat, and regulates your metabolic rate. It can make your heart beat faster or slower, can make you feel super energised or on the floor, and can even affect your stool transit time. Ideally we want all these things to be steady.

Parathyroid glands – these are like little spot patterns on the butterfly wings of your thyroid, and together with some of your thyroid hormones, trigger your body to either put more calcium into your bones or take it out.

Pituitary gland – seated in your brain behind the bridge of your nose, your pituitary is a bit like head office. It receives information from your nervous system via a brain structure called the hypothalamus, and then responds with a message to the appropriate endocrine gland, which then responds with a message of its own. So the HPA axis, for example, is where the **H**ypothalamus responds to a nerve message from your eyes telling you there's a tiger approaching, messaging (with a hormone) your **P**ituitary, which then sends another hormonal message to your **A**drenals, which then send out their own red alert stress hormones.

Pineal gland – in your "third eye" area between your eyebrows and back into your brain a bit, your pineal gland registers how much light is around and regulates your circadian rhythm, i.e. day/night cycle. This influences many of your hormonal cycles, so it's important to access as much daylight as possible during daylight hours, and avoid artificial light where feasible after dark.

All hormones tend to have their own natural cycles where they might peak and trough, but generally they maintain a sense of balance. Sometimes, however, you can get disruptions to their flow. This means they might be unable to tell your cells to do or stop doing the things necessary to keep you healthy; or they might over stimulate certain activities, or peak/trough at unhelpful times of the day. Either way, this can pan out badly, and certain things can get really out of kilter.

For example, Cushing's syndrome is a rare condition where the adrenals continuously send out excess cortisol, leading to symptoms such as central body obesity, glucose intolerance, high blood pressure, excess body hair, osteoporosis, menstrual problems, kidney stones and mood swings. Addison's disease, on the other hand, is where there is not enough cortisol being produced, and can cause weight loss, weakness, fatigue, low blood pressure, dizziness on standing, salt cravings, nausea and depression.

Ideally, you want to give your endocrine glands all the support and ingredients they need to stay focused and do their jobs well.

Endocrine System

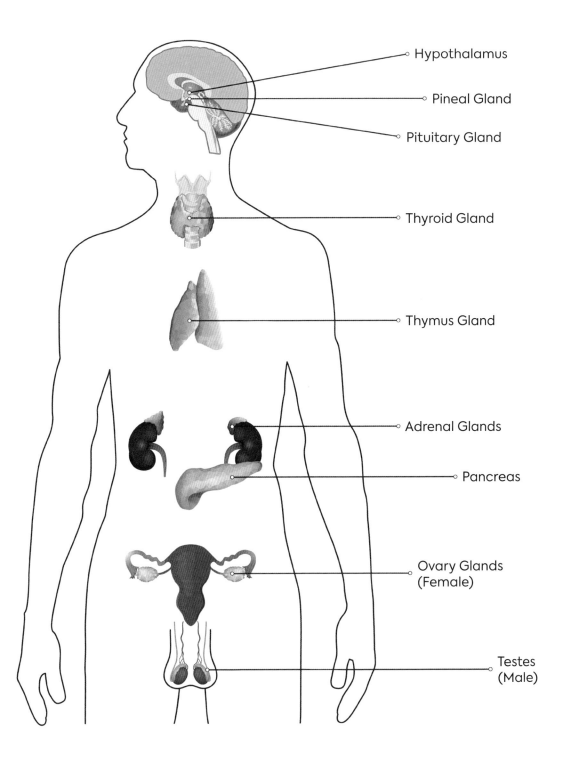

- Hypothalamus
- Pineal Gland
- Pituitary Gland
- Thyroid Gland
- Thymus Gland
- Adrenal Glands
- Pancreas
- Ovary Glands (Female)
- Testes (Male)

The good news

You already have the tools you need to do that!

Because we've spent so much (invaluable) time looking at *adrenal support*, you have the most important key to hormonal health. For the adrenals are the cornerstone of your endocrine system. By supporting them, you are putting in solid foundations that can give fundamental support to the rest. Equally, trying to reset other endocrine glands without giving time to your adrenals is like building your house on sand: it might not take much for it to topple over again.

The next crucial component is *blood sugar* stability, which we have also explored in depth. The blood sugar balancing advice in previous chapters is potentially beneficial not just for the pancreas, but for all the endocrine glands. Not least because they all require steady streams of energy to function well, and will be impeded by any stress or inflammation resulting from blood sugar crashes and disruptions to insulin pathways.

In addition, as you will see, you might find it useful to incorporate what we have already explored around nourishing your *liver, microbiome* and *gut health*. This is also a great time to remember how important *hydration* and *blood vessel integrity* are to healthy blood flow, so your hormones can travel easily enough to deliver their messages. In fact, putting together a hormonal health programme is a lovely way to draw together a lot of what you have learned throughout this book.

Two of the most common areas I get asked to provide nutritional advice around are menstrual health and thyroid, so I will go into them in a little more detail below. However, you can apply much of this to general hormonal balance. The classic analogy for the endocrine system is an orchestra: the melodies of each endocrine gland (and its set of hormones) harmonise with and influence each other to produce a wonderful overture.

Periods, pregnancy and menopause

Reproductive hormones, such as oestrogen and progesterone, are part of a magical dance that enables the absolute miracle of creating another human being. Studying the intricacies of how it all works is fascinating.

At the same time, the power they wield can have uncomfortable and sometimes unfortunate consequences if things aren't flowing smoothly. In addition, the shifts into and out of fertile years can be disruptive and demanding physically, mentally and emotionally – for men as well as for women. So although I'm focusing on female reproduction here, much of this is relevant for men too. We all have the same reproductive hormones, just in different amounts.

In an ideal world, we would transition effortlessly through puberty, between different phases of the month and then through menopause. There are many factors that seem to disrupt this natural flow, however, from toxicity to stress to poor nutrition. First of all, let's have a brief focus on oestrogen levels.

Oestrogen: the three wise women

I'm going to point out here that I'm nostalgically (and stubbornly!) fond of the old spelling of oestrogen, while most of the modern world has dropped the "o" to settle on estrogen. They are the same word, and I hope I don't confuse anyone.

Oestrogen's main job is to regulate inflammation and cell proliferation, as that triggers what is required in the womb to thicken the lining and prepare for potential pregnancy. Its main surge is just before ovulation. Progesterone will then take over, as its main role is to maintain the conditions required for pregnancy. If no egg is fertilized that month, progesterone levels will also drop, and that's when the period happens: a shedding of the extra womb lining (endometrium) that is no longer needed.

That's a very basic run down of menstrual cycles and their effect on womb tissue. If there is an overproduction of oestrogen, then this could contribute to conditions that involve inflammation and cell proliferation, such as fibroids,[269] endometriosis,[270] tumours[271] and other growths. This can happen in the womb area, or in other parts of the body. Actually, it might be more accurate to see this as an imbalance within oestrogen types. There are three main sorts of oestrogen:

E1 aka estrone   **E2 aka estradiol**   E3 aka estriol

E1 and E3 are weak versions, and E2, estradiol, is strong acting. We convert them into different forms, depending on where we're at. E1 and E3, the weakest, have particular roles to play in pregnancy and menopause. Although there is still much to learn about their interrelationships and impact, one thing we do know is that all three types of oestrogen are continually being broken down, recycled and put back together again. Supporting these pathways is one step towards enabling your body to keep reassessing what it needs, and making sure its options are fully open.

Hormone recycling

When your body is fine-tuning its balance of oestrogen, it uses its own recycling factory, involving your liver and microbiome. Your liver breaks down hormones – using methylation and glutathione – and sends them into your intestines;

your intestines do a quick check before getting rid of the waste products, and your microbiome puts them back together in the amounts and configurations you need.

So everything you have learned about nourishing your liver and your microbiome is incredibly relevant here. Also check the table below for some of the co-factors you need for making and regulating your main reproductive hormones. By ensuring a regular supply of all these nutrients, your body will have more of a chance to carry out its ideal scenario, whether that's making more of or breaking down each hormone.

Included in the table is a substance called indole-3-carbinol, which is helpful for regulating both oestrogen and testosterone. We obtain it from cruciferous vegetables, such as broccoli, cauliflower, cabbage and kale, and then convert it into a substance called diindolylmethane, or DIM. There's more in raw cruciferous vegetables, and in their sprouting seeds (e.g. sprouted broccoli seeds) – however, if your thyroid is sluggish (see below) you may want to just eat your cruciferous veg cooked.

Hormone	Co-factors for production and regulation
Testosterone	• Vitamin A, Vitamin D • Zinc, Magnesium, Boron • L-arginine • I-3-C (broccoli, cauliflower, cabbage, kale) • Omega 3 fatty acids
Progesterone	• Vitamin C • Vitamin E • Zinc • Magnesium
Oestrogen	• Magnesium • Methylators e.g. methylfolate, methylcobalamin (B12), B6 • Glutathione • Zinc • Vitamin D • I-3-C

Xenoestrogens

Xenoestrogens are substances that mimic the effects of oestrogen, and can be found in plastics, solvents, pesticides, hairsprays, cosmetics, perfumes, cleaning products and even in your tap water. They are "endocrine disruptors", which means they can have a direct impact on your hormonal balance and activity. They have been associated with cancer, fertility issues, autoimmune conditions and more.

There are also some natural hormone disruptors in some plant foods, such as genistein in soya. Whether genistein's impact is positive or negative seems to vary from person to person, and from study to study. The majority seem to find soya beneficial, but I would usually recommend avoiding a high intake.

As with most things, we still have a lot to learn about endocrine disruptors, both synthetic and natural. Logic seems to dictate that they are all to be avoided, while studies are inconsistent and confusing.

Until we unravel more, my best advice is to keep exposure as low as you can, especially to synthetic xenoestrogens, and give your liver as much support as you can to be able to deal with those you can't avoid. Avoiding synthetic xenoestrogens completely is impossible, but you can massively reduce your exposure by:

- Buying or growing organic food
- Buying or making cleaning products with more natural ingredients (bicarbonate of soda, lemon juice and white vinegar are amazing household essentials)
- Buying or making cosmetics and personal care products made from natural ingredients and materials
- Buying/storing mineral water in glass bottles or getting a reverse osmosis filter (preferably one that then remineralises the water, and perhaps reoxygenates it too).

Menstrual cycles

Some people seem to sail through their periods, while many others seem to have problems of one kind or another. If your periods are not the free and breezy affair you have been told is the norm – or the deeply connecting earth goddess experience you might be striving for – you are far from alone!

There are many factors involved, including xenoestrogen exposure, stress, diet (of course!) and even light exposure.

We have already seen how xenoestrogens might impact on your reproductive hormones and the menstrual cycles they help to trigger. The effects of stress can be immediate or slow acting. Firstly, some of your adrenal hormones, called DHEA, are also precursors to reproductive hormones; in long-term stress, DHEA levels often fall, and therefore so may oestrogen/progesterone/testosterone levels. In addition, fertility is very low on the list of priorities when you are being threatened by a tiger in the jungle or a shark in the ocean, so one of the first things your adrenals do in response to stress and trauma is to flick your reproductive switch from high to low. In some cases, your periods might stop completely; in other cases, they might become irregular, painful or difficult in other ways.

The same can also happen if you are lacking the nutrients you need to make reproductive hormones and healthy womb tissue – which is largely connective tissue. You need a bountiful supply of all the nutrients listed above, plus decent amounts of water, plus the ingredients required for connective tissue (see chapter 13 on this). Again, if you are short in any of these, or they are not being well digested or absorbed, then you might experience absent, irregular or painful, uncomfortable periods.

Light isn't really talked about enough, but it can't be a coincidence that most of the world starts procreating in springtime, when there's more light around. Each cell in your body has its own 24-hour clock that keeps on going even if it were isolated in a dark tunnel. In normal conditions, however, your cells adapt to monthly and seasonal changes, using clues from how much light is in your environment – gathered by your pineal gland. So that, for example, you might naturally sleep longer in the winter, and then rise earlier and be more active in the summer months. The amount and patterns of natural light you are exposed to directly influence your hormones and the activities they regulate, including those involved in stress and menstruation/fertility.

This all means that by making a few proactive adjustments to your lifestyle, you may notice significant shifts in your periods. Periods that are irregular, absent, painful, clotty, over-emotional, nausea inducing and/or exhausting can often be improved by:

- Ensuring you have and are absorbing all the nutrients you need
- Adequate hydration
- Liver support
- Microbiome support
- An anti-inflammatory diet, including reducing sugar and highly processed foods
- Stress management and adrenal support
- Regular sleep patterns and daily exposure to natural light (screens, artificial street lighting and even the lights in your home and workplace will all interfere with this, unfortunately, so try and compensate where you can)

This approach can be useful for menstrual health problems as well as to support fertility. In either case, I'd recommend you consult your GP to check your current hormone balance and rule out any diagnoses that may need to be addressed in other or additional ways.

Also be aware of whether or not your lifestyle is allowing you to rest and take time out around your actual period. You may not need to take a week off work or hide from the family for a week (however tempting that might feel!), but just schedule in some sofa time, or an extra gentle walk or two. Consider saying no to extra activities around that time, especially any that demand energy.

You can perhaps make up for it at that time in the month when you are potentially at your most outgoing and creative, which is usually around ovulation. For most women this is around two weeks after your period starts, but can vary somewhat.

Actually, you don't need to be menstruating to experience regular cycles of mood and energy. Some men and post-menopausal women notice that how they feel, their sleep patterns and other aspects of health and wellbeing fluctuate throughout the month.

Creative fire

Both physically and energetically, your reproductive organs are your creative centre. You can, of course, use them to make more human beings. You might also want to explore tuning into this area when creating art, or journaling, or any new projects. Nourishing your reproductive system might actually help your creative flow in other areas of life too, whatever life stage you are at.

In terms of Chinese Five Elements, your reproductive system relates to the warmth, passion and joy of the Fire Element. As such, your reproductive organs and function are also related to your heart and blood flow. Indeed, healthy blood flow is much more conducive to a happy period than stagnation, as well as testicular and prostate health. Regular exercise is usually helpful, as is hydration, mindful eating and anything that keeps you relaxed but warm and energised.

Your adrenals and thyroid relate to the Fire Element too. We've already looked at the adrenal link, and you can find out in previous chapters how to put in extra support there. In some cases, the thyroid gland also benefits from some attention and nourishment – see below for more on this.

Puberty and menopause

These transition times are sometimes straightforward, and sometimes really quite unpredictable. As reproductive hormones fluctuate and learn to settle into new patterns, there may be times when they affect your mental, physical and emotional health in ways that, for some people, can seem confusing, disturbing or out of control. It can affect different people in very different ways, so you can't assume you will have the same experience as your friends – but talking and sharing is still usually incredibly helpful. Note that male hormones also go through a menopause of sorts, where testosterone can start to drop more quickly than before – and we all go through puberty – so the more everyone can feel comfortable talking about all this, the better.

The balance of your reproductive hormones is intrinsically tied up with your identity, so both puberty and menopause can be times of loss, fear and confusion, as well as excitement, growth and self-discovery. In addition, the changes might affect energy levels, ability to concentrate and process new information, tolerance rates, sleep patterns, inflammatory processes, bone density and a whole lot more.

Remembering that there is a physical trigger for all of this can be helpful. Figuring out what you need to ease the process is easier for some than for others, but the same nourishing, hydrating approach, including particular support for your liver, adrenals and microbiome, will stand you in good stead. For some, it may take an all-important edge off, for others the whole process will feel deeply supported and much easier.

Remember:

- **Your liver** is your planner, regulating hormonal balance, shifts and changes.
- **Your liver** also helps to regulate blood sugar balance, hydration and what you do with nutrients, all of which are crucial to keeping your body, moods and mental focus in a great place.
- **Your adrenals** stimulate and then calm your stress responses, which then has a domino effect on hormonal activity throughout your body, including those involved in shifting through puberty and menopause.
- **Your stress response** can disrupt the flow of both nutrients and toxins, and so settling your adrenals and nervous system can assist your nourishment and detoxification processes.
- **Your microbiome** influences both how effectively you can calm down your stress response, as well as general inflammation and immune responses.
- **Your stress levels/adrenals and your microbiome** both influence your mood, behaviour and ability to deal with the kind of challenges that puberty and menopause often bring.
- **Your thyroid** may also be involved on some level, especially around menopause time – see below for more on this.

Also remember that you now have several chapters of information, tips and recipes in your hands that explore all of this.

A nutritional approach to smoothing the bumps in puberty and menopause need not be complicated – often simplicity works best – and the next chapter will hopefully help you plan your first steps. If it all seems a bit overwhelming, then ask for help: see your GP, a nutritional therapist and/or another therapist who has been recommended to you.

Thyroid hype

If your pituitary is sitting in head office dishing out commands, your thyroid is on the shop floor, making sure everything is in place to run a successful operation.

If energy is low, it can trigger you to release more from macronutrients; if energy is high it can slow down metabolism instead. It measures and adjusts your temperature, your heart rate, how quickly or slowly things move through your digestive system and your mood. Your thyroid also regulates muscle movement and how your brain develops.

If your thyroid is under functioning or hyperactive, things can really run amok. Usually a low thyroid (hypothyroidism) makes everything more sluggish, while an overactive thyroid (hyperthyroidism) makes everything speedy – but the opposite can sometimes happen too.

Common symptoms of hypothyroidism (underactive thyroid)	Common symptoms of hyperthyroidism (overactive thyroid)
• Tiredness • Sensitivity to cold • Weight gain • Constipation • Depression • Muscle aches, cramps and weakness • Dry and scaly skin • Brittle hair and nails • Loss of libido (sex drive) • Pain, numbness and tingling in hands and fingers (carpal tunnel syndrome • Irregular or heavy periods • Thinned or partly missing eyebrows • Low pitched or hoarse voice • Puffy-looking face • Slow heart rate • Anaemia See https://www.nhs.uk/conditions/underactive-thyroid-hypothyroidism/symptoms/ for complete list	• Nervousness, anxiety and irritability • Hyperactivity • Difficulty sleeping • Feeling tired all the time • Sensitivity to heat • Muscle weakness • Diarrhoea • Needing to pee more often than usual • Persistent thirst • Itchiness • Loss of interest in sex • Irregular or unusually fast heart rate (palpitations) • Twitching or trembling • Warm skin and excessive sweating • Patchy hair loss or thinning • Weight loss – often despite an increased appetite See https://www.nhs.uk/conditions/overactive-thyroid-hyperthyroidism/symptoms/ for complete list

I've come across way more people with underactive thyroid than those with hyperthyroid conditions. How people get to the point of an underactive thyroid can be varied and complex, but I'm not alone in noticing a history of adrenal stress, or a sizeable drain on resources, as a frequent contributing factor. So it might be someone who is working and/or playing hard to the point of adrenal fatigue – and then they just keep on pushing through. Or there might be a series of episodes of high stress, with little time or ability to support stress resilience. Alternatively, thyroid complaints might kick in after pregnancy, or in the approach to or during menopause. Or it may be as simple as a nutrient deficiency (see below).

Thyroid tests and what they mean

The main thyroid hormone we hear about is thyroxine, or T4. This is the one that is frequently prescribed in synthetic form to people with an underactive thyroid. Usually, if your body wants to speed things up, your pituitary sends a hormone called TSH (Thyroid Stimulating Hormone) to your thyroid, which triggers it to produce more T4. So some blood tests for thyroid activity will just measure TSH: if it's high, that means it's possibly trying to kick a sluggish thyroid into action.

Sometimes both TSH and T4 are measured, and a high TSH low T4 reading will suggest hypothyroidism, while the reverse might signify an overactive thyroid.

If your thyroid is being bombarded with TSH but can't make T4 (perhaps it doesn't have the right ingredients), then your thyroid might start to grow more thyroid tissue instead – this swelling at the front of the throat is called a goiter.

If TSH and T4 are within range, people are often told their thyroid is fine, even if they still have symptoms of thyroid imbalance. In some cases, it might be useful to then test T3 levels, which some consultants may do or you can have done privately. If T4 is in range but T3 is low, this can also produce the effects of hypothyroidism. This is because T4 is actually quite a weak-acting hormone, so ideally you convert a large proportion of it into the more strongly active T3.

If your T4 to T3 conversion is impaired, then you may also end up making more of a substance called reverse T3 (rT3) instead. Scientists have started to explore the implications of raised rT3, and while research is in its early stages, so far it looks like something you probably want to avoid.

Finally, TPO antibodies are sometimes measured in a blood test. TPO is thyroxine peroxidase, an enzyme that you need to make thyroid hormones. If you are producing antibodies against TPO, then you will struggle to produce thyroid hormones, and may be diagnosed with an autoimmune condition such as Hashimoto's disease. Some autoimmune diseases are triggered when you produce antibodies to a substance that is non-self, but that resembles a part of you. So people with Coeliac disease could potentially be producing antibodies to gluten (in wheat, spelt, kamut, rye and barley) that then also attack the thyroid tissue, which is very close in structure to gluten. In fact, people with Coeliac disease are three times more likely to have a thyroid condition, and people with Hashimoto's thyroiditis generally seem to benefit from a gluten-free diet, sometimes even to the point of disease remission.[272, 273]

Food for thyroid support

If you have a diagnosed thyroid condition that you are taking synthetic thyroid hormone medication for (e.g. Levothyroxine), then be cautious around adding in additional support nutritionally. Your doctor or consultant will be fine-tuning your dose according to your needs, and if you start making more natural thyroxine yourself, you'll end up with an imbalance. Equally, if you have an overactive thyroid, you may wish to avoid stimulating it even more.

However, if your TSH and/or T4 levels are within range but you want to give preventative support to your thyroid, it might be worth addressing your diet.

First of all, revisit the suggestions I have given around adrenal support. Then make sure your diet includes the ingredients you need to make thyroid hormones and convert as much T4 to T3 as your body requires.

The primary nutrients you need for this are:

- Tyrosine
- Iodine
- Selenium

Tyrosine is the amino acid that T4 and T3 is made from, and you can find it in seaweed, spirulina, eggs, turkey, game and soya protein (although note that genistein in soya can also act as a goitrogen, or iodine blocker, especially when iodine levels are already low).

The richest source of iodine is seaweed, especially kelp/kombu (there's not nearly as much in nori, unfortunately), and you can also find good levels in white fish and egg yolks.

Seaweed is also an excellent source of selenium and all the other co-factors you need to make T4 and then convert some of it to T3. Brazil nuts are notoriously rich in selenium, with oily fish, cod and chicken being the next best food sources.

If you want to keep things simple, then include seaweed as part of your daily diet. The recipe section in this book can give you some ideas how to do this. I also have a jar of mixed seaweed flakes that I sprinkle onto most savoury dishes, like a condiment. I use just a little, as too much makes everything taste of the sea! In addition, there is a little kelp powder in my favourite supergreen powder mix, which I add to smoothies, bircher muesli, chia pots, energy balls and sometimes salad dressings too.

Some foods are called goitrogens because they can interfere with iodine uptake. Cruciferous aka brassica vegetables (broccoli, cauliflower, cabbage, kale, Brussels sprouts etc.) as well as turnips, kohlrabi, radishes, mustard greens and some other vegetables are goitrogens *when raw*, so should generally be cooked if your thyroid is struggling. There is also an isoflavone in soya called genistein that is a known goitrogen. There is ongoing debate and research on how influential these foods can be, and my own experience is that different people notice varying impacts. So if you're unsure, at the very least keep soya (including edamame beans and tofu) and raw brassicas to a minimum.

Iodine belongs to a group of chemicals called halogens, and its uptake can also be blocked by the other halogens, including bromine, chlorine and fluorine. So if you swim a lot, or if there's a lot of chlorine and/or fluoride in your tap water, then you may need to compensate with more iodine-rich foods.

There have been recent trends in iodine supplementation, sometimes in fairly high doses, and there are strong arguments both for and against this. I have seen mixed outcomes, and so have always advised anyone wanting to take an iodine supplement to start very low and build up gradually and sensitively. For most people, introducing seaweed into the diet on a regular basis seems to make enough of a difference – especially as it contains not just the iodine but everything else you need too. I would not recommend regular seaweed – nor iodine supplementation – for people on thyroid medication, however, for the reasons given above.

Liver love

Finally, much of the T4 to T3 conversion and thyroid hormone regulation takes place in your liver, so once again you need to take the best care of your liver that you can. The same enzyme used here to produce T3 also helps clear excess reverse T3.[274]

Remember also that your liver is your planner, according to Traditional Chinese Medicine. It has a regulatory function, including that of regulating your hormones. So whether you want to improve your menstrual health, your fertility, your stress resilience, your energy levels, your blood sugar balance or you general thyroid health – give your liver some love!

Reflection time

- *Do you notice cycles of:*
  - *higher and lower energy through each month?*
  - *higher and lower levels of tolerance/stress/anxiety?*
  - *higher and lower levels of joy/creativity?*

- *Do those cycles seem smooth to you, or do levels seem to swing or be unpredictable?*

- *Have you noticed any recent changes to your levels or patterns of sleep, energy, mood or libido?*

- *Menstruating women:*
  - *How regular and easy are your periods?*
  - *Do they feel part of your natural life, or something you'd rather suppress or ignore?*

Recipes

Balancing your hormones has never been so flavoursome! These recipes all have vibrant flavours to match their powerful nutrient content. So you can just have a little alongside other dishes, or embrace the boldness of seaweeds, beetroot and ginger, and the creamy nuttiness of the cauliflower soup.

- **Kombu and ginger tea** *– p.293*
  A warming and deeply nourishing way to incorporate a daily dose of iodine-rich seaweed, for those who like a strong-tasting tea!

- **Bone strengthening carrot and seaweed salad** *– p.266*
  The sweet crunch of the carrot is the perfect sidekick to the deep saltiness of the sea spaghetti.

- **Methylating salad** *– p.263*
  The nutrients in this salad provide you with what your liver needs to regulate oestrogen and clear xenoestrogens. Choose a dressing with unfermented balsamic or apple cider vinegar, or yoghurt if non-vegan, for additional microbiome support.

- **Cauliflower and hazelnut soup** *– p.247*
  You could also substitute the hazelnuts for brazil nuts to superboost your selenium.

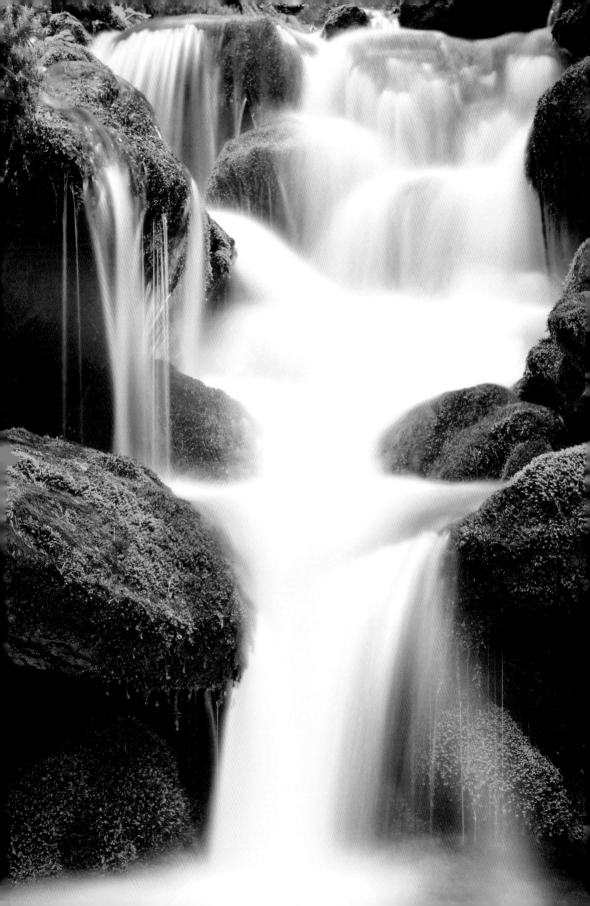

Chapter 20

Creating more flow
~ Putting together a personal action plan ~

So you may have gathered by now that I prefer a gentle approach. One that is based on self-love, and that aims to nourish you rather than make you feel stressed, deprived, anxious or resentful. This is your food, let it feed you!

In putting any kind of health plan together, we first need to acknowledge that we don't know everything. This is true even if you are a nutritional or medical "expert". The human body is far too complex, and there are too many different types of things that influence how it works.

You can't put your body or your health into a neat little box with black and white rules, however much in control that *seems* to help you to feel. But you can trust that, given the right fundamental support, your amazing body has the capacity to rebalance and rework itself to a remarkable extent. That it is much better at "being in control" than the limits of your current thought processes. It got you here so far, didn't it?

The second thing is to be clear with what you would like from your action plan. For example:

- "Have more energy"
- "Sleep better"
- "Feel less achy"
- "Improve my skin"
- "Eat fresher, more balanced meals"
- "Support my immune system"
- "Have a healthier, more joyful relationship with food and my body"
- "Feel more nourished"

To head towards any of these goals, the underlying principles will be similar, as it's often really about creating more flow. If everything is flowing well, then your body can make good use of incoming nutrients, as well as process and get rid of toxins and waste; it can communicate effectively via hormones and nerves, and then act appropriately to keep you safe and well; it can maintain a healthy turnover of high quality cells and tissue for as long as possible.

Where to begin!

Actually, you have already begun. Just by reading this far – and you may even have tried some of the suggestions at the end of each chapter. You may now want to bring some or all of it together into a cohesive programme, and here's how you can go about that.

If you are a practitioner yourself, then you may find it useful to now reflect on how you can incorporate any new insights, information or approaches into how you work.

Below is a reminder of the key areas we have looked at together during the course of this book, with an opportunity to try some gentle support in each area. You don't need to do everything all at once. In fact, that is often overwhelming and stressful for the body, and may just push you back in the opposite direction from where you want to go. Instead be realistic about what you can do, and what will fit in with your current work, family and other commitments.

My general advice for approaching tasks is:

- Make a list
- Aim to achieve the first three things on that list (or up to six if they're simple and you're sure you can manage them!)
- Acknowledge your achievement with pride when you have done so
- If you don't achieve them, rather than feel stressed or that you have failed, have a look at those 3-6 things and try to figure out what the issue is, and address that the best you can – asking for help if necessary
- Repeat the whole process

If you want to start with a super simple approach, then begin with this:

- Listen to your body
- Slow down
- Eat real food and enjoy it

Key areas for your personal action plan

As you can see in the folowing diagram, I have identified ten key areas that you can focus on – so perhaps choose three or so of these to begin with. Or you might even choose just one, and then identify three things you can address within that one area. When you have comfortably introduced those changes, assess where you're at, and try another three.

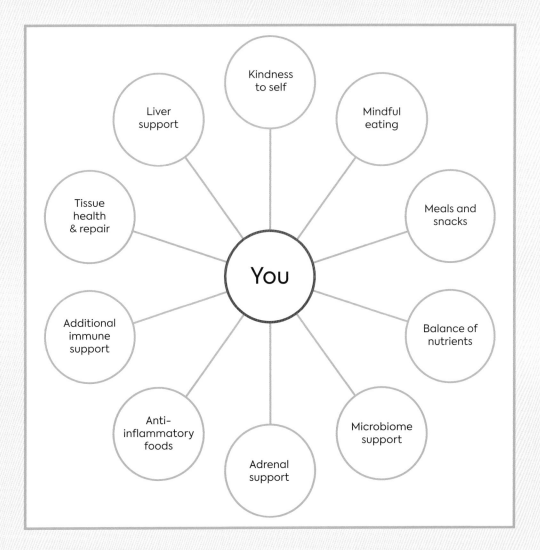

Always include "Kindness to self" as one of those things – even if you think you're already on top of that one. Activities for this might include:

- schedule in regular time each day/week/month where you do something you enjoy, that nourishes you deeply (this doesn't need to be expensive, it could just be a walk around the park, or an hour reading a novel)
- acknowledge every time you do something positive for yourself
- write a list of the things your body does well, the things you do well, the things you do to support yourself
- acknowledge when you're being self-critical, and read the above list to remind yourself!
- Put a note on the fridge/freezer door or biscuit jar saying "Enjoy each and every mouthful!" – instead of beating yourself up about reaching for snacks

Making time for change

You may need to make a few changes to your daily or weekly schedule, but do so in a way that frees you up rather than adds to your load. For example, if you don't usually find time to cook much, but want to start eating more home cooked food, then that cooking time isn't going to magically appear. You may find it useful to batch cook a few things on a day off. There are also plenty of recipes you can play with (including some at the end of this book), which are super quick and easy. The more you make them, the simpler they get, so that it really doesn't feel like an extra chore to prepare them.

On days where you have more time, you might want to slow down and really get into the creativity of what you're cooking. Immerse yourself in the tastes, smells and creative process, and experiment with new flavour and texture combinations. Play music, sing, or just enjoy a quiet, calm space while you're cooking. See this time as part of your self-nourishment.

Asking for help

If it all still seems overwhelming or unachievable, then ask for help. This could mean:

- *asking family members to do a little more* to free up some of your time, or to help with meal preparation

- *asking a friend or family member to go through your plan with you*, and help you find ways to implement it (make sure they understand what you're trying to achieve!)

- *working with a nutritional therapist* – I often spend time in consultations helping people find ways to implement what I'm recommending. In addition, a trained eye may be able to focus in more clearly on what kind of nutritional support you could benefit best from right now

- *working with a life coach or health coach*

- *going on a healthy cookery course* or a retreat that incorporates cookery classes – on the courses, workshops and retreats I have run and been involved with, not only have I been able to offer support, but participants have also been able to encourage each other, and share how they do things.

I appreciate some of these options aren't available to everyone, but you may be able to find other avenues of support within your community.

Ultimately, however, you need to take full responsibility for the changes you are going to make. This is your body, your health, your life. Asking for help is not the same as leaning on or handing over responsibility to someone else – it's about making sure you have what you need in place to embrace the responsibility yourself.

Listen to your body – and trust it

If anything you try doesn't feel beneficial, then don't do it! It may be that it's not the most appropriate thing for you right now. Or it may be that your body requires additional support in order to work with it. In this situation, I would recommend you seek professional advice.

If something you incorporate feels supportive, then that's fantastic. It may be something that will benefit you for the rest of your life, or it may be something that you need for a while and then can move away from at a later point. For example, your body may need more immune support in flu season, or during a time of extended stress.

Ultimately, everything is a guideline, rather than an absolute rule. Nobody understands the intricacies of your phenomenal body so much that they can tell you exactly what it needs – only your body can do that.

So what I'd really like you to get out of all this is an ability to more clearly hear what your body wants and needs right now. To find time to listen to it. To trust it. To be able to distinguish between cravings and requirements. And then to be able to make a decision free of self-judgement and criticism about what to eat.

This may take a lifetime of practice – I'll freely admit that I'm still practising this, and I don't always "get it right". But it's an approach that feels more nourishing than any other I've tried or witnessed.

So that's it now, over to you. Thank you for listening.

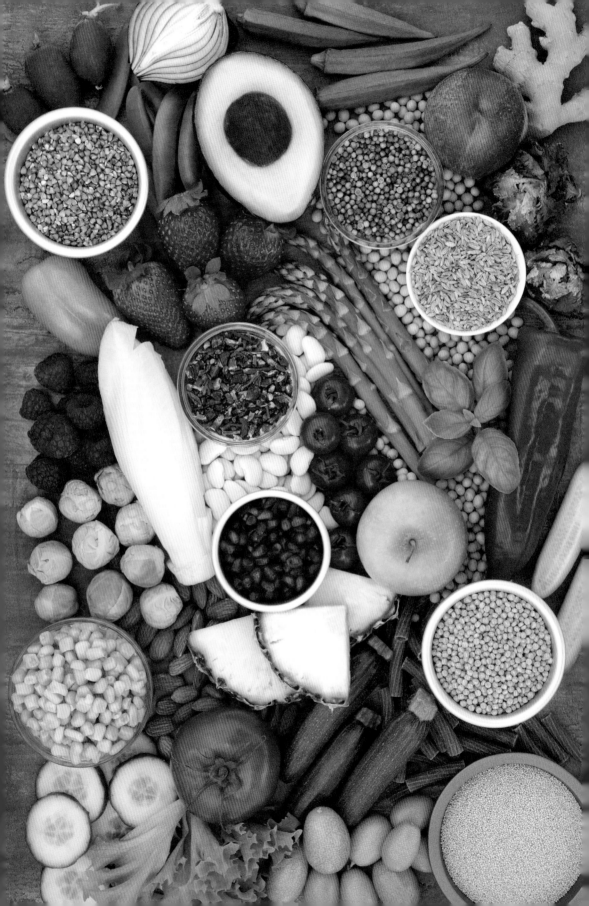

PART TWO

RECIPES

50 Delicious Recipes

Ironically I rarely follow recipes, but find them excellent for inspiration. If you're happiest following instructions, these recipes should work well for you, as they are all tried and tested.* However, you are welcome to tweak them to your own taste, or to match the ingredients in your cupboard – or if you just like playing with recipes to make them your own. All these recipes are vegan or vegetarian (***v*** = vegetarian, the rest are vegan). If you choose to eat meat and fish, please experiment with adapting these recipes accordingly, or using them to reduce the amount of animal produce and create more variety and balance in your diet. How you eat is your choice, but people seem to want help most with how to make delicious, healthy vegan and vegetarian meals. So here you go – enjoy!

Soups

Warm meals

Salads and wraps

Dressings, sauces and pastes

Snacks and dips

Desserts

Drinks and smoothies

---

* By me, my husband, friends and retreat guests I've cooked for, plus many people who have found some of these recipes on my website and social media pages, where you can find even more: **connectwithnutrition.co.uk**

Soups

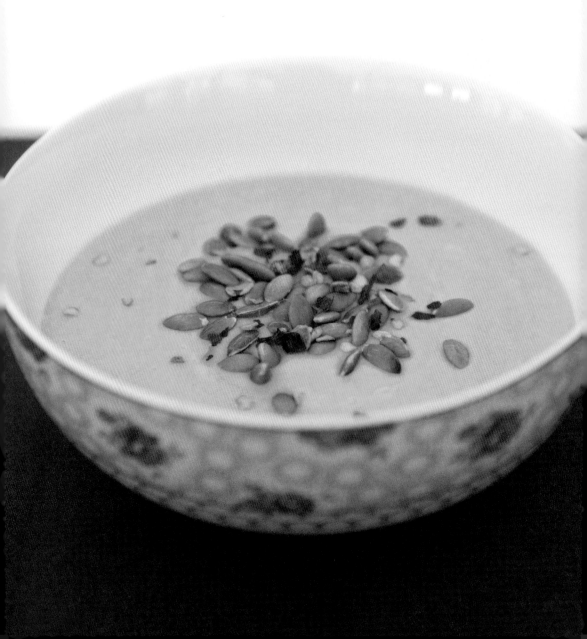

Earth Element soup

Deeply satisfying for breakfast, lunch or dinner, this soup nods to the principles of the Chinese Earth Element to help ease you warmly back into your body and ground you.

Ingredients *(serves 3-4)*
2 onions (red or white)
1 butternut squash
2-3 cloves garlic
150g orange lentils (preferably soaked overnight in water)
1-2 tsp turmeric powder or grated turmeric root
1-2 tsp ground coriander
½-1 tsp ground or grated nutmeg
1-2 tbsp coconut cream (the firmer bit in coconut milk) – optional
20g pumpkin seeds
handful fresh coriander
stock and seasoning

1. Heat the oven to 180 degrees C, or gas mark 5. Slice the butternut squash (or any squash) in half lengthways and scoop out the seeds. Place in the oven on a dish to roast.
2. When the squash is starting to soften (probably after about 20 minutes), add the onions and garlic.
3. Melt a little coconut oil in a pan and add the spices and some black pepper. Leave to simmer for a couple of minutes.
4. Thoroughly rinse the lentils, then add to the spices. Add enough stock/water to cover, and simmer till soft, topping up with fluid if necessary, so that it's always just covering the lentils.
5. When everything is cooked, blend it all together with the coconut cream, and season to taste.
6. Toast the pumpkin seeds by heating in a frying pan over a low to medium heat until they start to pop, perhaps stirring in a little tamari afterwards for extra taste.
7. Serve with a garnish of pumpkin seeds and chopped coriander leaves.

TIP: You can roast the butternut squash seeds to make a great savoury snack. Separate them from any squash flesh, give them a rinse, then toss in a little melted coconut oil with perhaps sea salt, black pepper and chilli flakes, or spices of your choice. Spread out on a baking tray and roast in a moderate to warm oven for about half an hour.

Wood Element soup

This vivid green soup aims to keep your liver happy, with plenty of ingredients for your phase 1 and phase 2 detoxification processes. Virtuous and surprisingly lovely. Serve with oatcakes and houmous to add some protein.

Ingredients *(serves 3-4)*
2 medium-sized potatoes (peeled) **OR** the equivalent amount of cauliflower
2 generous handfuls watercress
1 handful (approx. 100g) kale
1 handful (approx. 100g) cabbage (any type)
a few leaves of wild garlic (optional)
freshly ground nutmeg, seat salt and black pepper to season

1. Chop the potatoes or cauliflower (or mix of both) into cubes and boil in water or stock.
2. Chop the kale and cabbage, add to the pot, and simmer till all the veg is soft.
3. Add the watercress, wild garlic and seasoning. Blend and serve.

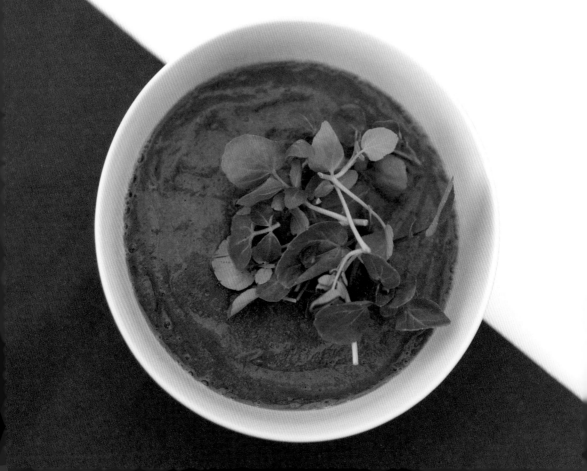

Broccoli and almond soup

This is a winner: light, tasty, really simple to make and full of amazing nutrients.

Ingredients *(serves 3-4)*
a few heads of broccoli
100g ground almonds
1-2 leeks
1 clove garlic, chopped
sea salt and black pepper to season
a little turmeric and nutmeg
the grated zest of a lemon (optional)
fresh mint

1. Steam the broccoli until almost cooked.
2. Meanwhile, simmer the leeks, garlic, black pepper and spices in a little coconut oil until soft.
3. Add the broccoli and enough water or stock to cover.
4. When cooked, add the ground almonds and lemon zest. Then blend and stir in the seasoning and spices. Serve and garnish with fresh mint.

Cauliflower and hazelnut soup

Ingredients *(serves 3-4)*
a head of cauliflower, cut into florets and chunks
100g ground hazelnuts (grind in a blender)
1-2 medium white onions
1 clove garlic, chopped
sea salt and black pepper
the grated zest of an orange (optional)
a few sprigs of fresh thyme or sage

1. Steam the cauliflower until almost cooked.
2. Meanwhile, simmer the onion and garlic in a little coconut oil until soft.
3. Add the cauliflower, nutmeg and seasoning, and enough water or stock to cover.
4. When cooked, add the ground hazelnuts, most of the orange zest and thyme or sage leaves, and blend. Garnish with the remaining thyme/sage and zest.

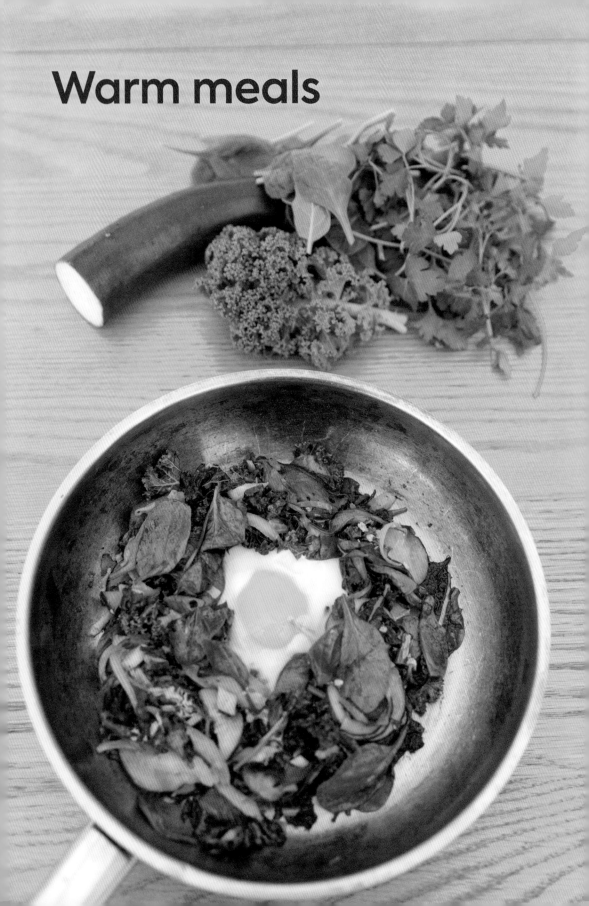

Warm meals

Soft egg omelette (v)

Ingredients *(serves 1-2)*
1 onion or leek – finely sliced
½ fennel bulb (optional) – thinly sliced
½ courgette – sliced
100g spinach and/or kale
1 handful of mushrooms (e.g. chestnut, portobello, shiitake)
1-2 eggs
½-1 tsp ground nutmeg
½-1 tsp ground coriander
1 tsp turmeric powder or grated turmeric root
black pepper
tamari (wheat-free soya sauce) or sea salt

1. Gently stir fry onion or leek in a little coconut oil plus the spices and black pepper.
2. Add the courgette, fennel and mushrooms, and stir till nearly cooked.
3. If the pan has dried out, add a little water or stock, plus tamari or sea salt to taste. Stir in the spinach until it starts to wilt.
4. Make one or two little nest-like dips in the vegetables, crack an egg in each, cover with a lid and cook till the white is firm but the yolk is still soft.

Green up your grains

Short grain brown rice and quinoa are both great to use as side dishes, in porridge (cook well until starting to go slushy and stir in a dollop of nut butter or tahini) and for salads (cook then stir in chopped salad vegetables, herbs, lemon juice and seasoning). If I'm using rice or quinoa as a side dish with a curry, stir-fry, some pulses and vegetables or maybe some fish and vegetables, then I'll often "green it up".
– N.B. Quinoa is technically a seed, but is easily used as a grain.

How to cook short grain brown rice
Use twice as much water as rice, bring it to the boil, and simmer for around 45 minutes or until soft.
– OR
I have a Schulte-Ufer thermal pot, so I bring it to the boil on the hob, put the saucepan in its thermal "coat" and let it sit for around 45 minutes, cooking itself with no additional heat source. You can also get similar alternatives to this.

How to cook quinoa
Use 1½ times as much water as quinoa, bring it to the boil, and simmer for around 20-30 minutes or until soft. You'll see the tiny quinoa seeds start to unfurl, and then swell as they rehydrate.

How to green up your grains

Ingredients
short grain brown rice or quinoa (or any grain) – cooked till soft (see above)
wild rocket and/or watercress and/or shredded raw spinach – approximately a handful raw per handful of cooked rice
green peas
pesto or fresh herbs – e.g. coriander, parsley, basil, thyme, oregano, chives, mint, etc. – see my **Pesto** recipe (*see p.275*) for unbeatable home made versions.

1. Stir it all together (the leaves will wilt in the warm rice), then season and serve.

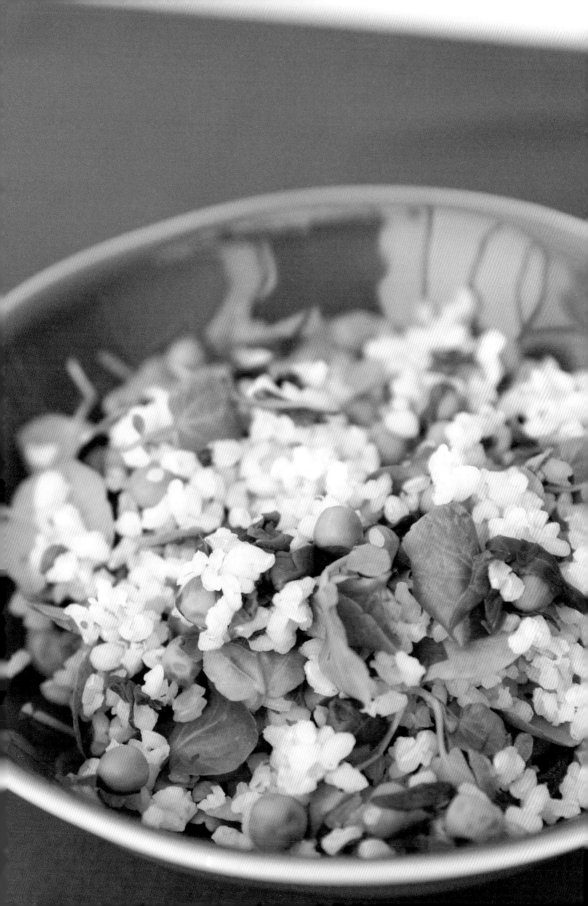

Rousing risotto

Most people think they need to use white arborio rice to make a risotto, but actually short grain brown rice works beautifully.

Arborio rice is essentially a short grain rice, anyway, but the beauty of short grain *brown* rice is you still get the creamy consistency, plus a slightly nuttier flavour, more nutrients and less of a potential blood sugar challenge.

Soaking your rice overnight (or even for a couple of days) and rinsing it really well ensures easier digestion.

As brown rice needs a longer cooking time than white, I usually cook the rice till it's soft before turning it into a risotto. Then the more you cook it, the softer and more risotto-like it becomes.

So the following recipe starts with cooked rice, a process that usually takes around 40 minutes.

Finally, this is a *rousing* risotto because it contains ingredients that help you to harness sunshine energy from all your foods.

Ingredients
2 cups short grain brown rice (cooked)
1 cup shiitake mushrooms (fresh or dried – if dried then soak first)
1 cup peas
2 large handfuls of spinach
2 red or white onions
2 cloves of garlic
stock or water
1-2 tbsp tahini
black pepper and sea salt or tamari to season

1. Finely slice the onions and garlic.
2. Gently fry the onions in a little coconut oil or butter until soft, and then add sliced shiitake mushrooms and seasoning.
3. When the mushrooms are nearly cooked, add the garlic.
4. Add the rice and enough stock or water to just cover, and keep stirring until the rice is very soft and there is just a little extra water/stock (add more if necessary).
5. Add in the peas and cook for a few minutes.
6. Stir in the tahini to make the risotto seem creamy, season further if necessary, and then stir in the spinach until it is wilted.
7. Serve with a drizzle of **Pesto** (*see p.275*).

Black bean and seaweed stew

Using classic ingredients to support the Chinese Water Element together with a complementary balance of vegetables, this just feels amazing on every level.

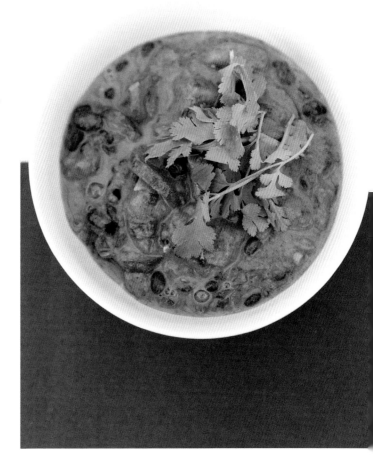

Ingredients *(serves 3-4)*
200g black beans – soaked overnight
2 strips kombu seaweed
handful dulse seaweed
2 sweet potatoes
2 courgettes
1 onion (red or white)
2-3 cloves of garlic
2-3 handfuls watercress
2 tbsp coconut block
OR ½-1 tin coconut milk
black pepper and tamari (wheat-free soya sauce) or sea salt to taste

1. Drain and rinse beans, cover with water, bring to boil, then add the kombu and simmer.
2. Finely chop the garlic, and leave to sit for 20 minutes (this activates the allicin that's good for your cardiovascular system).
3. Chop the sweet potatoes, courgettes and onions.
4. After simmering the beans for about an hour, fish out and discard the kombu. Then add the sweet potatoes, courgettes, onions, garlic and dulse.
5. Keep an eye on water levels and add more if necessary.
6. When almost ready (all ingredients are soft), add the coconut and seasoning.
7. Serve in bowls covered with chopped watercress.

Millet slice

This recipe is inspired by Infinity Foods' legendary millet slice. Infinity Foods is a thriving worker co-operative, situated in the heart of Brighton, dedicated to the provision of an extensive range of 100% vegetarian, natural & organic foods since 1971.

These are like savoury flapjacks and are incredibly versatile. They are melt-in-the-mouth delicious straight from the oven, and then improve as they rest. Then you can have the rest hot or cold – so perfect for lunchboxes and midweek meals when you don't want to cook. Below I have suggested serving with a tahini sauce and salad, but they work equally well with a tomato-based sauce or standard gravy, and with roasted or stir-fried vegetables.

Ingredients *(serves approx. 8)*
1-2 cups millet, preferably soaked overnight
1-2 tbsp tahini
1 large onion
1-2 cloves garlic
2-3 cups cooked vegetables – see below for ideas*
herbs, spices and seasoning

1. Bring millet to the boil in pan of water, and simmer until cooked.
2. Drain until there's just a little water left – just enough to stir the tahini into so it's a thick liquid, and stir thoroughly into millet.
3. Finley slice and gently fry the onions and garlic in a little coconut oil.
4. Stir in vegetables,* herbs/spices and seasoning.
5. Put into small, deep baking tray or dish (greased with coconut oil) as if making flapjacks.
6. Bake in a moderate oven until browning on top.
7. Cut into generous slices and serve with tahini sauce and salad.

* Vegetable options:

mushroom, courgette, red pepper, sun-dried tomatoes and basil
arame seaweed, onions, garlic and sunflower seeds
roasted sweet potato, beetroot and ginger (use plenty of ginger, fresh or dried)
pumpkin, pumpkin seed and ginger
spring onion, watercress, avocado and lemon
kale, onion and turmeric
...or try your own combinations – this is a perfect opportunity to use up leftovers and any vegetables you have a glut of.

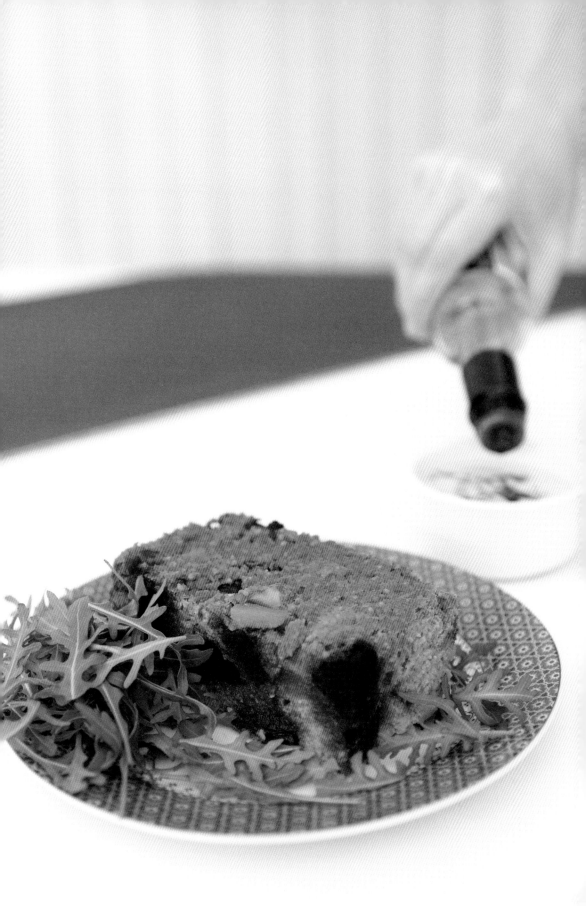

Mixed bean casserole

This is a very loose recipe as you can pretty much use whatever is in season and you have in your cupboard. A great opportunity to experiment and play with flavour combinations, as well as to batch cook something that will save you time and headspace in the days or weeks to come.

So you can make as much or as little as you like – just make sure there is a balance of beans and vegetables. If in doubt, add more vegetables! Sometimes I make this with lots of different vegetables, and sometimes I keep it simple with just two or three different kinds, but it will always be at least 2-3 veg.

I don't always use a tomato base for the sauce; I'll often just use well-seasoned water, maybe stirring in some tahini for extra taste and thickness. Oats also thicken the sauce – while upping the amino acid profile to make this a complete protein.

Ingredients
beans e.g. black beans, butter beans, mung beans, kidney beans, etc. – soaked overnight and rinsed well
allium vegetables e.g. onions, leeks, celery, fennel, garlic
root vegetables e.g. carrot, sweet potato, parsnip, swede, celeriac
cruciferous vegetables e.g. cauliflower, broccoli, kale, cabbage, Brussels sprouts
1-2 sticks kombu seaweed
fresh herbs e.g. parsley, rosemary, bay leaves, thyme
– **OR** spices e.g. cumin, coriander, paprika, turmeric
chopped or tinned tomatoes or passata – or just water – enough to cover the other ingredients
black pepper and tamari (wheat-free soya sauce) or sea salt to season
oats to thicken (I usually start with a handful and add more towards the end if necessary)

1. I like to at least partly cook the pulses first in water with the kombu strips to help make them more digestible.
2. Then add the rest of the ingredients, pop the lid on and simmer on a low heat, in a slow cooker, or in the oven in a casserole dish, for at least an hour until everything is well cooked and flavoursome. If you are using a slow cooker, you will need less liquid.
3. Stir from time to time, adjusting the seasoning and adding more oats if necessary towards the end.

Cruciferous curry

I frequently cook variations on this recipe and it always goes down well. This version focuses on the cruciferous family of vegetables, to help your body make the enzymes it needs for detoxification processes and regulating hormones. It also has a number of pungent spices that encourage sweating and other elimination processes. Together with the white onion, garlic and coconut milk, this provides ample support for the functions of the Chinese Metal Element.

Ingredients *(serves 3-4)*
1 handful of cauliflower florets
1 handful of broccoli florets
2 handfuls of chopped cabbage and/or kale
1 large white onion, chopped
1-2 cloves garlic, chopped
1-2 tsp each of freshly chopped ginger, turmeric powder (or chopped fresh turmeric), paprika, cumin seeds or powder, coriander powder, ground cinnamon, fennel seeds*
4-6 whole cloves and cardamom pods*
1 cup coconut milk
2 tbsp ground almonds or tahini
fresh green or red chilli, black pepper and tamari or sea salt to taste

* *Or you can keep it simpler with just coriander, cumin, turmeric and ginger.*

1. Finely chop the garlic and leave to sit (this allows the allicin to be activated before you cook it).
2. Gently dry fry the cumin and fennel seeds if you are using either of these.
3. Add a little coconut oil to the pan, and let the onions cook until soft in coconut oil.
4. Meanwhile, steam the cauliflower, broccoli and cabbage/kale until semi-cooked.
5. Add the rest of the spices to the pan, and then the vegetables.
6. Stir for a few minutes, then pour in the coconut milk.
7. Simmer on a low to moderate heat until vegetables have cooked and the sauce is full of flavour.
8. Stir in the ground almonds, and adjust seasoning if necessary.
9. Serve with short grain brown rice or quinoa (*see* **Green up your grains** recipe, *p.250*) and a garnish of fresh coriander or mint.

Roasted squash with lentils, seeds and rosemary

This meal is hearty and light all at the same time, and is super easy to make. It's one of the tastiest ways I know to support your immune system, with plenty of ingredients to make healthy white blood cells.

Ingredients *(serves 2)*
1 butternut squash
100g puy lentils (dry weight)
200g chopped or tinned tomatoes, or passata
1 large handful of spinach, chard, kale or similar green leaves
1 handful pumpkin seeds
1 large sprig rosemary
black pepper and tamari (wheat-free soya sauce) or sea salt to season

1. Soak the lentils overnight, rinse well and simmer in water until soft.
2. Meanwhile, bake the butternut squash whole in the oven at 180° or gas mark 4 until soft – this usually takes about an hour or so.
3. Pull the green needles off the rosemary and finely chop.
4. Drain the lentils, and add the tomatoes, green leaves, rosemary and seasoning. Simmer for another 5-10 minutes, stirring to help the leaves wilt. You may find you need to add more tomatoes if the mixture is too dry.
5. Slice the squash in half lengthways, scrape out the seeds, and spoon the lentil mix into the hollow and next to each half on the plate.
6. Dry toast the pumpkin seeds in a pan over a moderate heat until they start to pop, and sprinkle on top.

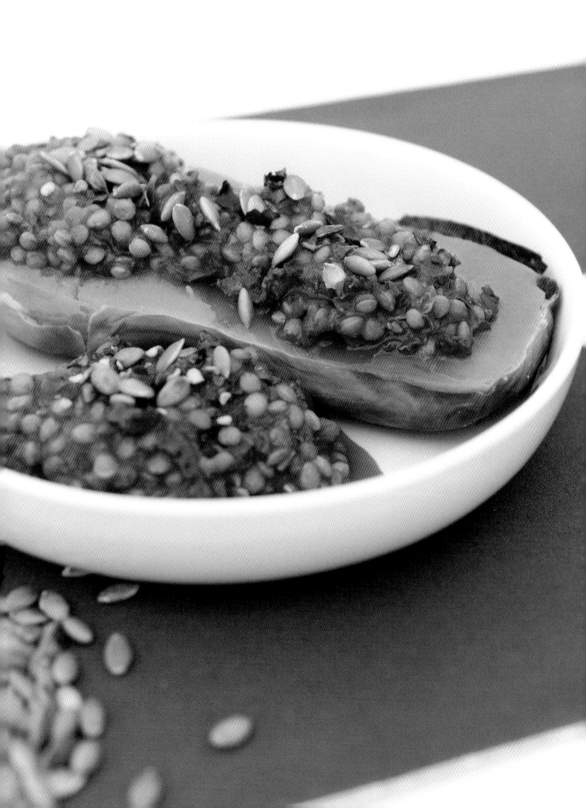

Salads and wraps

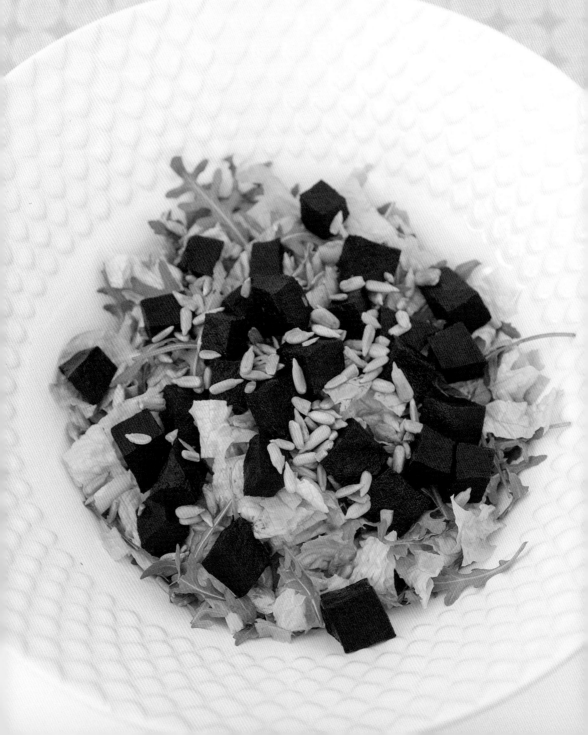

Methylating salad

As the name suggests, this colourful salad provides ingredients you need for methylation processes – which your liver uses as part of its detoxification protocol, and to help break down oestrogens.

So whether you want to help your liver combat pollution, maintain your reproductive health, or just eat a really tasty salad, this is for you.

Beetroot is easier to peel and chop once cooked. You can just chuck it in the oven while something else is cooking, maybe even the day before, and then just sit them in a covered bowl in the fridge until you're ready to use them.

Ingredients *(serves 2)*
½ romaine lettuce
1 large handful rocket
2 large or 4 small beetroot
1 handful sunflower seeds
yoghurt and mint, yoghurt and balsamic or tahini dressing (See **Dressings, sauces and pastes**, *p.273*)

1. Roast the beetroot in a moderate oven until soft (about 45 mins depending on size).
2. When cool enough, peel the beetroot, and slice into bite-sized chunks.
3. Gently toast the sunflower seeds over a low to moderate heat in a dry frying pan – they're done when they start to pop.
4. Combine the ingredients and serve with your dressing of choice.

Gram flour wraps with mushrooms and avocado

Wraps can be so deliciously satisfying – yet so disappointing when you buy them from a shop! This is a simple, gluten-free recipe with tasty, nourishing and immune-boosting ingredients. They're great for lunchboxes, and also served with salads and dips at home.

Ingredients *(for the pancakes)*
gram flour (chickpea flour)
water

In terms of quantities, it depends how much batter you want to make. I usually add about a cup of gram flour to a bowl, and then gradually stir or whisk in the water until it's a batter consistency, so like thick pouring cream.

    This batter will keep for 3-4 days in an airtight container in the fridge, so you can make fresh wraps at the drop of a hat.

1. Melt a little coconut oil, butter ghee or butter into a frying pan on a moderate heat.
2. Pour a little batter in as if making a pancake – swirl until it reaches the edge all around.
3. Patiently wait until it moves freely when you shake the pan.
4. Flip it over and cook the other side for a few minutes.

Filling your wraps:
There are so many delicious combinations you can fill your wraps with, you can get really creative with this. For a particularly immune-boosting wrap, I love mushroom and avocado:

Ingredients *(for the filling)*
Mushrooms – e.g. shiitake, chestnut, portobello, porcini (ceps), etc. – a small handful per wrap

1. Gently fry or bake sliced mushrooms with some tamari, coconut oil, black pepper and fresh thyme or parsley.
2. Fill wrap with mushrooms, salad and slices of avocado – you just need to make a 3-inch wide column of filling down the middle of the open wrap.
3. Optional: drizzle with **Tahini sauce** (*see p.274*).
4. Fold sides over, tucking the bottom under as you go, and wrap a napkin or piece of kitchen towel round the bottom to help hold it in place and catch any drips as you eat.

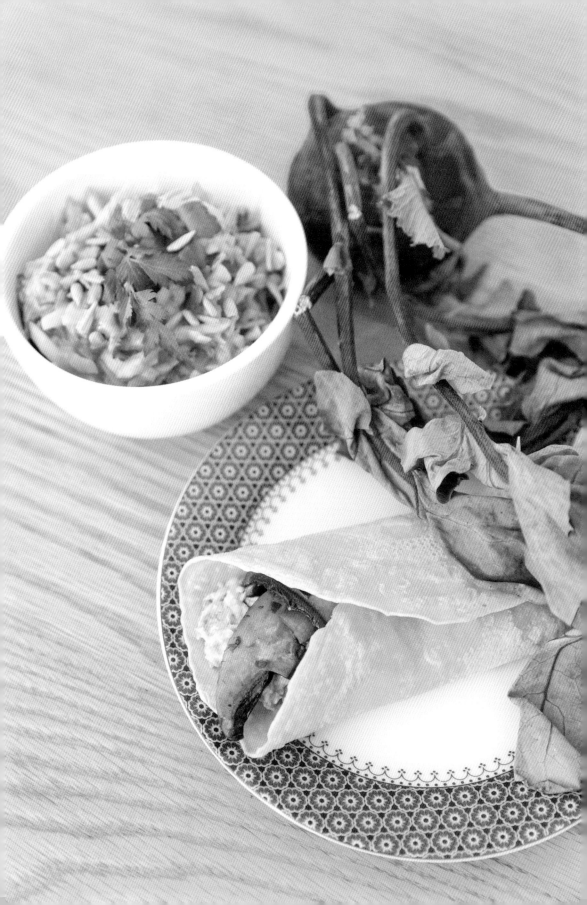

Energising salad

Salads often feel fresh and energizing, especially in summer, and this one contains the co-factors you need to make ATP, your energy batteries. When you eat, complex processes take the energy out of that food and put it into ATP, a form you can use. So to fuel up, you need a range of nutrients as well as the calories.

Ingredients
romaine lettuce
babyleaf spinach
avocado
cucumber
radishes
celery
sunflower seeds
walnuts
chickpeas, cooked (soaked overnight then simmered for 1-1½ hours until soft)

1. Roughly chop the lettuce and avocado, finely slice the cucumber, radishes and celery, add to a salad bowl with the babyleaf spinach and chickpeas.
2. Gently dry toast the sunflower seeds and walnuts in a pan over a moderate heat **OR** use walnuts and sunflower seeds soaked overnight in water, then rinsed and drained. Add to the salad together with the cooked chickpeas.
3. Dress with a **Salad dressing** of your choice (*see p.273*).

Nutty asparagus and brown rice salad

Salads don't have to be light and green – they can also be soulful and satisfying. This brown rice salad is great on its own, as a side dish or with a medley of other salads. Like the energizing salad, it contains the co-factor nutrients needed to convert energy from food into ATP, your energy batteries; plus, of course, the energy itself.

Ingredients
1 cup brown rice (soaked overnight, rinsed then cooked)
1-2 handfuls spinach
2 sweet potatoes
6-8 spears asparagus
2-3 tbsp hazelnuts or walnuts (soaked or toasted)
2-3 tbsp sunflower seeds (soaked or toasted)
sea salt and black pepper to season (plus optional garlic and fresh herbs)

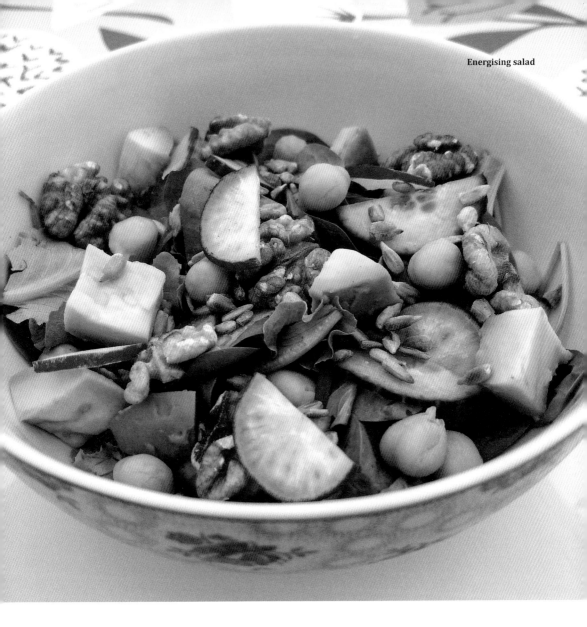

1. Add a little coconut oil to a baking tray or dish and put in the oven to warm at about 180 degrees C, or gas mark 4.
2. Chop the sweet potatoes into 2-3cm cubes and add to the baking tray, together with the asparagus, toss in the oil to coat, and roast for about half an hour, or until soft. You could also add some garlic, herbs and seasoning if you wish.
3. Remove from the oven and stir in the spinach until the spinach has wilted.
4. Mix together the vegetables, nuts, seeds and rice, and serve with a yoghurt and mint dressing.

Bone strengthening carrot and sea spaghetti salad

Sea spaghetti is a kind of seaweed I've been getting from a couple of local health food shops. It's usually from the Atlantic Ocean, is really easy to use and quite a palatable introduction to seaweed. It's not too strong tasting, but still adds a mineral flavour that works well with the sweetness of the carrot, especially when cut with the gentle acidity of the lemon juice.

Ingredients *(serves 2)*
2 carrots
1 sheet of sea spaghetti
2-3 tbsp raw tahini
½-1 lemon
tamari to taste

1. Soak the sea spaghetti in warm water for 20 minutes. Meanwhile...
2. Ribbon the carrots using a potato peeler: simply draw the peeler lengthways from carrot top to carrot tip, rotate the carrot slightly and repeat until you can't practically ribbon any more. (You can use the remainder of the carrot to dip into houmous, guacamole or almond butter as a snack later on.)
3. Stir the juice and zest of half to one lemon into 2-3 tbsp of raw or light tahini. Stir these ingredients vigorously until smooth, adding a little water to make a thick, creamy consistency. Season with a little tamari (wheat-free soya sauce).
4. Rinse and drain the seaweed and mix all the ingredients together.

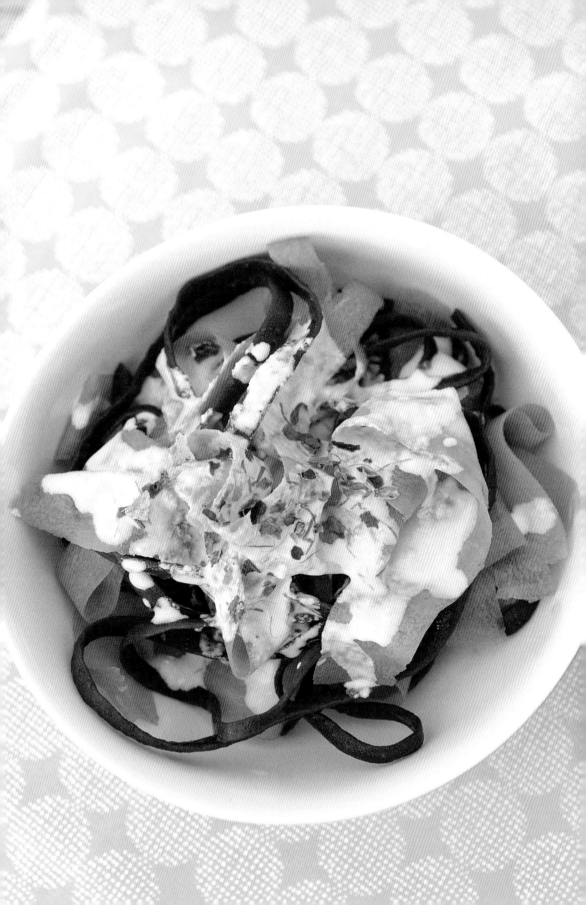

Mighty egg salad (v)

This is your superhero salad for strengthening your immune system. It contains ingredients to help you make really healthy white blood cells. At the same time, there are nutrients that will soothe your adrenals, help rebalance your cortisol levels, and so help your body resolve inflammation when it needs to. Plus it's really satisfying!

At the time of writing, eggs have finally been freed of their reputation for raising cholesterol levels. I'm still not going to advocate an excessively high egg intake, but unless you're vegan, they can be a useful addition to your weekly diet. In terms of animal welfare, note that "farm fresh" or even "free range" doesn't guarantee a great life for the chickens.

So research where your shop sources its eggs, or find a farm (or neighbour!) you know treats the chickens really well, gives them plenty of access to fresh air and pastures for foraging, and operates according to organic principles.

Ingredients *(serves 2)*
2-3 eggs
½ romaine lettuce
1 large handful watercress
1 handful chopped chives
1 avocado
¼ cucumber – sliced
1 handful brazil nuts – crushed, or soaked and thinly sliced
cucumber and yoghurt dressing (See **Dressings, sauces and pastes**, *p.273*)

1. Boil the eggs for 10-15 minutes, and cool in a bowl of cold water.
2. Roughly chop the lettuce and avocado, and mix with the other salad ingredients.
3. Peel the eggs, slice into quarters and add to the salad.
4. Drizzle over the dressing and serve.

Coleslaws

These are all twists on the classic coleslaw. All of them work well as side dishes, fillings and toppings, especially on a jacket sweet potato. They are vegan friendly, with vegetarian options, vibrantly coloured and a delight to have with any dish.

Sun slaw

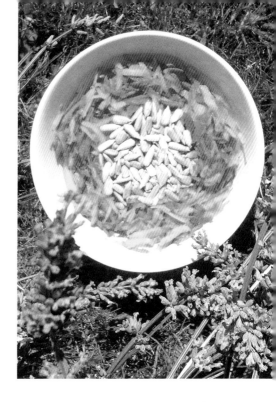

Sun slaw is perfect for nourishing your digestion. The Chinese Earth Element is represented by the colours orange and yellow. These colours, together with the natural sweetness of carrots and golden beetroot, gently soothe your stomach and spleen. Your digestive ability is said to be enhanced when you include such foods.

The "mother" in the apple cider vinegar is the ferment produced when vinegar is made. It helps top up your gut bacteria, and so supports your digestive functions as well as your immune system and general wellbeing.

The vitamin B6 and magnesium in the sunflower seeds are wonderful at soothing your adrenals and calming your nervous system. This directly impacts the health and activity of your digestive system – and your whole body.

Nourishing your Earth Element often helps you to feel grounded and connected. It may also help to reduce sugar cravings, especially together with the sour flavour of the apple cider vinegar.

Ingredients
equal amounts of:
golden beetroot
carrot
sunflower seeds
dressing: apple cider vinegar with mother

1. Grate the carrot and beetroot.
2. Lightly toast the sunflower seeds in a pan until they start to pop.
3. When the seeds have cooled, mix everything together and dress with the apple cider vinegar.

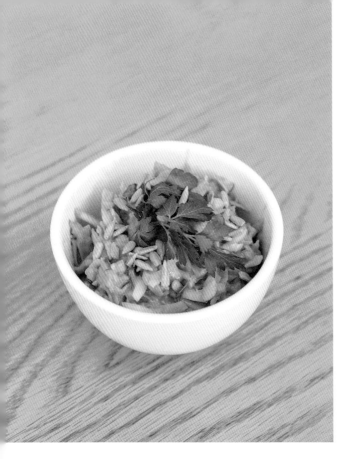

Super slaw

This is a totally invigorating, glorious rainbow of a superfood recipe, with various options to really make this your own.

Instead of mayonnaise, there is what I sometimes call avonnaise, an avocado-based paste to bring it all together. This makes the whole affair both vegan and super nourishing to your adrenals.

For a non-vegan option you could use mayonnaise instead (preferably home made with cold pressed oils and organic eggs) or mild and creamy sheep's yoghurt – or a blend of these with avocado.

Ingredients
equal amounts of:
carrot and/or beetroot
courgette
fennel or celery
celeriac or kohlrabi or squash
onions or spring onions
green leaves, e.g. rocket, spinach, watercress
½-1 ripe avocado
2 tbsp lemon or lime juice
2 tbsp cold pressed extra virgin olive oil
sea salt and black pepper to season
a handful of chopped, fresh herbs, e.g. coriander, parsley, basil, oregano or mint
optional: a handful of toasted sesame, sunflower or pumpkin seeds

1. Grate or finely slice the vegetables.
2. Blend the avocado, citrus juice, oil and seasoning – adjust the quantities if making a larger portion – also do a quick taste test and adjust to taste if necessary.
3. Mix everything together, including the herbs.

Warm slaw

A kind of play on words (although the original is coleslaw, not cold slaw!), warm slaw is essentially a warmed up version of the Super slaw. It's perfect for colder months, or if your digestion can't handle lots of raw food – or if you just fancy something a bit different. So the ingredients are the same as the super slaw. Just gently simmer the grated/finely sliced vegetables in a little water or stock until soft and warmed through. Then season and stir in everything else.

Sauerkraut

Sauerkraut is easy and satisfying to make, and will last for ages, especially as you only need to have about 1-2 spoonfuls a day.

You can buy excellent sauerkraut – make sure it's raw for its gut health benefits. Making your own, if you have the time and inclination to do so, is another great opportunity for creativity, however. There's nothing quite like eating or feeding people you love with something you've made yourself.

Ingredients
1 litre good quality water*
2 tbsp good quality sea or rock salt*
1 chopped cabbage

Optional extra ingredients
selection of other chopped vegetables e.g. cauliflower, sweet potato, carrot, fennel, cucumber, etc.
herbs and or spices, e.g. dill, thyme, coriander seeds, juniper seeds, peppercorns, fresh ginger, turmeric, etc.
a probiotic supplement to help the process along (empty in the capsule's contents)

1. Place vegetables in a clean glass storage jar with a sealable lid. If using herbs or spices, use these as a bottom layer.
2. Stir salt into water until well dissolved and add to vegetables.
3. Weigh vegetables down with a couple of large, clean stones or a small saucer. It is important that the vegetables are covered with fluid at all times.
4. Seal lid and store at room temperature for a few days. Once a day, open the lid for a few seconds and then replace. After about 3-7 days it should be ready and will keep refrigerated for a long time.

* Alternatively use freshly pressed cabbage juice or celery juice.

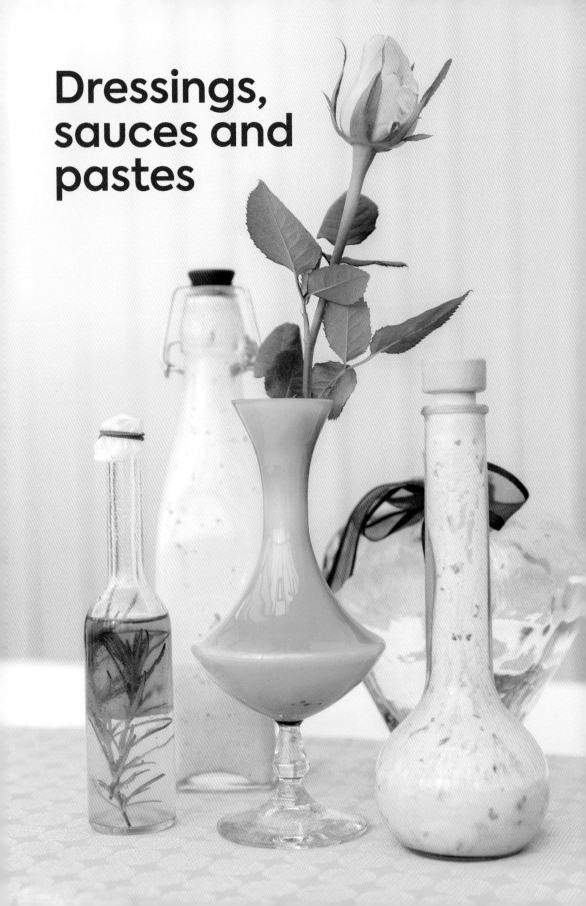

Dressings,
sauces and
pastes

Salad dressings

Salad dressings add bursts of flavour – and also a great deal of nutritional value. Apple cider vinegar "with mother" is the unfiltered version that contains the ferment, i.e. a colony of probiotic microbes. Unfiltered balsamic vinegar and yoghurt are similarly nourishing to your microbiome.

High quality cold pressed oils, such as extra virgin olive oil, are rich in fatty acids and polyphenols that keep your tissue healthy and help calm inflammation. Herbs and spices are also rich in anti-inflammatory and antioxidant compounds. You could also add minced garlic and/or root ginger to dressings for extra kick and health properties.

Essentially there are no rules when making a salad dressing, except to either use it all up or keep it in an airtight container for storage – preferably in a cool cupboard or the fridge. To make them, you just add the ingredients together and give them a stir or shake. If I'm really in a hurry, I'll add the ingredients straight into the salad and mix it all together there and then.

If I want the flavours to really permeate the oil, then I'll make the dressing in advance and leave it for at least 20 minutes before serving – I would definitely do this if adding a sprig of rosemary, and then might remove the rosemary before serving.

Apple cider vinaigrette (v)
6 tbsp cold pressed extra virgin olive oil
4-6 tbsp apple cider vinegar "with mother"
1 tsp raw (unpasteurized) honey – preferably local
1 tbsp finely chopped fresh basil, oregano or thyme, or a sprig of rosemary
Optional: 1 tsp mustard powder (as well as adding flavour, this will help to emulsify the dressing so you don't need to keep shaking it)

Yoghurt and balsamic dressing (v)
4 tbsp yoghurt (I use organic sheep's yoghurt, but you could use alternatives)
2 tbsp cold pressed extra virgin olive oil
3-4 tbsp unfiltered balsamic vinegar
1 tbsp finely chopped thyme

Yoghurt and mint dressing (v)
3-4 tbsp yoghurt (I use organic sheep's yoghurt, but you could use alternatives)
6-8 tbsp cold pressed extra virgin olive oil
2-3 tbsp freshly squeezed lemon juice
1 tbsp finely chopped mint

Rich tahini dressing

juice and zest of ½-1 lime or lemon

2 tbsp tahini (sesame seed paste), thinned by gradually stirring in no more than ½ pint of water

½ tsp freshly ground mustard seeds

¼ tsp finely chopped garlic

½ tsp finely chopped root ginger

1-2 tbsp finely chopped fresh herbs, e.g. parsley or oregano

½ tsp local, raw (unpasteurized) honey (optional)

You could also add finely chopped fresh chilli or dried chilli flakes for extra kick.

Sauces and pastes

Tahini sauce

Tahini sauce has been my go to for years. It's creamy, adds a great depth of flavour and is really easy to make. It replaces creamy and cheesy sauces really well to make any such recipe dairy-free, and works beautifully poured over steamed vegetables, roasted vegetables and millet slices.

Tahini is a sesame seed paste, and comes in varying guises: raw, roasted, light, dark… all of them work well according to your preference. If I'm in a real hurry, then I just add a little cold water and a little tamari to 2 tbsp tahini, stirring vigorously with a fork till it goes a little thinner. Then I gradually add the hot water from the vegetables I've been steaming, stirring all the time, until it's a thick pouring consistency.

When I'm in less of a hurry, I make a tahini roux:

Tahini roux

2 tbsp tahini

1 tbsp brown rice flour, corn flour or arrowroot flour

stock or water

tamari and black pepper to taste

Optional: freshly chopped herbs, lemon juice

1. In a small pan stir the flour into the tahini.
2. Over a low to medium heat, very gradually add the stock or water, stirring continuously to avoid lumps (a whisk is sometimes useful here).
3. When a good, thick, creamy consistency, season, then stir in herbs and/or lemon juice (optional).

Pesto

Pesto is one of the most versatile sauces you can make. It's obviously delicious run through pasta dishes (tip: check out brown rice pasta, it's surprisingly good). Also use it to **Green up your grains** (*see p.250*), liven up a wrap or drizzle on a soup.

Classic pesto is made from fresh basil, pine nuts, olive oil, garlic and parmesan, but you can make substitutions here to make really interesting pestos. Such as:

- rosemary and pumpkin seed
- sage, walnut and lemon zest
- thyme, cashew and orange zest
- coriander, sunflower seed and chili.

Parmesan is optional – in fact I don't recall ever making pesto with it. Softer nuts and seeds, soaked overnight, add an extra creamy hint that more than makes up for this. Plus if you pack it with flavour, the extra saltiness of the cheese isn't needed.

Ingredients
50-100g fresh herbs
4 tbsp nuts/seeds (preferably soaked overnight in water)
4 tbsp extra virgin olive oil
freshly ground black pepper and sea salt to season
Optional: lemon zest, orange zest, fresh or dried chili, garlic to taste

1. Blend all dry ingredients until small but not completely ground/minced.
2. Stir in olive oil and use or store for later use.

Turmeric paste

This is great just melted into sauces, casseroles, stir-fries, smoothies, etc. The curcuminoids in turmeric have great health benefits, but we don't absorb them well. The piperine in black pepper and the oil helps you get the most out of turmeric. Buy pure turmeric! Some cheaper turmeric powders on sale have been found to be laced with lead chromate to enhance the colour and flavour.

Ingredients
2 parts turmeric powder
9 part cold pressed coconut oil
1 part black pepper – or experiment with quantities according to your own taste

1. Gently melt the coconut oil if necessary – coconut oil is usually solid at room temperature, except in high summer.
2. Pour into a clean jar with the turmeric and black pepper, stirring from time to time as the oil cools and solidifies to keep the mix evenly spread – in high summer you may need to finish this off in the fridge.

Snacks and dips

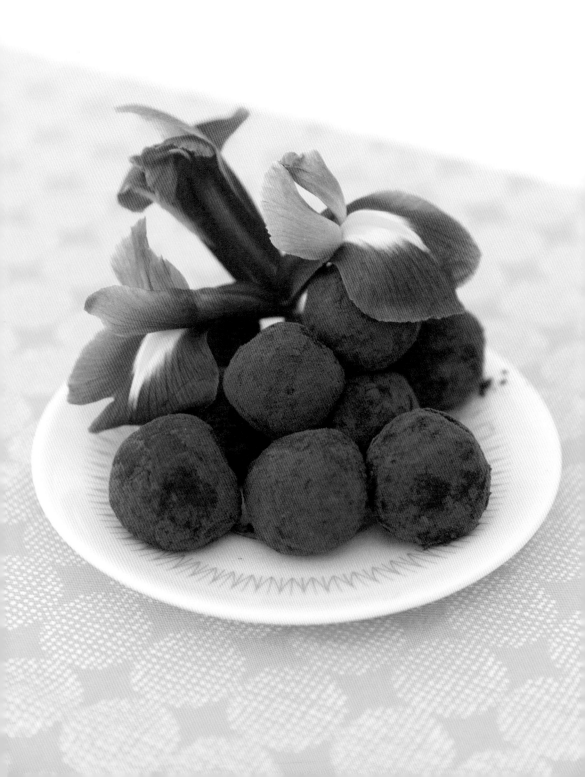

Energy balls

These are a perfect alternative to the sugar dense snack bars and energy balls you buy in the shops, they refrigerate and freeze well, and you can get creative with different flavour combinations. Here are a few I love that focus on energy.

For each recipe, use approximately *100g nuts/seeds/chestnuts* – preferably soaked overnight in water – with about *50g dried fruit* and *2-3tbsp coconut oil*. Add other spices and flavourings half a teaspoon at a time until it tastes just right. Note that I suggest a lot less of the sweet stuff that you get in shop bought versions, but they are still definitely sweet enough! Then you blend it all together, as smooth or as rough as you like, shape into truffle sized balls and roll in something like sesame seeds, desiccated coconut or cocoa powder to make them prettier.

- If the mixture is too dry to hold together, add a little more coconut oil
- If the mixture is too wet, add more nuts/seeds – remember the coconut oil will also harden a little when you put them in the fridge
- In winter, melt the coconut oil first by gently heating in a pan until liquid

Tropical truffles *(Rolled in desiccated coconut, or carob or cocoa powder)*
brazil nuts
dates
coconut oil
carob or cocoa powder
lime zest
supergreen powder (e.g. spirulina, wheatgrass powder, etc. – add a pinch at a time)

Decadent delights *(Rolled in carob or cocoa powder)*
boiled chestnuts
prunes
coconut oil
a little coconut cream or milk
carob or cocoa powder
supergreen powder

Winter warmers *(Rolled in carob or cocoa powder)*
NB: Also great for the kidneys.
walnuts and pumpkin seeds
cranberries (avoid the sugar sweetened one)
coconut oil
supergreen powder
ginger

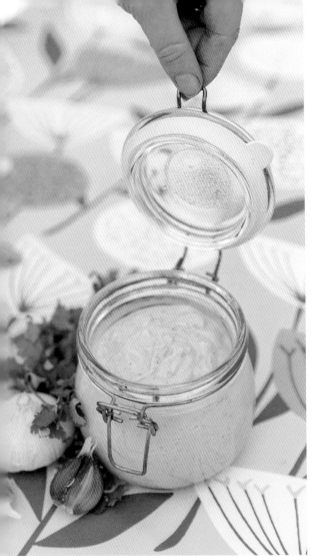

Coriander houmous

Houmous has to be the quickest and easiest thing to whizz up if you have a blender and the right ingredients. Spread on oatcakes, **Gluten-free pancakes** (*see p.282*), **Gram flour wraps** (*see p.262*) or sourdough rye bread. Use as a dip for carrot, celery, cucumber and courgette sticks. Or just dollop on a plate with some salad.

Houmous contains all the essential amino acids you need, and by making your own, you can ensure the quality of the oil used. Adding fresh coriander gives houmous a vibrancy of colour and flavour that I absolutely love, as well as extra vitamin K and phytonutrients.

Everyone likes their houmous a certain way, so keep tasting and testing as you go, and feel free to play around with this recipe. Keep it in an airtight container in the fridge and use within 2-3 days.

Ingredients
200g chickpeas, cooked (soaked overnight then simmered for 1-1½ hours until soft)
3-4 tbsp tahini
juice of 1 to 1½ lemons
garlic cloves to taste
extra virgin olive oil
black pepper and sea salt
1 handful fresh coriander leaves

1. Add everything except the coriander to your blender and blend till fairly smooth.
2. Taste and see if you need to add any more seasoning, lemon juice or garlic.
3. Add the coriander leaves and blend for just a couple of seconds.

Calm bars

These handy snacks are packed with ingredients for making acetylcholine to calm your nervous system, and soothe your adrenals. The protein and coconut oil they contain should help keep your blood sugar levels stable, too, so that you don't so easily dip into anxiety, irritability or fatigue. Make a batch to keep in the fridge or freezer, and pop one in a container to take out with you.

Ingredients
100g sunflower seeds – soaked overnight in water
½ carrot (grated if no blender)
2-3 unsulphured, dried apricots – adjust quantity for sweetness and to help mix stick together
½ tsp spirulina powder
½ tsp fresh (grated) or dried ginger
2-3 tsp lecithin granules
1 tbsp coconut oil

1. Blend the ingredients **OR** grate the carrot and ginger, finely chop the apricots and mix everything together in a bowl.
2. Spread thickly into a container, slice into small bar shapes and refrigerate.

Guacamole

This classic avocado dip is so quick to whip up. You can use it in wraps, with bean dishes, on pancakes and oatcakes, as a dip, sauce or dressing. So if you like avocado, you need to have this recipe up your sleeve.

Ingredients
1 avocado
juice and zest of ½ lime (or lemon if you're out of limes)
½-1 tsp ground cumin
1 handful freshly chopped coriander leaves
sea salt and black pepper to taste
Optional: 1-2 tomatoes, finely chopped
Optional: ½-1 tsp freshly chopped chili or dried chili flakes
Optional: 2 tsp coconut cream or sheep's yoghurt for a lighter guacamole

1. Mash the avocado with a fork, or blitz it in a blender.
2. Stir in the remaining ingredients – taste and adjust as necessary.

Superseed crackers with rosemary

Everybody needs a good cracker recipe in their life. This one ticks all my boxes: tasty, quick, easy, versatile and easy to remember: pretty much everything is 25g! (Or 50g or 75g if you want to make more). Plus gluten-free, vegan and packed full of nutrients.

You can substitute ingredients depending on what's in your cupboard. So if you're out of pumpkin seeds, use twice as many sunflower seeds. No poppy seeds? Use sesame instead. The flax seeds are fairly crucial, as they help hold the crackers together, but chia seeds will do a similar job.

Equally, you can play with different flour combinations (or just use 1), as well as different herbs and flavourings. That way, you will never get bored of these crackers.

They last for ages, but I'm not sure how long as they always get eaten up in a couple of days around here!

Ingredients
25g sunflower seeds
25g pumpkin seeds
25g poppy seeds
25g flax seeds
25g oats
25g buckwheat flour
25g brown rice flour
25g coconut oil
4 tbsp water
2 tsp tamari (wheat-free soy sauce)
1-2 tsp finely chopped fresh rosemary
black pepper to taste
pinch bicarbonate of soda

1. Mix all the ingredients together.
2. Smooth out onto a baking sheet lined with greaseproof paper.
3. Optional: temporarily cover with another sheet of greaseproof paper and roll out mixture until quite thin – then remove paper to bake.
4. Score with a knife to make easy to break apart when cooked – you can make squares, rectangles, triangles – whatever you like.
5. Bake in pre-heated oven at 150 degrees C for 20 minutes, until starting to brown.
6. When cool, gently snap apart.

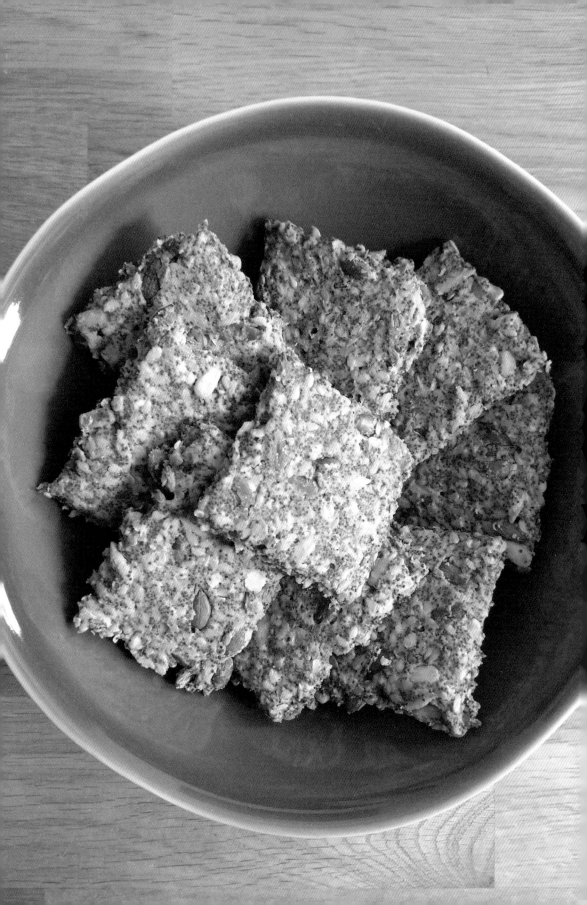

Gluten-free pancakes $^{(v)}$

Have I told you yet how much I adore pancakes? Classic Shrove Tuesday pancakes, paper thin crepes, fluffy scotch pancakes... I love them all. Sadly, gluten often doesn't love me.

It's difficult to replicate the pancakes of my childhood with gluten-free flour options, as part of their appeal was the gooeyness that only gluten can truly provide. However, buckwheat crepes are pretty much standard in France, and naturally gluten-free.

What I end up making most, however, are fluffy scotch pancakes, or drop scones as they are sometimes known. They work really well with buckwheat flour, brown rice flour and various gluten-free flour mixes. They need a thicker batter, and a pinch of bicarb to make them fluffy. I use them...

- instead of bread and crackers for houmous and other dips and spreads
- with poached eggs, mushrooms and watercress for a mouthwatering breakfast
- with berries and yoghurt or coconut cream as a breakfast or dessert
- with lemon juice, raw local honey and a few sultanas stirred into the batter for a sweet treat

...and in a host of other ways. See also the **Stewed Apple Pancake** recipe in the Desserts section (*p.289*).

To make them super digestible, make the batter the night before, cover with a cloth or paper towel and leave at room temperature overnight, and add the bicarbonate of soda and any extra ingredients just before cooking. This gives the flour a chance to ferment a little and reduce levels of phytates – adding a splash of lemon juice will help with this.

Then you can cook it all up in the morning, or keep the batter in an airtight container in the fridge for up to 3-4 days. If you batch cook them all at once, they usually freeze well – just pop them in the toaster or under the grill when you want to eat them. Or you could just mix up a small amount of batter, and cook and eat them there and then.

Ingredients
100-200g brown rice flour, buckwheat flour or a gluten-free flour mix
1-2 eggs
water, coconut milk or other plant-based milk – enough to make a thick batter
splash of lemon juice – if soaking overnight (see above)
pinch of bicarbonate of soda

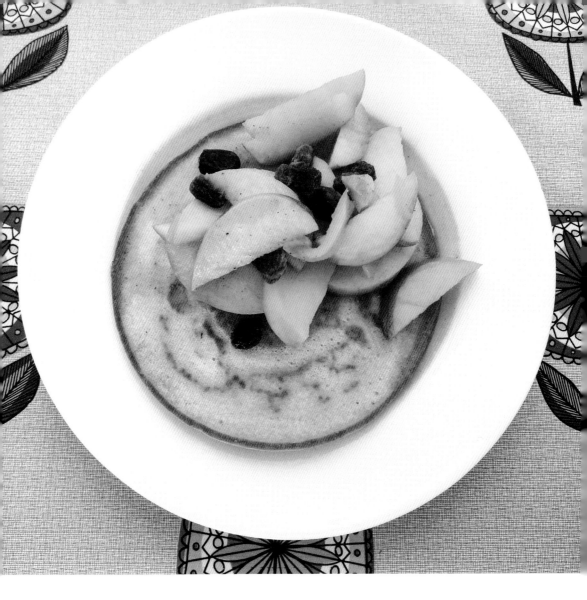

1. Stir the egg(s) into the flour, and then gradually whisk in the liquid until you have a thick batter.
2. Just before cooking, stir in a pinch of bicarbonate of soda.
3. Melt a little butter, ghee or coconut oil in a frying pan over a moderate heat.
4. Add 1tbsp batter to the pan, and watch it spread to about the size of your palm or a little smaller. You can probably fit two more into the pan if required.
5. When bubbles start to appear on the pancake(s), give the pan a little shake, and the pancake(s) should be able to move around the pan. They are now ready to flip over – you can use a fish slice to do this.
6. Cook for another couple of minutes, then serve.

Spiced fig and apple flapjacks

I designed this recipe when trying to make a healthier flapjack option, and it evolved into something really quite special. The flavours in this are amazing, and not a tub of golden syrup or margarine in sight!

Ingredients
200g oats
100g ground pumpkin seeds
2 cooking apples – grated (regular apples also work if that's all you have)
3 figs – preferably fresh, but if not available, then buy dried and soak them first
100g butter (or about 70g coconut oil)
2 tbsp blackstrap molasses
2-4 cardamom pods (split and crushed)
1-2 tsp cinnamon

1. Halve figs and cut into slices, then pan fry in a little of the butter until soft.
2. Add molasses, butter/coconut oil, spices and grated apples.
3. Stir in oats and pumpkin seeds.
4. Bake in a small greased square pyrex dish or baking tray for 30mins at 180 degrees C.
5. Leave to cool and slice into squares.

Like most of my recipes, this one is incredibly versatile, and I'd encourage you to experiment with different flavour combinations. To get your creative juices flowing, here are a few more flapjack ideas:

- Plum and ginger
- Pear and dark chocolate
- Hazelnut, orange zest and rosemary
- Pineapple and desiccated coconut
- Mango and chilli
- Lemon and rhubarb
- Banana and pecan
- Carrot, walnut and raisin

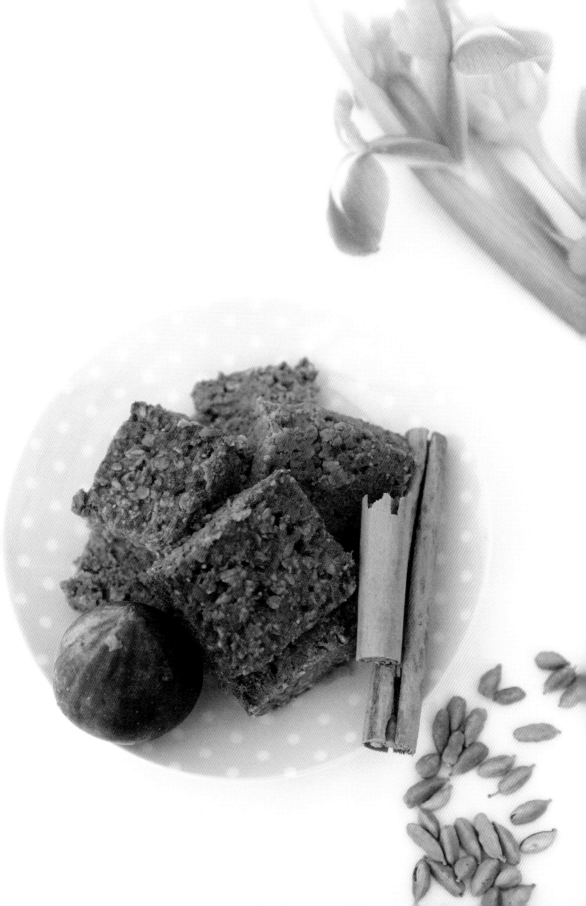

Desserts

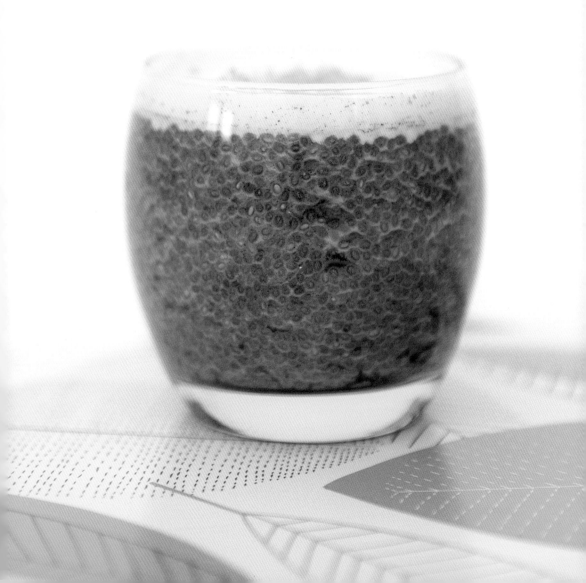

Superberry chia pot

This must be one of the lightest ways to start or end the day, and yet can be surprisingly filling. Chia seeds have been on trend for a while now, and are indeed nutrient-packed. Their omega 3:6 ratio is favourable, and when soaked, they form a kind of jelly that's great for a sluggish digestive system.

A chia pot usually has the seeds soaking in coconut milk, and is the superhealthy, vegan, modern equivalent of a milk pudding. You can add whatever extras you like: vanilla, cacao, cinnamon… but my favourite is with berries.

I also like to add my favourite supergreen powder, making this a supremely antioxidant-rich dessert. It also adds an intriguingly exotic green shimmer.

Ingredients: *(Serves 2-3)*
½ cup chia seeds
12 blueberries, chopped
12 raspberries or blackberries, chopped
2 tsp grated lemon zest
2 tsp supergreen powder
2 cups coconut milk
a few tbsp. coconut cream

1. Stir everything together except for the coconut cream and half the lemon zest and pour into glasses, ramekins or small bowls, leaving a few millimetres gap at the top.
2. Leave overnight, or for at least a couple of hours, in the fridge.
3. Pour the coconut cream over the top, and leave for another hour or two in the fridge.
4. Garnish with the rest of the lemon zest and serve.

Avochocolate mousse

Chocolate mousse made from avocados is no longer a surprise but it's still an absolute winner. It's a great one to have in your repertoire. Not only is it decadently delicious, it's one of the simplest things to whizz up. So perfect for dinner parties where other courses are taking up all your time and energy. And equally ideal when you just want something chocolatey, and you happen to have all the ingredients knocking around.

Ingredients
½ large avocado
3 tbsp cocoa powder
4 tsp raw honey or maple syrup
a few splashes of coconut milk
Optional extras: orange, lemon or lime zest and a little juice; ground cardamom and nutmeg; fresh or ground ginger

1. Blend REALLY thoroughly until completely smooth.
2. Pour or spoon into glasses, ramekins or small bowls, and refrigerate until needed.
3. Garnish beautifully and serve.

Lime zinger tart

This is a zesty, refreshing take on the avocado mousse with a crunchy base – a tart tart, if you will! It works equally well with lemon juice and zest, but the green colour of avocados lends itself to using lime. I've contrasted it here with dark chocolate – I love the bitter-sweet-sourness – but this recipe would work equally well without it.

Ingredients
2 medium avocados
juice and zest of 2 limes
2-3 tbsp raw honey or maple syrup
110g ground almonds
1 tbsp coconut oil (melt a little in winter to soften)
2-4 tbsp cocoa or carob powder (depending on its bitterness, taste to test and adjust accordingly)
Optional: 30-50g dark chocolate to garnish

1. Mix the ground almonds, coconut oil, cocoa/carob powder and ½-1 tbsp honey/maple syrup with a wooden spoon or in a blender.
2. Taste to make sure it's bitter, chocolatey and sweet enough to eat.
3. Press into four ramekins and refrigerate.
4. Blend the avocados, lime juice, half the zest and the rest of the honey/maple syrup together until completely smooth.
5. Taste to make sure zingy and tart, with enough sweetness to make it delicious.
6. Grate the chocolate. Sprinkle half of it onto the chocolate almond bases. This step is optional for those wanting to be sugar and chocolate free.
7. Spoon the filling on top, and finish with more grated chocolate and/or the other half of the lime zest. Refrigerate till ready to serve.

Stewed apple pancakes *(v)*

Anything with stewed apple in it has winter pudding written all over it. Pair it with pancakes, and there's your perfect comfort food, right there. Plus it ticks the easy-to-assemble boxes, the healthy eating boxes and the filling-but-not-heavy boxes. The additional spices are warming, anti-inflammatory and aid digestion. This is also my favourite breakfast. It feels like a treat, like I'm a child again getting excited about pancakes. It's warming and fresh at the same time, and keeps me going through the morning – with a huge smile on my face.

Ingredients *(serves 2)*
1 large cooking apple or 2 regular apples
1 tbsp sultanas
2 tsp ground cinnamon
2-3 cardamom pods (crush just enough to open the pods)
2-3 cloves
Optional: 1-2 tsp molasses to sweeten
Optional: coconut cream or sheep's yoghurt

1. Gently simmer all the ingredients in a little water (enough to just cover the apples) until the apples are soft.
2. Remove the cardamom and cloves, and strain off excess liquid.
3. Make scotch pancakes as per **Gluten-free pancake** recipe (*see p.282*).
4. Spoon apples over pancakes.
5. Optional: top with a dollop of sheep's yoghurt or pour a little coconut cream on top.

Drinks and smoothies

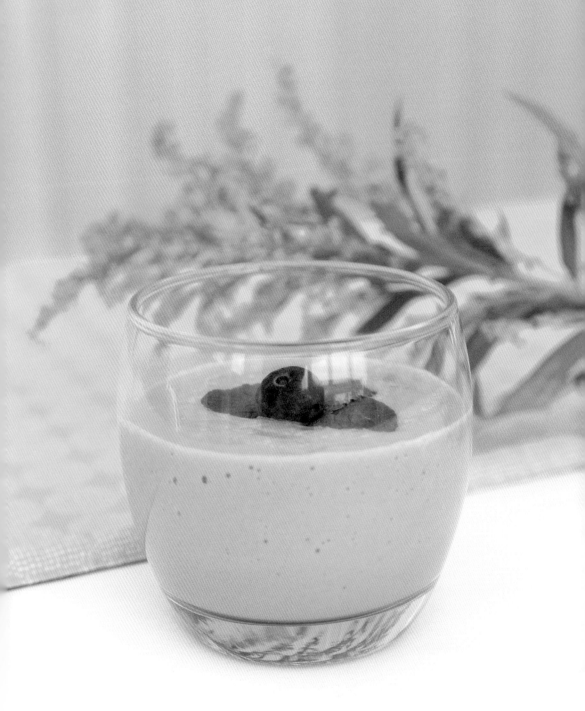

Avocado smoothie

Smoothies these days tend to be either all about the fruit, or rammed full of vegetables. This one is a little different, and has served me and many people I have worked with well over the years. It makes a great breakfast, post-workout drink, pre-morning run drink and general snack.

Note that a smoothie is where the ingredients are blended whole. A juice is where the juice and fibre are separated, and the fibre discarded. (Some blenders call themselves juice extractors, but unless the fibre comes out of a different hole and you get rid of it, then they're really just a type of blender, not a juicer, and so they make smoothies, not juice.)

Fruit smoothies can be delicious, but so much fructose crammed into one drink! Not quite as potentially inflammatory as a fruit juice, which takes out the fibre, but still more fruit than you would usually need to eat in one sitting, or even in one day.

Vegetable smoothies would seem to have the edge on this, and are high fibre to boot. However, so much fibre can for some people be just as constipating or irritating to the gut as not enough fibre. Especially if you're having more than one a day.

Some smoothie recipes have an overwhelming amount of superfoods, powders, vegetables and fruit in them– which may be why they make some people nauseous or cause digestive upset.

My avocado smoothie recipe aims to satisfy, sustain and soothe. I sometimes add half a carrot, or a few green leaves, but mostly I just keep it simple. Like all my recipes, play with the ingredients until it's just the way you like it, and makes you feel great.

Ingredients *(serves 1-2)*
¼-½ avocado
1 glass plant based milk (e.g. nut milk, oat milk, etc.)
1 tsp supergreen powder (e.g. a blend of really high quality spirulina, chlorella, barleygrass and wheatgrass)
1 tsp lecithin granules
1 tbsp pea protein powder, hemp protein powder or grass fed whey protein powder (optional)
You could also try adding mint, parsley, coriander, lemon zest (not juice), cinnamon and nutmeg, reishi mushroom powder or berries – but not all at once, as simple is often easier to digest.

1. Just blend and serve.

Golden milk

This is the most comforting, calming, soothing cup of love. The spices all have anti-inflammatory and antioxidant properties, making this drink great for your mental health and that of your gut, joints, cardiovascular system, and more. If the spices are too much for your digestion, or too warming in hot weather, then just use the turmeric, black pepper and one other spice. You can pretty much make this recipe up according to what's in your cupboard, but mine frequently contains:

Ingredients *(serves 2)*
2 cups plant-based milk (e.g. almond, oat, brown rice, coconut, hemp etc.)
3-4 tsp turmeric (organic powder or grated fresh)
2-3 tsp cinnamon powder or a large stick of cinnamon
3-4 cardamom pods (split open, scrape out the inside and use just that)
½-1 tsp nutmeg powder (best freshly grated)
a pinch of black pepper (important for turmeric absorption)
Occasionally I might also throw in a couple of cloves, or ½ tsp ginger powder if I need extra fire, but be cautious with using too much ginger, as it can be drying.

1. Simmer gently for 5-10 minutes, strain and serve.

Immune-boosting hot chocolate

There are two options for this: simple and decadent! Either way, savour every divine mouthful knowing you are giving your immunity a fantastic boost. The cocoa and medicinal mushrooms contain a wealth of nutrients for your immune system, and the decadent version takes this to another level of anti-inflammatory.

Ingredients *(serves 2)*
2 cups plant-based milk (e.g. almond, oat, brown rice, coconut, hemp etc.)
4 tsp unsweetened cocoa powder
1-2 tsp reishi mushroom powder – or any medicinal mushroom powder blend
1-2 tsp raw (unpasteurised) honey, preferably local (optional)

1. Make a paste by stirring together the honey, cocoa powder, mushroom powder and a splash of the milk – half in one mug, half in another.
2. Gently warm the rest of the milk in a small pan.
3. Pour the milk into the mugs, stir well and enjoy.

Decadent super-spiced version
Follow the recipe, adding **Golden milk** (*see top of this page*) instead of plain milk.

Linseed tea

This is the most soothing, hydrating drink I think I have ever come across. Drinking this makes my whole body smile and relax. It's best on an empty stomach, so nothing gets in the way of its golden caress. It seems like a faff to make, but it really isn't – it just takes a tiny amount of organizing. The process helps to release the super-soothing lignans from the flax seeds.

It will be different every time you make it: sometimes thick and gloopy, other times thin and watery. It doesn't really matter too much – but to avoid it getting unbearably gloopy, make sure you simmer it on a low heat with the lid on. You can add cinnamon sticks while it's simmering, or digestive herbs (such as chamomile, fennel or mint) while it's cooling – both to add even more anti-inflammatory properties and for flavour. Or just enjoy its simplicity.

Ingredients *(serves 4-6)*
2 tbsp golden linseeds
1½-2 litres water

1. Bring to boil then switch off IMMEDIATELY.
2. Leave for approximately 12 hours.
3. Simmer very gently for 1 hour with the lid on. Strain while still hot, discarding the seeds. I find the seeds usually sink to the bottom, so it's easy to pour the liquid into a glass kilner jar or jug, leaving the seeds behind.
4. Try a cup a day on an empty stomach, warm or cold (keeps for 3-4 days).

Kombu and ginger tea

Kombu seaweed is supremely mineral, vitamin and phytonutrient rich, and particularly nourishes the kidneys and thyroid.* Its strong taste can only really be matched with ginger, which provides a warming boost especially to the kidneys. So this is a great winter elixir for those who love strong flavours!

* It contains iodine and other ingredients you need to make thyroid hormones, so avoid if you are taking a synthetic thyroid hormone such as Levothyroxine.

Ingredients (makes a pot)
1 strip of kombu seaweed, cut into small pieces (I use kitchen scissors)
4 slices fresh ginger

1. Add hot water and steep for 5-15 minutes, then strain and serve.

Refreshing infusions and cold drinks

Your main drink through the day will ideally be water. If you "don't like the taste" or find it difficult to drink, then I strongly suggest you try a good water filter – it can make all the difference.

In addition, both warm and cold infusions can make a refreshing change and bring all kinds of benefits of their own. If you're used to squashes, fruit juices and fizzy drinks, then this is a way to add delightful flavours to your day without the sugars and additives.

Cold infusions are also wonderful to serve to guests and can look so pretty in a glass jug.

Mint and cucumber

This is a great cooling summer infusion, and best enjoyed cold or at room temperature. If you are having it with food, then room temperature will be more helpful to your digestive processes.

Simply add a few sprigs of fresh mint and a few slices of cucumber to a jug of water.

Chamomile and lemon zest

There has been such a craze for adding lemon juice to warm water in the mornings, and yet the zest is far more nutritious and less damaging to the enamel on your teeth. The oils, vitamins, minerals and polyphenols in citrus zest have countless health benefits, including protecting and repairing your DNA and various types of tissue.

This infusion balances feisty lemon with calming chamomile to give you a gentle start or end to your day.

Simply steep dried chamomile flowers – or good quality chamomile teabags – and grated lemon zest or slices of lemon peel in hot water. Boil the water in a kettle, but leave it to cool a little, perhaps a few minutes, before using.

Rosemary, thyme and orange zest

Rosemary and thyme are both very cleansing herbs, and pair beautifully with orange to make the most delicious hot or cold infusion.

I prefer this one cold, so I just add sprigs of rosemary and/or thyme to a jug of water together with pretty coils of orange peel.

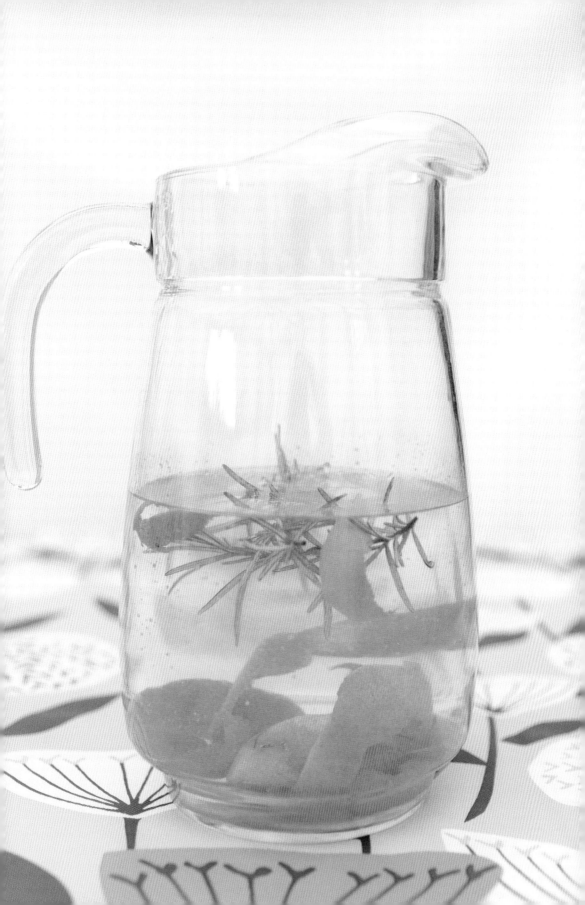

Endnotes

1 Power, M.L. and Schulkin, J., 2011. Anticipatory Physiological Regulation in Feeding Biology. Handbook of Behavior, Food and Nutrition (pp. 829-844). Springer, New York, NY.

2 Beal, M.F. (2004). Mitochondrial dysfunction and oxidative damage in Alzheimer's and Parkinson's diseases and coenzyme Q10 as a potential treatment. Journal of bioenergetics and biomembranes, 36(4), 381-386.

3 Anssi H Manninen, Metabolic Effects of the Very-Low-Carbohydrate Diets: Misunderstood "Villains" of Human Metabolism, Journal of the International Society of Sports Nutrition 2004, 1:7-11 doi: 10.1186/1550-2783-1-2-7.

4 Danial, N.N., Hartman, A.L., Stafstrom, C.E. and Thio, L.L., 2013. How does the ketogenic diet work? Four potential mechanisms. Journal of child neurology, 28(8), pp.1027-1033.

5 Schwartz, K.A., Noel, M., Nikolai, M. and Chang, H.T., 2018. Investigating the ketogenic diet as treatment for primary aggressive brain cancer: challenges and lessons learned. Frontiers in nutrition, 5, p.11.

6 Thomas N. Seyfried and Purna Mukherjee, Targeting energy metabolism in brain cancer: review and hypothesis, Nutrition & Metabolism 2005, 2:30 doi: 10.1186/1743-7075-2-3.

7 Ho, M.W. The Rainbow and the Worm: The Physics of Organisms. Singapore: World Scientific 1993.

8 Sinatra, S.T., Oschman, J.L., Chevalier, G. and Sinatra, D., 2017. Electric nutrition: The surprising health and healing benefits of biological grounding (Earthing). Altern Ther Health Med, 23(5), pp.8-16.

9 Vooijs M.A. et al, Hypoxic regulation of metastasis via hypoxia-inducible factors. Current molecular medicine 8.1 (2008): 60-67.

10 DeBerardinis R.J., Is cancer a disease of abnormal cellular metabolism? New angles on an old idea. Genetics in Medicine 10.11 (2008): 767-777.

11 Baba, N., Bracco, E.F., Seylar, J., Hashim, S.A. Enhanced thermogenesis and diminished deposition of fat in response to overfeeding with diets containing medium chain triglycerides. J Am Soc Clin Nutrition, 1981, 34: 624.

12 Approximate calorie calculations taken from www.nutritiondata.self.com – in actual fact, we can never rely on calorie labelling as the amounts given, while appearing precise, are rarely accurate and can be quite different to what is in the actual food.

13 Monica L. Assunção Affiliated with Faculdade de Nutrição, Universidade Federal de Alagoas, Haroldo S. Ferreira, Aldenir F. dos Santos, Cyro R. Cabral Jr, Telma M.M.T. Florêncio, Effects of Dietary Coconut Oil on the Biochemical and Anthropometric Profiles of Women Presenting Abdominal Obesity, July 2009, Volume 44, Issue 7, pp 593-601, First online: 13 May 2009.

14 Montague, C.T. and O'Rahilly, S., The perils of portliness: causes and consequences of visceral adiposity, Diabetes June 2000 vol. 49 no. 6 883-888, doi: 10.2337/diabetes.49.6.883.

15 André Tchernof, Jean-Pierre Després, Pathophysiology of Human Visceral Obesity: An Update, Physiological Reviews Published 1 January 2013 Vol. 93 no. 1, 359-404 doi: 10.1152/physrev.00033.2011.

16 ibid.

17 Kenneth C.H. Fearon, David J. Glass, Denis C. Guttridge Cancer Cachexia: Mediators, Signaling, and Metabolic Pathways, Cell Metabolism Volume 16, Issue 2, 8 August 2012, Pages 153-166.

18 Gerald M Reaven, Role of Insulin Resistance in Human Disease, Diabetes December 1988 vol. 37 no. 12 1595-1607.

19 Muntoni S., Muntoni S., Draznin B., Effects of chronic hyperinsulinemia in insulin-resistant patients, Curr Diab Rep. 2008 Jun;8(3):233-8.

20 Talbot, Konrad et al. Demonstrated Brain Insulin Resistance in Alzheimer's Disease Patients Is Associated with IGF-1 Resistance, IRS-1 Dysregulation, and Cognitive Decline. The Journal of Clinical Investigation 122.4 (2012): 1316-1338. PMC. Web. 11 Nov. 2015.

21 A. Christine Könner, Jens C. Brüning, Selective Insulin and Leptin Resistance in Metabolic Disorders, Cell Metabolism, Volume 16, Issue 2, 8 August 2012, Pages 144-152.

22 Meghana D. Gadgil et al, The Effects of Carbohydrate, Unsaturated Fat, and Protein Intake on Measures of Insulin Sensitivity, Diabetes Care May 2013 vol. 36 no. 5 1132-1137.

23 Penny M. Kris-Etherton, Monounsaturated Fatty Acids and Risk of Cardiovascular Disease, Circulation. 1999; 100: 1253-1258.

24 Lustig, R.H., Mulligan, K., Noworolski, S.M., Tai, V.W., Wen, M.J., Erkin-Cakmak, A., Gugliucci, A. and Schwarz, J.M. (2015), Isocaloric fructose restriction and metabolic improvement in children with obesity and metabolic syndrome. Obesity. doi: 10.1002/oby.21371.

25 Richard D. Feinman and Eugene J. Fine, Fructose in perspective, Nutrition & Metabolism 2013 10:45.

26 Welty F.K. How do elevated triglycerides and low HDL-cholesterol affect and atherothrombosis? Curr Cardiol Rep. 2013 Sep; 15(9):400.

27   George A. Bray, How bad is fructose? Am J Clin Nutr October 2007 vol. 86 no. 4 895-896.

28   ibid.

29   Michael Alderman; Kala J.V. Aiyer, Uric Acid: Role in Cardiovascular Disease and Effects of Losartan, Curr Med Res Opin. 2004;20(3).

30   Lustig, R.H., Mulligan, K., Noworolski, S.M., Tai, V.W., Wen, M.J., Erkin-Cakmak, A., Gugliucci, A. and Schwarz, J.M. (2015), Isocaloric fructose restriction and metabolic improvement in children with obesity and metabolic syndrome. Obesity. doi: 10.1002/oby.21371.

31   Richard D. Feinman and Eugene J. Fine, Fructose in perspective, Nutrition & Metabolism 2013 10:45.

32   ibid.

33   Bolton, R.P., Heaton, K.W. and Burroughs, L.F., The role of dietary fiber in satiety, glucose, and insulin: studies with fruit and fruit juice, Am J Clin Nutr February 1981 vol. 34 no. 2 211-217.

34   Joanne L. Slavin, Carbohydrates, Dietary Fiber, and Resistant Starch in White Vegetables: Links to Health Outcomes, Advances in Nutrition, Volume 4, Issue 3, May 2013, Pages 351S-355S, https://doi.org/10.3945/an.112.003491.

35   Jaroslawska, J., Wroblewska, M., Juskiewicz, J., Brzuzan, L. and Zdunczyk, Z. (2015), Protective effects of polyphenol-rich blackcurrant preparation on biochemical and metabolic biomarkers of rats fed a diet high in fructose. Journal of Animal Physiology and Animal Nutrition. doi: 10.1111/jpn.12321.

36   Fortuna, J.L., Sweet preference, sugar addiction and the familial history of alcohol dependence: shared neural pathways and genes, J Psychoactive Drugs. 2010 Jun;42(2):147-51.

37   Michael Moss, The extraordinary science of addictive junk food, New York Times, Feb 2013.

38   Buosi, W., Bremner, D.M., Horgan, G.W., Fyfe, C.L., & Johnstone, A.M. (2015). Effect of High-Protein Breakfast Meals on Within-Day Appetite and Food Intake in Healthy Men and Women. Food and Nutrition Sciences, 6(03), 386.

39   Crowder, C., Neumann, B., Johnson, D., & Baum, J. (2015). The Effect of Breakfast Protein Source on Postprandial Hunger and Glucose Response in Women. The FASEB Journal, 29(1 Supplement), 599-3.

40   Glanzman, M.M. (2009). ADHD and nutritional supplements. Current Attention Disorders Reports, 1(2), 75-81.

41   Sugars intake for adults and children, World Health Organisation, 2015.

42   Mäkinen KK, Sugar alcohol sweeteners as alternatives to sugar with special consideration of xylitol, Med Princ Pract. 2011;20(4):303-20. doi: 10.1159/000324534. Epub 2011 May 11.

43   Mäkinen KK et al, Effect of erythritol and xylitol on dental caries prevention in children, Caries Res. 2014;48(5):482-90. doi: 10.1159/000358399. Epub 2014 May 21.

44   Although many would argue that blaming sugar alone is far too simplistic.

45   Chua, L.S., et al. Effect of thermal treatment on the biochemical composition of tropical honey samples. Inter. Food Res. J 21.2 (2014): 773-778.

46   Report to the Officers and Board of Directors of the Committee for the Promotion of Honey and Health (from The First International Symposium on Honey and Human Health), January 17, 2008.

47   ibid.

48   Wang, Rui et al. Honey's Ability to Counter Bacterial Infections Arises from Both Bactericidal Compounds and QS Inhibition. Frontiers in Microbiology 3 (2012): 144. PMC. Web. 22 Dec. 2015.

49   Ranzato, Elia, Simona Martinotti, and Bruno Burlando. Epithelial mesenchymal transition traits in honey-driven keratinocyte wound healing: Comparison among different honeys. Wound Repair and Regeneration 20.5 (2012): 778-785.

50   Demling, R.H., & Desanti, L. (2001). Effects of silver on wound management. Wounds, 13(1), 4-15.

51   Report to the Officers and Board of Directors of the Committee for the Promotion of Honey and Health January 17, 2008.

52   Avena, N.M., Rada, P., & Hoebel, B.G. (2008). Evidence for sugar addiction: behavioral and neurochemical effects of intermittent, excessive sugar intake. Neuroscience & Biobehavioral Reviews, 32(1), 20-39.

53   Model, S.A. (2015). Behavioral Evidence of Addiction. Hedonic Eating: How the Pleasurable Aspects of Food Can Affect Our Brains and Behavior. pp187-195.

54   Mindfulness meditation is essentially a calm space where you can practise being in the here and now. You might focus on or even count your breaths to help keep you centred. Most people – even apparently the Dalai Lama – find that all kinds of thoughts will regularly come to distract and tie up the mind. The aim is to allow these thoughts to come and go without getting involved in them. They will pull you off centre, either into the past or into the future. Mindfulness meditation is an opportunity to practise staying in the present moment.

55   Mittal, Ravinder K., and Raj K. Goyal. Sphincter mechanisms at the lower end of the esophagus. GI Motility online (2006).

56   ibid.

57   Smith, James L. The role of gastric acid in preventing foodborne disease and how bacteria overcome acid conditions. Journal of Food Protection® 66.7 (2003): 1292-1303.

58   Yoon, Saunjoo L., et al. Management of irritable bowel syndrome (IBS) in adults: conventional and complementary/alternative approaches. Altern Med Rev 16.2 (2011): 134-51.

59   Trauner, Michael, and James L. Boyer. Bile salt transporters: molecular characterization, function, and regulation. Physiological reviews 83.2 (2003): 633-671.

60   Hamann, Jason J., Kevin M. Kelley, and L. Bruce Gladden. Effect of epinephrine on net lactate uptake by contracting skeletal muscle. Journal of Applied Physiology 91.6 (2001): 2635-2641.

61 Godfraind, T., and A. Kaba. Blockade or reversal of the contraction induced by calcium and adrenaline in depolarized arterial smooth muscle. British journal of pharmacology 36.3 (1969): 549-560.

62 e.g. Pitchford, Paul. Healing with whole foods: Asian traditions and modern nutrition. North Atlantic Books, 2002 or Connelly, Dianne M. Traditional acupuncture: the law of the five elements. Centre for Traditional Acupuncture, 1979.

63 Rick Hanson, Buddha's Brain: the practical neuroscience of happiness, love and wisdom, with Richard Mendius, New Harbinger Publications 2009, p.51.

64 University of Colorado at Boulder. Your brain on imagination: It's a lot like reality, study shows. ScienceDaily. www.sciencedaily.com/releases/2018/12/181210144943.htm.

65 Rick Hanson, Buddha's Brain: the practical neuroscience of happiness, love and wisdom, with Richard Mendius, New Harbinger Publications 2009, pp.85-86.

66 Dalen, Jeanne, et al. Pilot study: Mindful Eating and Living (MEAL): weight, eating behavior, and psychological outcomes associated with a mindfulness-based intervention for people with obesity. Complementary therapies in medicine 18.6 (2010): 260-264.

67 Timmerman, Gayle M., and Adama Brown. The effect of a mindful restaurant eating intervention on weight management in women. Journal of nutrition education and behavior 44.1 (2012): 22-28.

68 Miller, Carla K., et al. Comparative effectiveness of a mindful eating intervention to a diabetes self-management intervention among adults with type 2 diabetes: a pilot study. Journal of the Academy of Nutrition and Dietetics 112.11 (2012): 1835-1842.

69 Hepworth, Natasha S. A mindful eating group as an adjunct to individual treatment for eating disorders: A pilot study. Eating Disorders 19.1 (2010): 6-16.

70 Wanden-Berghe, Rocío Guardiola, Javier Sanz-Valero, and Carmina Wanden-Berghe. The application of mindfulness to eating disorders treatment: a systematic review. Eating disorders 19.1 (2010): 34-48.

71 Kristeller, Jean L., and Ruth Q. Wolever. Mindfulness-based eating awareness training for treating binge eating disorder: the conceptual foundation. Eating disorders 19.1 (2010): 49-61.

72 Daubenmier, Jennifer, et al. Mindfulness intervention for stress eating to reduce cortisol and abdominal fat among overweight and obese women: an exploratory randomized controlled study. Journal of obesity 2011 (2011).

73 Reiner, Keren, Lee Tibi, and Joshua D. Lipsitz. Do Mindfulness-Based Interventions Reduce Pain Intensity? A Critical Review of the Literature. Pain Medicine 14.2 (2013): 230-242.

74 Ong, Jason C., et al. A randomized controlled trial of mindfulness meditation for chronic insomnia. Sleep 37.9 (2014): 1553.

75 Bailey, Neil W., et al. Asthma and Mindfulness: an Increase in Mindfulness as the Mechanism of Action Behind Breathing Retraining Techniques? Mindfulness (2016): 1-7.

76 Fogarty, Francesca A., et al. The effect of mindfulness-based stress reduction on disease activity in people with rheumatoid arthritis: a randomised controlled trial. Annals of the rheumatic diseases 74.2 (2015): 472-474.

77 Zernicke, Kristin A., et al. Mindfulness-based stress reduction for the treatment of irritable bowel syndrome symptoms: a randomized wait-list controlled trial. International Journal of Behavioral Medicine 20.3 (2013): 385-396.

78 Chen, Yu, et al. A randomized controlled trial of the effects of brief mindfulness meditation on anxiety symptoms and systolic blood pressure in Chinese nursing students. Nurse education today 33.10 (2013): 1166-1172.

79 Borovikova, Lyudmila V., et al. Vagus nerve stimulation attenuates the systemic inflammatory response to endotoxin. Nature 6785 (2000): 458-462.

80 Critchley, Hugo D., and Neil A. Harrison. Visceral influences on brain and behavior. Neuron 77.4 (2013): 624-638.

81 Fanselow, Michael S. Fear and anxiety take a double hit from vagal nerve stimulation. Biological psychiatry 73.11 (2013): 1043.

82 Vonck, Kristl, et al. Vagus nerve stimulation… 25 years later! What do we know about the effects on cognition? Neuroscience & Biobehavioral Reviews 45 (2014): 63-71.

83 Hurst, Katryn. Singing Is Good for You: An Examination of the Relationship between Singing, Health and Well-Being. Canadian Music Educator 55.4 (2014): 18-22.

84 He, F., and H.B. Ai. Effects of electrical stimulation at different locations in the central nucleus of amygdala on gastric motility and spike activity. Physiological research/ Academia Scientiarum Bohemoslovaca (2016).

85 Leclercq, Sophie, Paul Forsythe, and John Bienenstock. Posttraumatic Stress Disorder Does the Gut Microbiome Hold the Key? The Canadian Journal of Psychiatry (2016): 0706743716635535.

86 Yen, Samuel SC. Dehydroepiandrosterone sulfate and longevity: new clues for an old friend. Proceedings of the National Academy of Sciences 98.15 (2001): 8167-8169.

87 Ohlsson, Claes, Liesbeth Vandenput, and Åsa Tivesten. DHEA and mortality: What is the nature of the association? The Journal of steroid biochemistry and molecular biology 145 (2015): 248-253.

88 Grant, Jon E., et al. Introduction to behavioral addictions. The American journal of drug and alcohol abuse 36.5 (2010): 233-241.

89 Lyte, M. Probiotics function mechanistically as delivery vehicles for neuroactive compounds: Microbial endocrinology in the design and use of probiotics. Bioessays. doi: 10.1002/bies.201100024.

90 Dinan, Timothy G., et al. Collective unconscious: how gut microbes shape human behavior. Journal of psychiatric research 63 (2015): 1-9.

91 ibid.

92   Dinan, Timothy G., and John F. Cryan. Regulation of the stress response by the gut microbiota: implications for psychoneuroendocrinology. Psychoneuroendocrinology 37.9 (2012): 1369-1378.

93   Messaoudi, Michaël, et al. Beneficial psychological effects of a probiotic formulation (Lactobacillus helveticus R0052 and Bifidobacterium longum R0175) in healthy human volunteers. Gut microbes 2.4 (2011): 256-261.

94   Dinan, Timothy G., and John F. Cryan. Regulation of the stress response by the gut microbiota: implications for psychoneuroendocrinology. Psychoneuroendocrinology 37.9 (2012): 1369-1378.

95   Kelly, Gregory S. Pantothenic acid. Altern Med Rev 16, no. 3 (2011): 263-74.

96   Stough, C., Scholey, A., Lloyd, J., Spong, J., Myers, S. and Downey, L.A., 2011. The effect of 90 day administration of a high dose vitamin B-complex on work stress. Human Psychopharmacology: Clinical and Experimental, 26(7), pp.470-476.

97   Brody, S., Preut, R., Schommer, K. and Schürmeyer, T.H., 2002. A randomized controlled trial of high dose ascorbic acid for reduction of blood pressure, cortisol, and subjective responses to psychological stress. Psychopharmacology, 159(3), pp.319-324.

98   Seelig MS, et al Latent tetany and anxiety, marginal magnesium deficit, and normocalcemia. Dis Nerv Syst. Aug1975 www.ncbi.nlm.nih.gov/pubmed/1164868.

99   Dr Carolyn Dean The Miracle of Magnesium Ballantine Books 2003.

100   Fantidis, P., Sanchez, E., Khan, I., Tarhini, I. and Pineda, T., 2015. Is there a Role of Intracellular Magnesium in Prevention of Heart Failure. Angiology, 3, p.148.

101   ibid.

102   Brandão-Neto J. Zinc acutely and temporarily inhibits adrenal cortisol secretion in humans. A preliminary report, Biol Trace Elem Res. 1990 Jan;24(1):83-9. http://www.ncbi.nlm.nih.gov/pubmed/1702662.

103   Barbadoro P, Annino I, Ponzio E, Romanelli RM, D'Errico MM, Prospero E, Minelli A (2013) Fish oil supplementation reduces cortisol basal levels and perceived stress: a randomized, placebo-controlled trial in abstinent alcoholics. Mol Nutr Food Res 57(6):1110-1114.

104   Jäger, R., Purpura, M. and Kingsley, M., 2007. Phospholipids and sports performance. Journal of the International Society of Sports Nutrition, 4(1), p.5.

105   Pompei, Anna, et al. Folate production by bifidobacteria as a potential probiotic property. Applied and environmental microbiology 73.1 (2007): 179-185.

106   Skosnik, Patrick D., and Jose A. Cortes-Briones. Targeting the ecology within: The role of the gut-brain axis and human microbiota in drug addiction. Medical Hypotheses 93 (2016): 77-80.

107   Leclercq, S., Forsythe, P., and Bienenstock, J. Posttraumatic Stress Disorder: Does the Gut Microbiome Hold the Key? The Canadian Journal of Psychiatry 61.4 (2016): 204-213.

108   Anderson, George, et al. Gut Permeability and Microbiota in Parkinson's Disease: Role of Depression, Tryptophan Catabolites, Oxidative and Nitrosative Stress and Melatonergic Pathways. Current Pharmaceutical Design 22.40 (2016): 6142-6151.

109   Krack, Andreas, et al. The importance of the gastrointestinal system in the pathogenesis of heart failure. European heart journal 26.22 (2005): 2368-2374.

110   Khosravi, Arya, et al. Gut microbiota promote hematopoiesis to control bacterial infection. Cell host & microbe 15.3 (2014): 374-381.

111   Uronis, Joshua M., et al. Modulation of the intestinal microbiota alters colitis-associated colorectal cancer susceptibility. PloS one 4.6 (2009): e6026.

112   Arthur, Janelle C., et al. Intestinal inflammation targets cancer-inducing activity of the microbiota. science 338.6103 (2012): 120-123.

113   Mager, D.L., et al. The salivary microbiota as a diagnostic indicator of oral cancer: a descriptive, non-randomized study of cancer-free and oral squamous cell carcinoma subjects. Journal of translational medicine 3.1 (2005): 27.

114   Dicksved, Johan, et al. Molecular characterization of the stomach microbiota in patients with gastric cancer and in controls. Journal of medical microbiology 58.4 (2009): 509-516.

115   Farrell, James J., et al. Variations of oral microbiota are associated with pancreatic diseases including pancreatic cancer. Gut (2011): gutjnl-2011.

116   Zitvogel, Laurence, et al. Cancer and the gut microbiota: an unexpected link. Science translational medicine 7.271 (2015): 271ps1-271ps1.

117   Pawlak, Roman, S.E. Lester, and T. Babatunde. The prevalence of cobalamin deficiency among vegetarians assessed by serum vitamin B12: a review of literature. European journal of clinical nutrition 68.5 (2014): 541-548.

118   Neis, Evelien PJG, Cornelis HC Dejong, and Sander S. Rensen. The role of microbial amino acid metabolism in host metabolism. Nutrients 7.4 (2015): 2930-2946.

119   Zitvogel, Laurence, et al. Cancer and the gut microbiota: an unexpected link. Science translational medicine 7.271 (2015): 271ps1-271ps1.

120   Hary J. Flint and Nathalie Juge. Role of microbes in carbohydrate digestion. The Journal of the Institute of Food Science and Technology (March 2015).

121   Jumpertz, Reiner, et al. Energy-balance studies reveal associations between gut microbes, caloric load, and nutrient absorption in humans. The American journal of clinical nutrition 94.1 (2011): 58-65.

122   Collen, A. 10% Human. How you body's microbes hold the key to health and happiness. William Collins (2016) 78-81

123   Ghaisas, Shivani, Joshua Maher, and Anumantha Kanthasamy. Gut microbiome in health and disease: Linking the microbiome-gut-brain axis and environmental factors in the pathogenesis of systemic and neurodegenerative diseases. Pharmacology & therapeutics 158 (2016): 52-62.

124 Evans, Simon J., et al. The gut microbiome composition associates with bipolar disorder and illness severity. Journal of Psychiatric Research 87 (2017): 23-29.

125 Tilg, Herbert, Christoph Grander, and Alexander R. Moschen. How does the microbiome affect liver disease? Clinical Liver Disease 8.5 (2016): 123-126.

126 Maalouf, Naim M., et al. Low urine pH: a novel feature of the metabolic syndrome. Clinical Journal of the American Society of Nephrology 2.5 (2007): 883-888.

127 Welch, Ailsa A., et al. Urine pH is an indicator of dietary acid-base load, fruit and vegetables and meat intakes: results from the European Prospective Investigation into Cancer and Nutrition (EPIC)-Norfolk population study. British Journal of Nutrition 99.06 (2008): 1335-1343.

128 Macdonald, Helen M., et al. Low dietary potassium intakes and high dietary estimates of net endogenous acid production are associated with low bone mineral density in premenopausal women and increased markers of bone resorption in postmenopausal women. The American journal of clinical nutrition 81.4 (2005): 923-933.

129 Welch, Ailsa A., et al. More acidic dietary acid-base load is associated with reduced calcaneal broadband ultrasound attenuation in women but not in men: results from the EPIC-Norfolk cohort study. The American journal of clinical nutrition 85.4 (2007): 1134-1141.

130 Odvina, Clarita V. Comparative value of orange juice versus lemonade in reducing stone-forming risk. Clinical Journal of the American Society of Nephrology 1.6 (2006): 1269-1274.

131 Shepherd, Susan J., and Peter R. Gibson. Fructose malabsorption and symptoms of irritable bowel syndrome: guidelines for effective dietary management. Journal of the American Dietetic Association 106.10 (2006): 1631-1639.

132 Tosun, Ilkay, N. Sule Ustun, and Belkis Tekguler. Physical and chemical changes during ripening of blackberry fruits. Scientia agricola 65.1 (2008): 87-90.

133 GutiéRrez, Margarita, et al. Postharvest changes in total soluble solids and tissue pH of cherimoya fruit stored at chilling and non-chilling temperatures. Journal of Horticultural Science 69.3 (1994): 459-463.

134 Han, Ting-Li, Richard D. Cannon, and Silas G. Villas-Bôas. The metabolic basis of Candida albicans morphogenesis and quorum sensing. Fungal Genetics and Biology 48.8 (2011): 747-763.

135 Maintz, Laura, and Natalija Novak. Histamine and histamine intolerance. The American journal of clinical nutrition 85.5 (2007): 1185-1196.

136 Johnston, C.S. (1996). The antihistamine action of ascorbic acid. In Subcellular Biochemistry (pp. 189-213). Springer US.

137 Martner-Hewes, P.M., Hunt, I.F., Murphy, N.J., Swendseid, M.E., & Settlage, R.H. (1986). Vitamin B-6 nutriture and plasma diamine oxidase activity in pregnant Hispanic teenagers. The American journal of clinical nutrition, 44(6), 907-913.

138 Fukudome, I., Kobayashi, M., Dabanaka, K., Maeda, H., Okamoto, K., Okabayashi, T., ... & Hanazaki, K. (2013). Diamine oxidase as a marker of intestinal mucosal injury and the effect of soluble dietary fiber on gastrointestinal tract toxicity after intravenous 5-fluorouracil treatment in rats. Medical molecular morphology, 1-8.

139 Ji, Y., Sakata, Y., Li, X., Zhang, C., Yang, Q., Xu, M., ... & Tso, P. (2013). Lymphatic diamine oxidase secretion stimulated by fat absorption is linked with histamine release. American Journal of Physiology-Gastrointestinal and Liver Physiology, 304(8), G732-G740.

140 Rumessen, Juri Johannes, et al. Fructans of Jerusalem artichokes: intestinal transport, absorption, fermentation, and influence on blood glucose, insulin, and C-peptide responses in healthy subjects. The American journal of clinical nutrition 52.4 (1990): 675-681.

141 Langlands, S.J., Hopkins, M.J., Coleman, N. and Cummings, J.H. (2004) Prebiotic carbohydrates modify the mucosa-associated microflora of the human large bowel. Gut 53, 1610-1616.

142 McFarland, Lynne V. Systematic review and meta-analysis of Saccharomyces boulardii in adult patients. World J Gastroenterol 16.18 (2010): 2202-2222.

143 Bhagat, Shivani, Monika Agarwal, and Vandana Roy. Serratiopeptidase: a systematic review of the existing evidence. International Journal of Surgery 11.3 (2013): 209-217.

144 Mine, Yoshinori, Ada Ho Kwan Wong, and Bo Jiang. Fibrinolytic enzymes in Asian traditional fermented foods. Food Research International 38.3 (2005): 243-250.

145 Lister, Jessica L., and Alexander R. Horswill. Staphylococcus aureus biofilms: recent developments in biofilm dispersal. Biofilm formation by staphylococci and streptococci: Structural, functional and regulatory aspects and implications for pathogenesis (2015). p82.

146 Longhi, Catia, et al. Protease treatment affects both invasion ability and biofilm formation in Listeria monocytogenes. Microbial pathogenesis 45.1 (2008): 45-52.

147 Singh, Pradeep K., et al. A component of innate immunity prevents bacterial biofilm development. Nature 417.6888 (2002): 552-555.

148 Lönnerdal, Bo. Nutritional roles of lactoferrin. Current Opinion in Clinical Nutrition & Metabolic Care 12.3 (2009): 293-297.

149 Marsh, Philip D. Dental plaque as a biofilm and a microbial community-implications for health and disease. BMC Oral health 6.1 (2006): S14.

150 Yonezawa, Hideo, Takako Osaki, and Shigeru Kamiya. Biofilm formation by Helicobacter pylori and its involvement for antibiotic resistance. BioMed research international (2015).

151 Motta, Jean-Paul, et al. Hydrogen sulfide protects from colitis and restores intestinal microbiota biofilm and mucus production. Inflammatory bowel diseases 21.5 (2015): 1006-1017.

152 Rowan, F.E., et al. Sulphate-reducing bacteria and hydrogen sulphide in the aetiology of ulcerative colitis. British Journal of Surgery 96.2 (2009): 151-158.

153 Schleip R, Lehmann-Horn F, Klingler W (2006). Fascia is able to contract in a smooth muscle-like manner and thereby influence musculoskeletal mechanics. In: Liepsch D: Proceedings of the 5th World Congress of Biomechanics, Munich, Germany, 2006, pp51-54.

154 Schleip, Robert. Faszien und nervensystem. Osteopathische Medizin 1 (2003): 20-30.

155 De Luca, Luigi, et al. Maintenance of epithelial cell differentiation: the mode of action of vitamin A. Cancer 30.5 (1972): 1326-1331.

156 Fenech, Michael. The role of folic acid and Vitamin B12 in genomic stability of human cells. Mutation Research/Fundamental and Molecular Mechanisms of Mutagenesis 475.1 (2001): 57-67.

157 Theaker, Jeffrey M., Stephen R. Porter, and Kenneth A. Fleming. Oral epithelial dysplasia in vitamin B12 deficiency. Oral surgery, oral medicine, oral pathology 67.1 (1989): 81-83.

158 Pawlak, Roman, et al. How prevalent is vitamin B12 deficiency among vegetarians? Nutrition reviews 71.2 (2013): 110-117.

159 Watanabe, Fumio, et al. Vitamin B12-containing plant food sources for vegetarians. Nutrients 6.5 (2014): 1861-1873.

160 Assa, Amit, et al. Vitamin D deficiency promotes epithelial barrier dysfunction and intestinal inflammation. Journal of Infectious Diseases (2014): jiu235.

161 Fischer, Kimberly D., and Devendra K. Agrawal. Vitamin D regulating TGF-β induced epithelial-mesenchymal transition. Respiratory research 15.1 (2014): 146.

162 Meeker, Stacey, et al. Increased dietary vitamin D suppresses MAPK signaling, colitis, and colon cancer. Cancer research 74.16 (2014): 4398-4408.

163 Liu, Fan, et al. Selenium and vitamin E together improve intestinal epithelial barrier function and alleviate oxidative stress in heat-stressed pigs. Experimental physiology 101.7 (2016): 801-810.

164 Jaspers, Ilona, et al. Selenium deficiency alters epithelial cell morphology and responses to influenza. Free Radical Biology and Medicine 42.12 (2007): 1826-1837.

165 Selenium Dietary Supplement Factsheet, National Institutes of Health Office of Dietary Supplements, https://ods.od.nih.gov/factsheets/Selenium-HealthProfessional/.

166 Cario, Jung, Harder d'Heureuse, Schulte, Sturm, Wiedenmann, Goebell and Dignass (2000), Effects of exogenous zinc supplementation on intestinal epithelial repair in vitro. European Journal of Clinical Investigation, 30: 419-428. doi:10.1046/j.1365-2362.2000.00618.x.

167 Wang, Xuexuan, et al. Zinc supplementation modifies tight junctions and alters barrier function of CACO-2 human intestinal epithelial layers. Digestive diseases and sciences 58.1 (2013): 77-87.

168 Venturi, M. Iodine, PUFAs and Iodolipids in Health and Diseases: An Evolutionary Perspective. Human Evolution 29.1-3 (2014): 185-205.

169 Xu, Jiqu, et al. Flaxseed lignan secoisolariciresinol diglucoside ameliorates experimental colitis induced by dextran sulphate sodium in mice. Journal of Functional Foods 26 (2016): 187-195.

170 Zarepoor, Leila, et al. Dietary flaxseed intake exacerbates acute colonic mucosal injury and inflammation induced by dextran sodium sulfate. American Journal of Physiology-Gastrointestinal and Liver Physiology 306.12 (2014): G1042-G1055.

171 Cao, Min, et al. Amelioration of IFN-γ and TNF-α-induced intestinal epithelial barrier dysfunction by berberine via suppression of MLCK-MLC phosphorylation signaling pathway. PloS one 8.5 (2013): e61944.

172 Wang, Bin, et al. Glutamine and intestinal barrier function. Amino Acids 47.10 (2015): 2143-2154.

173 Campbell McBride, Natasha. Gut & Psychology Syndrome. Medinform Publishing, 2010.

174 Pasquali, Marzia, et al. Abnormal formation of collagen cross-links in skin fibroblasts cultured from patients with Ehlers-Danlos syndrome type VI. Proceedings of the Association of American Physicians 109.1 (1997): 33-41.

175 Ringsdorf, W.M., and E. Cheraskin. Vitamin C and human wound healing. Oral Surgery, Oral Medicine, Oral Pathology 53.3 (1982): 231-236.

176 Boraldi, Federica, et al. Magnesium Modifies the Structural Features of Enzymatically Mineralized Collagen Gels Affecting the Retraction Capabilities of Human Dermal Fibroblasts Embedded within This 3D System. Materials 9.6 (2016): 477.

177 Newnham, Rex E. Essentiality of boron for healthy bones and joints. Environmental health perspectives 102. Suppl 7 (1994): 83.

178 Shaw, Gregory, Ann Lee-Barthel, Megan LR Ross, Bing Wang, and Keith Baar. Vitamin C-enriched gelatin supplementation before intermittent activity augments collagen synthesis. The American journal of clinical nutrition 105, no. 1 (2016): 136-143.

179 Ge, Dan, et al. Poly-ion Complex of Chondroitin Sulfate and Spermine and Its Effect on Oral Chondroitin Sulfate Bioavailability. Chemical and Pharmaceutical Bulletin 64.5 (2016): 390-398.

180 Smith, T.J., 2002. Fibroblast biology in thyroid diseases. Current Opinion in Endocrinology, Diabetes and Obesity, 9(5), pp.393-400.

181 Castiglioni, Sara, et al. Magnesium and osteoporosis: current state of knowledge and future research directions. Nutrients 5.8 (2013): 3022-3033.

182 Asmus, Hans-Gernot, et al. Two year comparison of sevelamer and calcium carbonate effects on cardiovascular calcification and bone density. Nephrology Dialysis Transplantation 20.8 (2005): 1653-1661.

183 Schurgers, L.J., et al. Role of vitamin K and vitamin K-dependent proteins in vascular calcification. Zeitschrift für kardiologie 90.15 (2001): III57-III63.

184   Shiraki, Masataka, et al. Vitamin K2 (menatetrenone) effectively prevents fractures and sustains lumbar bone mineral density in osteoporosis. Journal of bone and mineral research 15.3 (2000): 515-521.

185   Castiglioni, Sara, et al. Magnesium and osteoporosis: current state of knowledge and future research directions. Nutrients 5.8 (2013): 3022-3033.

186   ibid.

187   Sripanyakorn, Supannee et al. The Comparative Absorption of Silicon from Different Foods and Food Supplements. The British journal of nutrition 102.6 (2009): 825-834. PMC. Web. 6 Apr. 2017.

188   Rondon, L.J., et al. Magnesium attenuates chronic hypersensitivity and spinal cord NMDA receptor phosphorylation in a rat model of diabetic neuropathic pain. The Journal of physiology 588.21 (2010): 4205-4215.

189   Table adapted from Amino-acid content of foods and biological data on proteins, Food Policy & Food Science Service, Food and Agriculture Organisation of the United Nations (1981) – with additional data supplied by nutritiondata.self.com, traditionaloven.com and varying sources. Note that the actual levels in the fish/oats/chickpeas etc. you are eating will be different, according to soil conditions, growing and harvesting methods and so on.

190   Khan, Muhammad Altaf, et al. Comparative Nutritional Profiles of Various Faba Bean and Chickpea Genotypes. International Journal of Agriculture and Biology 17.3 (2015): 449-457.

191   Messina, Virginia. Nutritional and health benefits of dried beans. The American journal of clinical nutrition 100. Supplement 1 (2014): 437S-442S.

192   Steck, Susan E., and James R. Hebert. GST polymorphism and excretion of heterocyclic aromatic amine and isothiocyanate metabolites after Brassica consumption. Environmental and molecular mutagenesis 50.3 (2009): 238.

193   Oz, F., G. Kaban, and M. Kaya. Effects of cooking methods and levels on formation of heterocyclic aromatic amines in chicken and fish with Oasis extraction method. LWT-Food Science and Technology 43.9 (2010): 1345-1350.

194   Turesky, Robert J., and Loic Le Marchand. Metabolism and biomarkers of heterocyclic aromatic amines in molecular epidemiology studies: lessons learned from aromatic amines. Chemical research in toxicology 24.8 (2011): 1169.

195   Shabbir, Muhammad Asim, et al. Effect of thermal treatment on meat proteins with special reference to heterocyclic aromatic amines (HAAs). Critical reviews in food science and nutrition 55.1 (2015): 82-93.

196   Lewandowska, Anna, et al. Isothiocyanates may chemically detoxify mutagenic amines formed in heat processed meat. Food chemistry 157 (2014): 105-110.

197   Steck, Susan E., and James R. Hebert. GST polymorphism and excretion of heterocyclic aromatic amine and isothiocyanate metabolites after Brassica consumption. Environmental and molecular mutagenesis 50.3 (2009): 238.

198   Steel, Caroline Joy, et al. Thermoplastic extrusion in food processing. Thermoplastic elastomers. InTech, 2012.

199   Qi, Lu, and Frank B. Hu. Dietary glycemic load, whole grains, and systemic inflammation in diabetes: the epidemiological evidence. Current opinion in lipidology 18.1 (2007): 3-8.

200   Willett, W.C. (2012), Dietary fats and coronary heart disease. Journal of Internal Medicine, 272: 13-24. doi:10.1111/j.1365-2796.2012.02553.x.

201   Dobarganes, Carmen, and Gloria Márquez-Ruiz. Possible adverse effects of frying with vegetable oils. British Journal of Nutrition 113.S2 (2015): S49-S57.

202   Mendick, Robert. Cooking with vegetable oils releases toxic cancer-causing chemicals, say experts. The Telegraph, 7 November 2015.

203   Esterbauer, Hermann. Cytotoxicity and genotoxicity of lipid-oxidation products. The American journal of clinical nutrition 57.5 (1993): 779S-785S.

204   Grootveld, Martin, et al. In vivo absorption, metabolism, and urinary excretion of alpha, beta-unsaturated aldehydes in experimental animals. Relevance to the development of cardiovascular diseases by the dietary ingestion of thermally stressed polyunsaturate-rich culinary oils. Journal of Clinical Investigation 101.6 (1998): 1210.

205   Claxson, Andrew WD, et al. Generation of lipid peroxidation products in culinary oils and fats during episodes of thermal stressing: a high field 1H NMR study. FEBS letters 355.1 (1994): 81-90.

206   Budwig, J. Flax Oil as a True Aid against Arthritis, Heart Infarction and Cancer. Apple Publishing December 1994 (lectures delivered in 1959, 1972 and 1976).

207   Ravnskov, U. The Cholesterol Myths. New Trends Publishing, September 2001.

208   Kendrick, M. The Great Cholesterol Con. John Blake Publishing, July 2008.

209   Teicholz Nina. The scientific report guiding the US dietary guidelines: is it scientific? BMJ 2015;351:h4962.

210   de Souza, Russell J., et al. Intake of saturated and trans unsaturated fatty acids and risk of all cause mortality, cardiovascular disease, and type 2 diabetes: systematic review and meta-analysis of observational studies. BMJ 351 (2015): h3978.

211   Information taken from Guillén, Natalia, et al. Knowledge of the biological actions of extra virgin olive oil gained from mice lacking apolipoprotein E. Revista Española de Cardiología (English Edition) 62.3 (2009): 294-304.

212   de Silva, Punyanganie SA, et al. Dietary arachidonic and oleic acid intake in ulcerative colitis etiology: a prospective cohort study using 7-day food diaries. European journal of gastroenterology & hepatology 26.1 (2014): 11-18.

213   Escrich, Eduard, Montserrat Solanas, and Raquel Moral. Olive oil and other dietary lipids in breast cancer. Advances in Nutrition and Cancer. Springer Berlin Heidelberg, 2014. 289-309.

214   Schwingshackl, Lukas, and Georg Hoffmann. Monounsaturated fatty acids, olive oil and health status: a systematic review and meta-analysis of cohort studies. Lipids in health and disease 13.1 (2014): 154.

215   Fabiani, R. Anti-cancer properties of olive oil secoiridoid phenols: a systematic review of in vivo studies. Food & Function 7.10 (2016): 4145-4159.

216   Fabiani, R. Anti-cancer properties of olive oil secoiridoid phenols: a systematic review of in vivo studies. Food & Function 7.10 (2016): 4145-4159.

217   Bassani, Barbara, et al. Potential chemopreventive activities of a polyphenol rich purified extract from olive mill wastewater on colon cancer cells. Journal of Functional Foods 27 (2016): 236-248.

218   Rossi, T., et al. Effect of a purified extract of olive mill waste water on endothelial cell proliferation, apoptosis, migration and capillary-like structure in vitro and in vivo. J. Bioanal. Biomed. S 12 (2015): 006.

219   Barbaro, Barbara, et al. Effects of the olive-derived polyphenol oleuropein on human health. International journal of molecular sciences 15.10 (2014): 18508-18524.

220   Mahabaleshwar V. Hegde, Anand Arvind Zanwar, Sharad P. Adekar Omega 3 Fatty Acids: keys to nutritional health. Humana Press, 3 Oct 2016 Chapter 7, p.343.

221   DISCLAIMER: I am not at Star Wars geek or expert in any way, and have just a superficial understanding that I hope aficionados will forgive me for.

222   Guo, Yanxia, et al. Leukocyte homing, fate, and function are controlled by retinoic acid. Physiological reviews 95.1 (2015): 125-148.

223   Mizee, Mark R., et al. Astrocyte-derived retinoic acid: a novel regulator of blood-brain barrier function in multiple sclerosis. Acta neuropathologica128.5 (2014): 691-703.

224   Schwager, Joseph, et al. Ascorbic acid modulates cell migration in differentiated HL-60 cells and peripheral blood leukocytes. Molecular nutrition & food research 59.8 (2015): 1513-1523.

225   Bikker, A., et al. Ascorbic acid deficiency impairs wound healing in surgical patients: Four case reports. International Journal of Surgery Open 2 (2016): 15-18.

226   Pludowski, Pawel, et al. Vitamin D effects on musculoskeletal health, immunity, autoimmunity, cardiovascular disease, cancer, fertility, pregnancy, dementia and mortality – a review of recent evidence. Autoimmunity reviews12.10 (2013): 976-989.

227   Gombart, Adrian F., Niels Borregaard, and H. Phillip Koeffler. Human cathelicidin antimicrobial peptide (CAMP) gene is a direct target of the vitamin D receptor and is strongly up-regulated in myeloid cells by 1, 25-dihydroxyvitamin D3. The FASEB journal 19.9 (2005): 1067-1077.

228   Hata, Tissa R., et al. Administration of oral vitamin D induces cathelicidin production in atopic individuals. The Journal of allergy and clinical immunology 122.4 (2008): 829.

229   Kamen, Diane L., and Vin Tangpricha. Vitamin D and molecular actions on the immune system: modulation of innate and autoimmunity. Journal of Molecular Medicine 88.5 (2010): 441-450.

230   Holick, Michael F., and Arash Hossein-Nezhad. The D-lemma: narrow-band UV type B radiation versus vitamin D supplementation versus sunlight for cardiovascular and immune health. The American Journal of Clinical Nutrition 105.5 (2017): 1031-1032.

231   Steinbrenner, Holger, et al. Dietary selenium in adjuvant therapy of viral and bacterial infections. Advances in Nutrition: An International Review Journal 6.1 (2015): 73-82.

232   Haase, Hajo, and Lothar Rink. Multiple impacts of zinc on immune function. Metallomics 6.7 (2014): 1175-1180.

233   Prasad, A.S., 2013. Discovery of human zinc deficiency: its impact on human health and disease. Advances in nutrition, 4(2), pp.176-190.

234   Sazawal, Sunil, et al. Zinc supplementation reduces the incidence of acute lower respiratory infections in infants and preschool children: a double-blind, controlled trial. Pediatrics 102.1 (1998): 1-5.

235   Chacko, S.A., Song, Y., Nathan, L., Tinker, L., de Boer, I.H., Tylavsky, F., Wallace, R., Liu, S. Relations of dietary magnesium intake to biomarkers of inflammation and endothelial dysfunction in an ethnically diverse cohort of postmenopausal women. Diabetes Care 2010, 33, 304-310.

236   Nielsen, Forrest H. Effects of magnesium depletion on inflammation in chronic disease. Current Opinion in Clinical Nutrition & Metabolic Care 17.6 (2014): 525-530.

237   Simopoulos, A.P., 2016. An increase in the omega-6/omega-3 fatty acid ratio increases the risk for obesity. Nutrients, 8(3), p.128.

238   Simopoulos, A.P., 2016. Evolutionary Aspects of the Dietary Omega-6/Omega-3 Fatty Acid Ratio: Medical Implications. In Evolutionary Thinking in Medicine (pp. 119-134). Springer, Cham.

239   ibid.

240   Justo, Oselys Rodriguez, et al. Evaluation of in vitro anti-inflammatory effects of crude ginger and rosemary extracts obtained through supercritical CO 2 extraction on macrophage and tumor cell line: the influence of vehicle type. BMC complementary and alternative medicine 15.1 (2015): 390.

241   S Bisen, P. and Emerald, M., 2016. Nutritional and therapeutic potential of garlic and onion (Allium sp.). Current Nutrition & Food Science, 12(3), pp.190-199.

242   S Bisen, P. and Emerald, M., 2016. Nutritional and therapeutic potential of garlic and onion (Allium sp.). Current Nutrition & Food Science, 12(3), pp.190-199.

243   Chassard, C., Dapoigny, M., Scott, K.P., Crouzet, L., Del'homme, C., Marquet, P., Martin, J.C., Pickering, G., Ardid, D., Eschalier, A. and Dubray, C., 2012. Functional dysbiosis within the gut microbiota of patients with constipated-irritable bowel syndrome. Alimentary pharmacology & therapeutics, 35(7), pp.828-838.

244   Kalaras, M.D., Richie, J.P., Calcagnotto, A. and Beelman, R.B., 2017. Mushrooms: A rich source of the antioxidants ergothioneine and glutathione. Food chemistry, 233, pp.429-433.

245   Li, X., Wu, Q., Xie, Y., Ding, Y., Du, W.W., Sdiri, M. and Yang, B.B., 2015. Ergosterol purified from medicinal mushroom Amauroderma rude inhibits cancer growth in vitro and in vivo by up-regulating multiple tumor suppressors. Oncotarget, 6(19), p.17832.

246   Tan, W., Pan, M., Liu, H., Tian, H., Ye, Q. and Liu, H., 2017. ergosterol peroxide inhibits ovarian cancer cell growth through multiple pathways. OncoTargets and therapy, 10, p.3467.

247   Nowak, R., Drozd, M., Mendyk, E., Lemieszek, M., Krakowiak, O., Kisiel, W., Rzeski, W. and Szewczyk, K., 2016. A new method for the isolation of ergosterol and peroxyergosterol as active compounds of Hygrophoropsis aurantiaca and in vitro antiproliferative activity of isolated ergosterol peroxide. Molecules, 21(7), p.946.

248   Kang, J.H., Jang, J.E., Mishra, S.K., Lee, H.J., Nho, C.W., Shin, D., Jin, M., Kim, M.K., Choi, C. and Oh, S.H., 2015. Ergosterol peroxide from Chaga mushroom (Inonotus obliquus) exhibits anti-cancer activity by down-regulation of the β-catenin pathway in colorectal cancer. Journal of ethnopharmacology, 173, pp.303-312.

249   Sankaran, M., Isabella, S. and Amaranth, K., 2017. Anti proliferative Potential of Ergosterol: A Unique Plant Sterol on Hep2 Cell Line. Int J Pharma Res Health Sci, 5(4), pp.1736-42.

250   Hodges, R.E. and Minich, D.M., 2015. Modulation of metabolic detoxification pathways using foods and food-derived components: a scientific review with clinical application. Journal of nutrition and metabolism, 2015.

251   ibid.

252   ibid.

253   ibid.

254   ibid.

255   ibid.

256   ibid.

257   Tchounwou, P.B., Yedjou, C.G., Patlolla, A.K. and Sutton, D.J., 2012. Heavy metal toxicity and the environment. In Molecular, clinical and environmental toxicology (pp. 133-164). Springer, Basel.

258   Hodges, R.E. and Minich, D.M., 2015. Modulation of metabolic detoxification pathways using foods and food-derived components: a scientific review with clinical application. Journal of nutrition and metabolism, 2015.

259   Boyer, J.L., 2013. Bile formation and secretion. Comprehensive physiology.

260   Jarrar, B.M. and Al-Rowaili, M.A., 2011. Chemical composition of gallstones from Al-jouf province of saudi arabia. The Malaysian journal of medical sciences: MJMS, 18(2), p.47.

261   Shabanzadeh, D.M., Sørensen, L.T. and Jørgensen, T., 2016. Determinants for gallstone formation – a new data cohort study and a systematic review with meta-analysis. Scandinavian journal of gastroenterology, 51(10), pp.1239-1248.

262   Ortega, R.M., Fernández-Azuela, M., Encinas-Sotillos, A., Andres, P. and Lopez-Sobaler, A.M., 1997. Differences in diet and food habits between patients with gallstones and controls. Journal of the American College of Nutrition, 16(1), pp.88-95.

263   ibid.

264   Ridlon, J.M., Kang, D.J., Hylemon, P.B. and Bajaj, J.S., 2014. Bile acids and the gut microbiome. Current opinion in gastroenterology, 30(3), p.332.

265   Madden, A.M., Trivedi, D., Smeeton, N.C. and Culkin, A., 2017. Modified dietary fat intake for treatment of gallstone disease. The Cochrane Library.

266   Nassuato G, Iemmolo RM, et al. Effect of silibinin on biliary lipid composition. Experimental and clinical study. J Hepatol 1991;12:290-5.).

267   Gaby, A.R., 2009. Nutritional approaches to prevention and treatment of gallstones. Alternative medicine review, 14(3), p.258.

268   Sies CW, Brooker J. Could these be gallstones? Lancet 2005;365:1388.

269   Borahay, M.A., Asoglu, M.R., Mas, A., Adam, S., Kilic, G.S. and Al-Hendy, A., 2017. Estrogen receptors and signaling in fibroids: Role in pathobiology and therapeutic implications. Reproductive Sciences, 24(9), pp.1235-1244.

270   Han, S.J., Jung, S.Y., Wu, S.P., Park, M.J., Qin, J., Lydon, J.P., Tsai, S.Y., Tsai, M.J., DeMayo, F.J. and Bert, W.O., 2018, February. The pathogenic role of estrogen receptor beta drives in endometriosis. In Nuclear Receptors: New Roles for Nuclear Receptors in Development, Health and Disease Conference 2018 (Vol. 54). BioScientifica.

271   Brinton, L.A., Trabert, B., Anderson, G.L., Falk, R.T., Felix, A.S., Fuhrman, B.J., Gass, M.L., Kuller, L.H., Pfeiffer, R.M., Rohan, T.E. and Strickler, H.D., 2016. Serum estrogens and estrogen metabolites and endometrial cancer risk among postmenopausal women. Cancer Epidemiology and Prevention Biomarkers.

272   Sategna-Guidetti, C., Volta, U., Ciacci, C., Usai, P., Carlino, A., De Franceschi, L., Camera, A., Pelli, A. and Brossa, C., 2001. Prevalence of thyroid disorders in untreated adult celiac disease patients and effect of gluten withdrawal: an Italian multicenter study. The American journal of gastroenterology, 96(3), p.751.

273   Liontiris, M.I. and Mazokopakis, E.E., 2017. A concise review of Hashimoto thyroiditis (HT) and the importance of iodine, selenium, vitamin D and gluten on the autoimmunity and dietary management of HT patients. Points that need more investigation. Hell J Nucl Med, 20(1), pp.51-56.

274   Peeters, R.P. and Visser, T.J., 2017. Metabolism of thyroid hormone.

Index

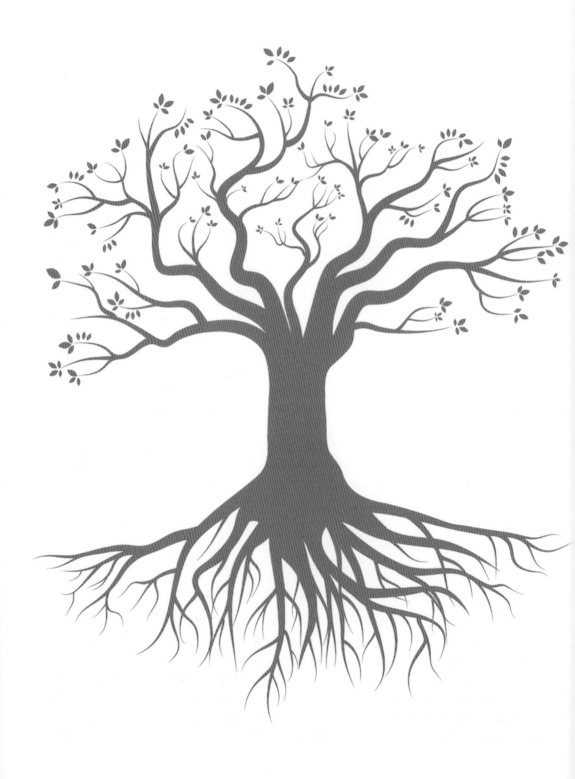

Acknowledgements

This book has its roots and support in so many teachings, friendships and inspirations.

Firstly, I'd like to thank Deborah & Harvey at Alchimia for giving me free rein alongside focus and deadlines to actually get this book written.

Heartfelt gratitude also:
To my husband and best friend Andy for buying me my first ever nutrition book and so planting the seed of this whole journey – and for dragging me kicking and screaming into self-care at a time when I needed it most.

To Kitty Cava, Barbara Wren, Bob and Lee Nitsch and many others for your insights, wisdom and guidance as I healed from cancer and developed as a practitioner.

To Hayley North for your sistership, creativity and fire in the many years we have worked together on retreats and workshops. You have undoubtedly inspired some of my recipes, too, and your work as a holistic chef has been pioneering.

To each and every nutrition client and student over the past 17 years for sharing your stories, experiences and insights, and letting me walk alongside you for a while as you explore how nutrition might work for you.

Thanks also to the photographers and artists who have helped make this book so beautiful:

Cover artwork: Kristen Meyer (KM Salvage Design)

Food photography: Lesley Burdett Photography, Kirsten Chick (pp. 265, 269, 281, 283)

Author portrait photography: Anna Strickland (Heardinlondon Photography)

Other credits (page): alexzrv (141), Marilyn Barbone (6, 240), Bondd (166), Kirsten Chick (34, 183, 237), Coolgraphic (96), Double Brain (221), Evart (86), Harvey Fenton (171), Freepik (310), Robert Adrian Hillman (116), Sonya Kamoz (10), Axel Kock (108), LadyofHats (60), Neail Langan (182), Leung Cho Pan (16), Macrovector (126), Stuart Miles (204), Ike Louie Natividad (54), Pixabay (20, 72, 190), Anastasiya Rutkovskaya (42), Shots Studio (142), Subbotina Anna (1), Chanikarn Thongsupa (156), Vencav (218, 234), Wake up (69), Yingko (32).

NOTES